FALSE ALARM

W9-ATE-642

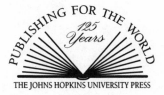

THE JOHNS HOPKINS UNIVERSITY PRESS

Recent and related titles from the Johns Hopkins University Press

Stuart H. Altman and David I. Schactman, eds.
Policies for an Aging Society

Robert H. Binstock, Leighton E. Cluff, and Otto von Mering, eds.
The Future of Long-Term Care: Social and Policy Issues

Tom Hickey, Marjorie A. Speers, and Thomas R. Prohaska, eds.
Public Health and Aging

Robert B. Hudson, ed.
The Future of Age-Based Public Policy

Leslie Walker, Elizabeth H. Bradley, and Terrie Wetle, eds.
Public and Private Responsibilities in Long-Term Care: Finding the Balance

Carol S. Weissert and William G. Weissert
Governing Health: The Politics of Health Policy, 2d ed.

Robert H. Binstock
CONSULTING EDITOR IN GERONTOLOGY

"/2011

368.43
W58

FALSE ALARM

Why the Greatest Threat to Social Security and Medicare Is the Campaign to "Save" Them

Joseph White

Luxenberg Family Professor of Public Policy, Department of
Political Science, and Director, Center for Policy Studies
Case Western Reserve University
Cleveland, Ohio

A Century Foundation Book

The Johns Hopkins University Press
Baltimore and London

© 2001, 2003 The Century Foundation
All rights reserved. Published 2001
Printed in the United States of America on acid-free paper

Johns Hopkins Paperbacks edition, 2003
2   4   6   8   9   7   5   3   1

The Johns Hopkins University Press
2715 North Charles Street
Baltimore, Maryland 21218-4363
www.press.jhu.edu

The Library of Congress has cataloged the hardcover edition of this book as follows:

White, Joseph, 1952–
False alarm : why the greatest threat to social security and
medicare is the campaign to "save" them / Joseph White.
p.   cm.
"A Century Foundation book."
Includes bibliographical references and index.
ISBN 0-8018-6665-0
1. Social security—United States.   2. Medicare—United
States.   I. Title.
HD7125 .W473 2001
368.4′3′00973—dc21   00-011529

ISBN 0-8018-7449-1 (pbk.)

A catalog record for this book is available from the British Library.

The Century Foundation, formerly the Twentieth Century Fund, sponsors and supervises timely analyses of economic policy, foreign affairs, and domestic political issues. Not-for-profit and nonpartisan, it was founded in 1919 and endowed by Edward A. Filene.

Board of Trustees of The Century Foundation

H. Brandt Ayers
Peter A. A. Berle
Alan Brinkley, *Chairman*
Joseph A. Califano, Jr.
Alexander Morgan Capron
Hodding Carter III
Edward E. David, Jr.
Brewster C. Denny
Christopher Edley, Jr.
Charles V. Hamilton
Matina S. Horner
Lewis B. Kaden
James A. Leach
Richard C. Leone

Jessica Tuchman Mathews
Alicia H. Munnell
P. Michael Pitfield
John Podesta
Richard Ravitch
Alan Sagner
Arthur M. Schlesinger, Jr.
Harvey I. Sloane, M.D.
Theodore C. Sorensen
Kathleen M. Sullivan
David B. Truman
Shirley Williams
William Julius Wilson

Richard C. Leone, *President*

To honor the legacy of Aaron Wildavsky

CONTENTS

FOREWORD

One of the more notable characteristics of the ongoing debate about how to carve up the anticipated federal budget surplus has been the underlying preoccupation with fears about the future. The driving force behind this concern is the aging of the population—a shift in the share of Americans age 65 and older from about one in ten to one in five. This shift is in large part a result of the graying of the baby-boomer cohort born between 1946 and 1964. Somewhat to the surprise of those who believe foresight is virtually impossible in a society that thinks short-term, our politicians are arguing about where we will be in seventy-five years and about whose plan will be better far into the future. While current needs are not being completely ignored in these debates about the surplus, woe be it to the politician deemed guilty of neglecting our grandchildren and "future generations."

Unfortunately, the seeming nobility of a debate oriented toward sacrificing today for the future is deceptively artificial. It is carried on as though preserving the Social Security surplus or committing future funds to Medicare involves storing up goods and services that will be delivered at some point in the future when they are needed by a larger, older population. In fact, of course, the productive capacity of the economy at those future dates and the political decisions made by voters between now and then will be the main determinants of how "burdensome" sustaining Social Security and Medicare will be in 2050, or 2075, or whenever.

Moreover, in public deliberations about how to deal with problems twenty, thirty, or seventy-five years in the future, voters are being asked to make a highly sophisticated choice involving a great deal of guesswork. There is no crystal ball providing experts and other prominent observers with reliable predictions—although one would think so given the way they confidently bandy about precise, gargantuan numbers intended to quantify government programs some half-century or more in the future. It is important to keep in mind that seventy-five years ago, when neither Social Security nor Medicare existed, no one in his or her right mind could have imagined either the Great Depression or the unprecedented economic progress that followed. For that matter, not a single respectable economist predicted as recently as four years ago that the federal budget would move into the black.

The shortcomings of long-term forecasting are not confined to the vagaries of economics. Political trends can be just as confounding. Over the past two decades, the collapse of Communism, the ascent of Ronald Reagan, and the end of Democratic control of the U.S. House of Representatives astounded most prognosticators. Because political choices will shape the contours of federal programs as forcefully and unpredictably as will the economy itself, most doomsayers and Panglossians should be given equally little credibility. A little more modesty about our ability to see the future should be coupled with a little more reasonableness in assessing public behavior today as either unequivocally virtuous or selfish when it comes to the allocation of goods and services tomorrow.

Joseph White's foremost contribution in these pages is to cut through the thicket of political rhetoric and fuzzy thinking. It goes to the heart of the choices that must be made, demonstrating that there are any number of reasonable options available. White, a professor of political science at Case Western Reserve University, is a master of both number crunching and political science. That rare combination is ideally suited to parsing the debates over Social Security and Medicare, where the gap is so wide between the accounting tables and the political rhetoric. By simply investigating the etymology of entitlement, which is used as a description for the two programs, White demonstrates how that single word has steered the political debate in a direction that downplays the importance of social insurance to the public.

Of necessity, this book is replete with numbers. Because these programs constitute nearly a third of the federal budget, White devotes considerable attention to sorting out how that money is spent, how those amounts compare with those spent on other government activities and in the economy as a whole, and how changing demographics could affect those allocations. But throughout his explanations, White devotes far more care than you will find elsewhere to distinctions among certainties, likelihoods, possibilities, and pure speculation. In the process, he subjects the most prominent proposals for reform—including his own—to a level of scrutiny that will benefit all readers who care about the future of these programs.

The issues covered in this book became central to the agenda of The Century Foundation during the 1990s. Concerned about the same shortcomings in political discourse that motivated this book, the Foundation's trustees encouraged the sponsorship of activities and publications related to the connections between public policy and the aging of the population. On Social Security, our publications include Robert M. Ball's *Straight Talk about Social Security;* the late Robert Eisner's *Social Security: More, Not Less;* and, perhaps most important, *Countdown to Reform: The Great Social Security Debate,* by Henry J. Aaron and Robert D. Reischauer. We also operate a popular Web site on the subject (www.socsec.org), which includes a wide range of information explaining the program and proposals for reforming it. Many of the highlights of our work are included in an edited volume—*Social Security Reform: Beyond the Basics.* On Medicare, we have sponsored a task force under the chairmanship of Richard Ravitch and Shoshanna Sofaer that will release a report in 2001 with recommendations for the program's future. We also have launched a new Web site—www.medicarewatch.org.

The 2000 elections may well lead to changes in Social Security and Medicare. But any such changes are sure to be followed by further reforms in the years and decades hence. Although no one can predict what those changes will be, in this book White provides a way for all sides in the debate to think more intelligently about the choices facing the nation.

Richard C. Leone, President
The Century Foundation
October 2000

PREFACE TO THE PAPERBACK EDITION

Analysis of proposed policy reforms should begin with the world as it is, as best we can understand it, and try to project how policy changes will alter that world. But what should readers think if the world has changed since the analysis was completed?

Three years have passed since I completed the hardcover edition of this book. I began that work in an era of seemingly unending federal budget deficits and finished at a time when surpluses were projected almost as far as the eye could see. Now we are back to deficits again (probably). I began writing at a time when private payers were constraining health insurance costs far better than the federal government, finished at a time when that pattern had reversed; and now Medicare costs have accelerated but private payers' costs have accelerated even more. I wrote this book during a great stock market boom, but since its completion broad market indexes have declined and then stagnated, while values in some sectors have nearly collapsed. All of these factors arguably could affect the merits of the policies discussed here, and certainly alter some of the data provided in the text.

Yet much of the point of this book is that short-term and even long-term trends do not alter the basic case for Social Security and Medicare. The budget numbers used in chapters 5 and 12 are out of date, but they still serve to illustrate important points about both the scale of possible benefits from incremental changes and the difficulty of predicting the future. Events in the financial and health care markets, if anything, have strengthened the case for skepticism about radical reforms, but my argument does not depend on short-term trends in the Dow or Standard & Poor's indexes. The advantages of social insurance as opposed to relying on individual savings to protect against life's risks have not changed since 1999, or indeed since 1939. Therefore, I have altered the original text only by adding an Afterword, in which I discuss some of the policy developments during the years 2000 through 2002 and how they could alter some specific conclusions but not the basic argument and recommendations that I made.

Another change since I first wrote, the election of George W. Bush as president, when combined with Republican control of Congress by even a slim margin, makes radical reform of Social Security, Medicare, or both a serious possibility. Yet the narrow Republican ascendancy in U.S. politics is only one reason for those prospects. For many years, Social Security was viewed by Washington pundits as the "third rail of American politics"—touch it and you die. Early in his campaign for the presidency, however, Bush announced his support for partial privatization of the system. Bush's position immediately set off speculation about the political calculation he might be following ("Social Security Politics" 2000; Calmes 2000; Gigot 2000). In that context, three points should be remembered.

First, Bush had room to suggest radical reforms because of an elite consensus that a coming financing crisis made Social Security, in the *Washington Post*'s words, "a major issue not just for the campaign but beyond" ("Social Security Politics" 2000). This consensus extended to Medicare because whatever concerns might be raised about Social Security—affordability, fairness across generations, fairness within generations—apply equally plausibly (which does not mean accurately) to Medicare. In this context, defenders of the status quo, who raised legitimate questions about the risks of change, could be denounced as conducting "fear campaigns" that lacked a positive agenda to "save" the programs.

Second, practical politicians give their policies attractive labels. Thus, Bush promised to "build a bipartisan consensus to save Social Security."[1] He emphasized, "Social Security is a defining American promise, and we will not turn back," while promising to "reform and strengthen Medicare" as well.[2]

Third, political debate rarely enlightens anyone. Vice President Gore's campaign challenged the Bush rhetoric, even though some commentators believed that it did not do so effectively enough.[3] But the press could poke holes in both parties' positions ("Campaigning on Social Security" 2000; Samuelson 2000) and, while Gore's objections were right in principle, they were wrong on some significant details. After watching the campaign, few Americans were likely to have learned much about the central empirical or even value questions posed by reform proposals. What might the return on private investments be? What might Medicare vouchers accomplish? What do Medicare and Social Security really do, so what might be the real stakes in the political battle? In what sense is "reform" necessary to avoid "bankruptcy" of the programs?

This book seeks to answer those and other questions. It begins with the developments that made then-Governor Bush's campaign position politically conceivable. At some point, in much of public debate, Social Security and Medicare became not specific programs with specific merits and demerits but a dangerous thing called "entitlements."

My argument has four stages. Part I, "The Stakes: What Social Security and Medicare Do," addresses the incrementalist's, or even the conservative's, first question: how much should I value the status quo? Chapter 2, "Why Americans Trust Social Insurance and Distrust Entitlements," explains the logic of social insurance. The benefits of social insurance, which is what Social Security and Medicare really are, tend to be ignored or understated in the standard critiques. There are legitimate arguments for devoting more of society's product to those benefits. The chapter contrasts those arguments for social insurance with the presumptions of the attack on "entitlements." Chapters 3 and 4, which explain the basics of Social Security and Medicare, also discuss some important disagreements about how the programs work.

Part 2, "Challenges That Are Not Crises," deals with the three major claims used to make the status quo seem unbearable. Chapter 5 debunks the most important of these claims, that the costs of Social Security and Medicare threaten grievous harm to the national economy. Chapter 6 considers the specific problem of health care costs. It shows that there is little reason to believe costs will expand as much as is claimed by some analysts; that some cost increases may be desirable; and that, if there is a cost problem, it is likely to be as severe for private insurance as for public. Chapter 7 refutes the assertion that Social Security and Medicare will be grossly unfair, burdening "our grandchildren" to the benefit of "greedy geezers."

Even though there are no crises, some reforms might still be appropriate. Reforms can be designed to make the world a happier place, not just to avoid misery. Advocates of versions of Medicare and Social Security privatization claim not only that they will be saving the country from the costs of the current systems but also that the results will be better for everyone. If the outcome will be better, then no crisis is needed to justify change. Part 3 therefore discusses "Reforms That Would Not Be Improvements." Chapter 8 addresses the most heavily promoted idea, replacing a portion of traditional Social Security with mandatory individual retirement accounts. Such "privatization" probably would eventually, very eventually, have benefits, on average. Unfortunately, the possible average benefits are so far in the future, and privatization would so greatly increase the risk that many individuals would not receive adequate pensions, that privatization is not advisable for a program whose purpose is to guarantee a basic pension. Private investment is a fine idea, and people should do it for themselves, but something close to the current Social Security system should be the floor on which people build their private savings.

Chapter 9 explains why Medicare vouchers are "Not Ready for Prime Time." Maybe someday they will be a good idea, but so far there is little evidence that they would save any money, never mind provide decent health care at a reasonable price, far into the future. Instead of abandoning a system that works pretty well now, policy makers should focus on reforms and experiments that might make competition more likely to work later.

Chapter 10 considers three widely promoted reforms within the frameworks of the traditional programs, arguing that all three are dangerous. One is to raise the ages of eligibility for Social Security and Medicare. Another is to "means test" those programs in some way. The third is to permanently reduce inflation adjustments for Social Security benefits. Although I reject the standard proposals, I argue that other changes might address legitimate concerns behind suggestions to alter the ages of eligibility and create mean tests.

The final section of the book, "Responsible Reform," suggests a package of moderate, incremental, but hardly modest reforms. Chapter 11 describes each of the proposals. Chapter 12 describes how they could have been fit together as part of a policy agenda for the administration that took office in 2001 and how they could have affected future budget conditions. The chapter argues that, starting from the world as it seemed to be at that time, incremental reforms seemed likely to leave the federal budget in tolerable shape until around 2050, so that no further action might be required until sometime in the 2040s. In the Afterword I discuss how budgetary developments during the Bush administration have made prospects somewhat less positive. But it is still possible to have responsible policies that preserve Social Security and Medicare so our children and grandchildren can make their own choices, when they must know more about the facts and values of their time than we could ever know today.

ACKNOWLEDGMENTS

Any work of intended scholarship is the product not just of its author but of a host of collaborators. In a real sense, everyone whose work is cited in the bibliography and endnotes of this book has contributed to this analysis, whether by providing information and arguments or by provoking me to clarify the reasons why I dissagree with them. Some no doubt would be horrified to receive that kind of credit, and perhaps some would be pleased. All those who have helped me, willingly or unwillingly, deserve no blame for any dermerits or infelicities of either my argument or its expression.

While the bibliography and endnotes are an acknowledgment of a sort, some individuals and institutions deserve a special share in any credit this work may receive. Pride of place must go to The Century Foundation, which provided funding, a place to work, and intellectual support as well as guidance for the work. Within TCF I owe special debts to Richard C. Leone, Greg Anrig Jr., Sarah Ritchie, Bernard Wasow, and Leif W. Hasse for both support and counsel over the course of this project.

Other institutions provided congenial locales for work and intellectual stimulation. I began this project as a Visiting Fellow at the Brooklings Institution and would like to thank Tom Mann for that opportunity. Brooklings has provided a superb collection of scholars on subjects related to this book, and I benefitted over many years from discussions with its staff and visiters, who account for much of my more detailed citations. The record will show that we have not always agreed, but I have learned much from, and appreciated the collegiality of, Henry Aaron Barry Bosworth, Gary Burtless, Bob Reischauer, and R. Kent Weaver. I did much of my writing while on the faculty of Tulane University and final editing at Case Western Reserve University. Individual scholars such as Dick Culbertson, Dahlia Remler, Ken Thorpe, and Bob Binstock contributed to my understanding; more generally, I tried not to bore colleages in either place too much with discussions of arcane aspects of Social Security, Medicare, or the budget, but they tolerated the exceptions.

Certain scholars contributed directly by critiquing drafts of this manuscript or of related articles. I especially want to thank Eric Kingson, who read and commented on the entire first draft. Others who were especially helpful at stages of this intellectual journey include Dean Baker, Peter Diamond, Gordon Fisher, Eric Patashnik, Paul Posner, Allen Shick, and Bruce Vladeck. Anonymous reviewers for *Health Affairs* and *Public Budgeting & Finance* contributed to my analysis of subjects on which I also prepared separate articles for those journals. I thank all for their time and effort and insight.

The production of any book requires a great deal of cooperation, sometimes grudging, between author and publisher. In this case I have felt no desire to grudge: Wendy Harris of the Johns Hopkins University Press, Lois Crum, who edited the manuscript, and all other staff have been continually not only helpful but right, making and suggesting changes that only improved the work.

Any student of a subject becomes part of a network, with particular guides into and through a chosen field. In the field of social insurance, my guide has been Theodore R. Marmor. Through his own writing, introduction to other scholars, and conversation, Ted has provided ideas and criticism and opportunities for me to learn more. No one has done a better job of explaining the importance of social insurance to Americans. Readers who wish to learn more than I have told should turn to his work next.

Some may live purely for their work, but of late, at least, that has not been my fate, much as I care about ideas and policy. I need only to come home and see my wife, Sydelle Zinn, and daughter, Abigail, to know that I care about much more. I thank them for far more than this book.

The greatest influence on this book, however, was someone who could give no advice or council on this particular project and whom I can no longer thank in person. Aaron Wildavsky was my teacher, my collaborator, my friend. Throughout my work on this project, I have attempted to provide a policy analysis of the subject of Social Security and Medicare reform which meets the standards that he set in his own scholarship.

The spirit and practice of Aaron's work included a quizzical attitude toward conventional wisdom, careful attention to how problems are defined and who is favored by their definition, explicitness about the values at stake in any policy dispute, a willingness to seek any data that could illuminate the question at hand, and especially an emphasis on what it is reasonable to ask human policy makers to do. I would like to believe that my analysis here reflects all those methods and lessons, especially the last. We neither know nor could know enough today to "save" Social Security and Medicare for the next seventy-five years. But we can use careful analysis not only to set a general direction for policies but also to protect against grievous errors and to enable future policy makers to learn from our choices and use them to inform their own decisions. This book makes a case for incremental and experimental reform of two of the most important parts of not just American government but American life. I have no idea whether Aaron Wildavsky would agree with my conclusions. I dearly wish he were still here to be asked. But I hope he would recognize his lessons in the spirit of this book.

FALSE ALARM

ONE

Introduction: Saving What, from What?

The United States has faced many challenges in its history. It has won its freedom, peopled and developed much of a continent, and built a nation from the efforts of people from many different lands. America has created and confronted the conflicts of an industrial economy, faced massive depressions, fought in two world wars, and borne the costs of the Cold War. Throughout, it has had to find ways to balance individual freedom and yet a tolerably coherent society, within the context of pervasive divisions over race.

As the 1996 election approached, David Broder of the *Washington Post*, perhaps the most respected political journalist in the country, wrote a column with rhetoric appropriate for only the most serious of conditions. "There may be a brief window of opportunity . . . in 1997–98," he proclaimed, "for Congress and the president to step up to the growing challenge of entitlement reform. Fundamental changes will be needed in Medicare, Medicaid and Social Security if we are to avert the fiscal calamity that the retirement of the baby-boom generation poses for the early years of the next century and avoid the political upheaval of all-out generational war." Predictions of "calamity" and "war" are strong enough, but Broder further suggested that failure to meet the challenge of entitlements could "force a political realignment" in which one of the two major parties could be replaced by a third (Broder 1996). To put that in perspective, political scientists agree that the last two clear realignments occurred with the Great Depression of the 1930s and the financial panics and massive socioeconomic change of the 1890s. The last time an issue caused the replacement of one major party, the issue was slavery; and its other major consequence was the Civil War.

There were no "fundamental changes" in Medicare, Medicaid, and Social Security by the time of the 2000 election. Yet President Clinton's second term saw continual rhetoric about "saving" Social Security and Medicare. And behind that rhetoric, as we shall see, lurked a conviction by which David Broder and much of the rest of semiofficial Washington have been gripped for years.

Could "entitlements" really rank with the Great Depression and slavery as threats to the nation? I argue in this book that they cannot and do not. Yet the most important political fact about Broder's analysis is that he was not viewed as some sort of hysteric. Few in Washington would expect a partisan realignment because of the entitlement issue, but many may have agreed with his implicit assumption that if the parties did not "solve" the entitlement problem quickly, one or both of them would deserve to be realigned out of existence.

From the perspective of Washington policy types, that statement should not be surprising. But for the sake of the proverbial woman from Mars or the college sophomore, it may be useful to show the extent of the consensus. We can look through the lens of commentary on the election of 1996 and the federal budget battles in the first half of 1997.

The "Entitlement Monsters"

As the 1996 election approached, Joe Klein of *Newsweek* editorialized that, though the press "harps on the entitlement monster," President Clinton and his challenger, former Senate Majority Leader Robert Dole, were ducking the issue. He wrote that the only hope of a road "back towards sanity" lay in the chance that after his reelection, "Bill Clinton, deeply concerned with his legacy to history and to his daughter's generation," might reverse field and provide the necessary leadership (Klein 1996). David Gergen, a Republican Reagan and Ford administration aide whose service as a senior assistant to President Clinton was viewed as part of Clinton's effort to move to the responsible center, chimed in that entitlements were a matter of "national character and honesty." Their solution demanded "immediate, significant changes not only in Washington but in our own personal lifestyles as well" (1996).

Clinton's reelection was followed by many efforts to remind him of his, and the nation's, supposed duty. The *National Journal,* the superb weekly newsmagazine widely read by policy elites who can afford the price ($1,197 per year in 2000), reported that "the most menacing problem Clinton has ahead of him, policy experts say, is the exploding financial burden of federal entitlement programs." It quoted Robert Reischauer, a senior fellow at the Brookings Institution and former director of the Congressional Budget Office, who referred to the "demographic tsunami of the baby boom generation's retirement" (Solomon 1996). The cover article of *Time* preceding Clinton's second inauguration was titled "No Guts, No Glory," with a subhead declaring that "on the eve of his Inauguration, Clinton is thinking in lowercase terms. But the big issues—like Social Security and Medicare—need bigger action by far." Those programs were described as "the middle-class entitlement monsters that will consume the budget if left unchecked" (Pooley 1997).

The reelected president had joined his congressional Republican opponents in promising to balance the budget by 2002. As the year's budget debates began, the *Wall Street Journal*'s Jackie Calmes reported that even if those efforts succeeded, politicians would "know better" than to "claim to have solved the nation's fiscal problems," for "normally myopic politicians actually have begun focusing on the longer term, when unprecedented fiscal and demographic pressures could push the deficit to unthinkable depths. . . . As in any chronic addiction, publicly acknowledging the problem is an important step, but there is no consensus about how to cure it" (1997a). Jonathan Rauch of the *National Journal* declared that "prospects for a balanced budget deal are relatively bright this year, but so what? That achievement won't solve the government's biggest fiscal headache—the need to make huge structural reforms in entitlements." He quoted economist John Makin's opinion that "getting the deficit down to zero in 2002 is a nonproblem that is enabling us to avoid dealing with the real issues" (Rauch 1997).

Progress toward a budget agreement, such as the announcement of agreement between the two parties' leaders on May 5, was met by further reminders that the long-term crisis was more important. Even the president's chief of staff, Erskine Bowles, emphasized that "now, having solved the short- and intermediate-term problems with Medicare, we do have to face the generational problems and go forward with some kind of bipartisan process that really will solve the long-term problems associated with Medicare and Social Security" (Vobejda 1997; see also Passell 1997b; Wessel 1997b).

Though some of these commentators are Republicans, it is important to note that many are not. They represent a spectrum of "responsible opinion" in Washington, and all were engaged in raising fears about entitlements. Some would acknowledge that the rhetoric was overstated and yet argue, in Reischauer's words, that "hyperbole is necessary to jar an apathetic public and calcified political system into action before a serious problem deteriorates into a major societal catastrophe" (1997a). They succeeded in making the existence of an entitlement crisis something that was taken for granted by journalists in their news reporting and by nonjournalists in their political analysis.[1]

Two Sets of Fears

By 1999, for a series of political reasons, some of this rhetoric of fear was pushed to the background as advocates of taming the "entitlement monsters" rephrased their campaign as "saving" Social Security and Medicare. Yet common rhetoric about that seemingly popular goal should not be allowed to disguise the cleavage that is at the heart of debate about the future of those programs. We need to distinguish two different fears.

Technical Bankruptcy

The first fear is that Social Security or Medicare, or both, will "go bankrupt" and cease to deliver their necessary benefits. This fear is based on the specific ways that federal law finances those programs. There is a very high probability that funds currently earmarked for the Old Age and Survivors Insurance (OASI), Disability Insurance (DI), and Hospital Insurance (HI) trust funds will, eventually, be insufficient to meet those programs' expenses. OASI and DI combined (OASDI) are Social Security, and HI is half of Medicare.

These programs have trustees who in March 2000 reported that in or about 2036 for OASDI and 2023 for HI, the programs would be short of funds (Board of Trustees 2000b). Around those times, the revenues dedicated to those funds will need to be increased, or benefits cut, or some other budgetary adjustments made—perhaps a combination of such measures. These forecasts alone, however, do not justify cries of crisis. Chapter 2 explains why the financing of Social Security and Medicare is important. Yet the specific financing of these programs should not be confused with either whether the government can afford them or whether their future is secure.

Social Security and Medicare are government programs, financed by the taxing and borrowing power of the federal government. I have asked college students how many expected Social Security benefits to be available when they retire. After all the publicity about Social Security's long-term crisis, as you might expect, less than half of these students raise their hands. Then I ask how many expect governments to still be providing public education. I get blank looks—why would I be asking that?—shrugs, and then almost all the students raise their hands (those who do not fear there is some sort of trick).

Why, I ask, should there be a difference? We are talking about two government functions, education for the young and a basic pension for the old. Both are not only well accepted but also extremely popular. Both have huge constituencies and have been around for a long time. Both are among governments' largest expenses.[2] As government programs, each basically depends on the willingness of citizens and politicians to vote for them. So why would anyone imagine that education is secure and pensions are not?

The main difference is that Social Security has a dedicated source of financing (the "trust funds") that is likely, under current law, to prove insufficient at some point. But to assume that the level of contributions would not be changed when necessary, or even new revenue sources found, contradicts both the sixty-year history of the program and common sense. Governments find ways to pay for their most popular programs. That may include shaving them at the margins; but when a program is as popular as Social Security or public education (or Medicare), it does not disappear.

This does not mean there is no point in thinking about the future. Sometimes there are advantages to acting sooner rather than later; some measures have to be enacted well in advance of their effects in order to be effective at all; and debate is always appropriate. But it is for many reasons absurd to say that projected shortfalls in Medicare or Social Security financing in 2023 or 2037 require action now, in order to "save" those programs. If we really want to "save" them, we may choose to do so later.

Nor do the forecast shortfalls in Social Security and Medicare finance justify some definitions of "solutions." Many of the proposals to "save" Social Security and Medicare, particularly versions of privatization, would change the programs so fundamentally that many of their current supporters would believe they had been destroyed, not saved. That is why many supporters of Social Security and Medicare, although agreeing that cost control for Medicare and improving the financing of Social Security are worthwhile goals, reject the rhetoric of crisis. They want to help, not "save," the programs. In this book I explain much of their position. But first it must be distinguished from the alternative.

Saving the Country from Social Security and Medicare

The fundamental assumption behind the campaign for immediate, radical action on Social Security and Medicare is that America cannot afford to pay for the benefits those programs currently promise. The demand for immediate action is not about saving Social Security and Medicare but about saving the country from Social Security and Medicare. That is what all the rhetoric concerning "middle-class entitlement monsters," what Bill Clinton owes to his daughter, Chelsea, and the like, was about. Nobody worries about threats to monsters; they worry about threats from monsters. The worry about "entitlements" defines Social Security and Medicare not as threatened, but as threats to the nation.

Unless you assume not only that current benefits cannot be afforded but also that fairly modest benefit cuts would not be enough, there can be no "need" for immediate action. After all, relatively modest cuts (say, 10% in Social Security) could be phased in, if necessary, years from now (say, 1% a year from 2020 to 2030). So what is the hurry?

The heart of the matter, then, is whether Social Security and Medicare are "affordable." Arguments that they are not affordable are closely related to claims that the programs are inequitable—what we will discuss as the "generational inequity" claim. From these perspectives, radical reforms that greatly reduced the protection that these programs currently provide would indeed be responsible public policy. But it is simply doublespeak to define them as "saving" Social Security and Medicare.

Positions and Rationales

By distinguishing the two types of fear, we can understand the three basic positions in the present and coming battles over Social Security and Medicare reform. One group, consisting of much of the Republican party, has never much liked Social Security and Medicare; people in that group see the concern about entitlements as a chance to pursue their longtime desire to fundamentally alter those programs. I seek to eliminate their excuse. The second group is made up of what might be called traditional liberals, including many or most congressional Democrats. They have been on the defensive because the weight of conventional wisdom has been against them. This book may strengthen their resolve by showing that the "liberal" position is eminently respectable, even responsible.

But the audience that I most want to reach is the third group, individuals normally considered centrists, both in the public and in Washington. Moderate Democrats, the few remaining moderate Republicans, and many independents may be less set in their views: they value Social Security and Medicare but are indeed worried by what they have heard about the dangers of entitlements.

Among politicians, my target audience is especially the large portion of Democratic legislators who at a minimum worry that entitlements for the elderly might be unaffordable yet fear the consequences of the most heavily promoted reforms. I argue that, since the crises are exaggerated, there is a practical middle way, in which moderate reforms would improve budget prospects without sacrificing what Social Security and Medicare accomplish. Within the wider world of political debate, my argument above all is with the reporters and commentators and think-tank scholars who set the tone in this chapter's first pages.

The positions of moderate or conservative Democrats and elite commentators are likely to be especially crucial if Governor Bush becomes president. He positioned himself during his campaign as a candidate who could break the "gridlock" in Washington by leading in a "bipartisan" manner. But what is bipartisan? Does bipartisan reform include his proposed changes in Social Security and Medicare? There can be no doubt that Governor Bush, as president, would argue that his proposals are bipartisan responses to urgent national needs. If even a small number of Democratic politicians agree, and the elite commentators go along, those initiatives will be presented to the public as coming not from a president with a tenuous electoral mandate seeking to use his power to enact a radical agenda, but from a president seeking to do the responsible thing in a bipartisan manner. The analysts and politicians who seek to preserve traditional Social Security and Medicare will be described not as defenders of important national responsibilities but as cynical seekers of partisan advantage—people using, as perhaps-President Bush put it in his campaign, "scare tactics" to prevent needed change.

In this case as in many others, beliefs about policy can be transmuted into characterizations of individuals who support certain positions. The conventional wisdom that has defined support for the current Social Security and Medicare programs as irresponsible likely helped Governor Bush define opposition to his proposals as the politics of fear. Yet it would be at least as fair to characterize the campaign against entitlements, with its rhetoric about economic disaster, as a fear campaign. I hope with this book to show reporters and experts and opinion leaders that incremental change of Social Security and Medicare is not only a possible course but also the most responsible one. They have done the country no favors by attempting to panic citizens into supporting more radical steps.

There are some good recent books that explain why citizens should not be seduced by the rhetoric of alarm about Social Security in particular.[3] But the alarmists claim that though the Social Security problem can be made to seem relatively small (mainly because it is), voters would be more worried if they considered Social Security and Medicare together. This book is in the much smaller group that challenges the alarm about entitlements on all fronts, including Medicare. I do not deny the many legitimate concerns that are mixed up with the undue panic. But I argue that the idea that Social Security and Medicare must be "saved" soon is a greater danger.

The Financing Challenge

There is reason for concern about future financing of those programs. Yet *it is reasonable to view the challenges as something to be addressed in incremental steps, so that policies can be adjusted as we learn about the condition of the world and the possible alternatives.*

Any case for incrementalism, as opposed to radicalism, is likely to have certain components. First, the incrementalist values the status quo more than the radical does. In the context of this argument, I (and I suspect most Americans) am more impressed by what Social Security and Medicare do well than the radical reformers are. We fear losing those benefits.

Second, the incrementalist believes that policymakers rarely have enough information to justify radical moves; smaller steps are less likely to backfire badly. In this case, that is especially true of proposed Medicare reforms but also true of many Social Security options. We simply do not know how to make a Medicare voucher system work. Nor do we know how to administer a national system of mandatory private pension accounts. Nor do we know what the return on investments in accounts would be, or even how much future citizens will want to spend on health care for senior citizens. Under these circumstances, making decisions about such matters is irrational: it requires leaps of faith, whereas there might be opportunities for more informed decisions if we move more slowly.

Third, the incrementalist tends to be less worried that the world is on a path to some horrible result than the radical is. So the incrementalist feels less need to take drastic action to avoid disaster. In this case the forecast fiscal challenges will look more manageable to the incrementalist than to the radical. We will see that some of the expected spending increases might even seem desirable; some of them might be offset by policy changes outside Social Security and Medicare; some of the rest might be dealt with by legislation that does not go so far as the radical proposals.

Fourth, the incrementalist is likely to feel that he does not have to save the world. There are always problems and challenges. If they are reduced to a level that makes choices manageable for future citizens, that should be enough. Absent a real disaster very different from the challenges posed by financing Social Security and Medicare, it should be possible to reduce the difficulties of paying for those programs to a level that future citizens can be allowed to address.

Incrementalism is not inaction. I recommend a substantial amount of change in both Social Security and Medicare. But incrementalism recognizes that smaller, more frequent steps are often better than a policy "big bang." In the case of Social Security and Medicare reforms, big bangs are more likely to blow up things that we value than to make the world a better place.

The numbers created to forecast future spending for Social Security and Medicare do give reason for concern. There are four separate trust funds whose trustees report on their condition (though the same individuals serve as trustees of all four funds). Old Age and Survivors' Insurance (OASI) and Disability Insurance (DI) are parts of Social Security. Hospital Insurance (HI) is the part of Medicare paid for by payroll taxes, and Supplementary Medical

TABLE I.1
Year of Trust-Fund Exhaustion as Estimated in March 2000

Set of Assumptions	OASI	DI	OASDI	HI
Alternative I (low cost)	never	never	never	never
Alternative II (intermediate estimate)	2039	2023	2036	2023
Alternative III (high cost)	2029	2012	2026	2012

SOURCE: Board of Trustees 2000b: 8.

TABLE I.2
OASI, DI, HI, and SMI Spending as a Percentage of Gross Domestic Product
(2000 Intermediate Estimates)

Trust Fund	2000	2025	2050	2074
OASI	3.62	5.34	5.65	5.90
DI	0.58	0.92	0.92	0.92
OASDI	4.20	6.26	6.57	6.82
HI	1.39	2.00	2.63	2.91
SMI	0.94	1.95	2.17	2.36
Medicare	2.33	3.95	4.80	5.27
TOTAL	6.53	10.21	11.37	12.09

SOURCE: Board of Trustees 2000b: 10.

Insurance (SMI) is the part of Medicare paid basically by individuals' premiums (which cover about a quarter of the costs) and general revenues. Tables 1.1 and 1.2 provide the trustees' summaries of their estimates of the funds' conditions as of March 2000.

These figures are subject to a great many uncertainties. Demographic trends, which shape the proportion of the population who benefit from, and the proportion that pay for, the programs, may be different. Economic and wage growth, which determine the relationship between taxes that pay for the programs and their benefits, may be higher (good) or lower (bad). The Medicare projections depend on assumptions about the relative growth of medical spending and the rest of the economy. When even small differences in these assumptions are compounded over decades, they can turn into big differences in the projected results.

Table 1.1 therefore shows that the condition of the OASI, DI, and HI trust funds, as conventionally projected, depends significantly on the assumed values of these variables.[4] The trustees adopt three packages of economic and demographic assumptions: one more optimistic ("low cost"), one more pessimistic ("high cost"), and one intermediate. On balance, it is best to focus on the intermediate estimates (Alternative II). But the table shows one reason for incrementalism: if the actual values are different from those projected, policy choices based on the long-term forecasts could be badly mistaken. On the one hand, if conditions are better than forecast, then policymakers might make entirely unnecessary cuts. On the other hand, if conditions turn out to be more dire than forecast, they might have wanted to cut or reform differently than they actually did. Basing policy on a worst-case scenario would make the latter error less likely but the former one probable.

Supplementary Medical Insurance (SMI) was excluded from table 1.1 because SMI does not depend on payroll taxes and cannot legally go broke. It is included in table 1.2, however, because that table expresses program costs as a share of the economy, or gross domestic product (GDP). Expressing costs as a share of GDP allows us to compare periods when comparisons in dollar figures, because of inflation and economic growth, would be meaningless. It also presents spending in a way that makes intuitive sense as a measure of "burden": how much of the total product of the economy would be needed for these programs.

These 2000 projections show Medicare and Social Security costs, combined, growing substantially. They would increase by about 3.7 percent of GDP from 2000 to 2025, as the baby boom retires, and by another 1.2 percent of GDP over the following twenty-five years. These forecasts clearly justify some concern. Yet they are, as we shall see, only part of the story.

Some portion of the projected costs might be met with a mix of higher contributions and lower spending for other government functions. That is essentially how increased Social Security and Medicare costs have been financed in the past. Federal spending as a share of GDP, for example, was at the same level in fiscal year 1998 as in fiscal year 1972. Yet Medicare and Social Security spending had risen from a total of 4 percent of GDP to 7 percent (CBO 1999: tables F-9, F-13).[5] The federal budget has to be seen as a whole in order to assess claims of crisis. Chapter 5 discusses why there are good reasons to believe that two categories of federal spending, "discretionary" programs and payments of interest on the federal debt, will decline as shares of GDP in the future (though not as much as in the common estimates as of 1999).

There are good reasons to believe that higher future costs for Social Security and Medicare, as a share of GDP, would not entirely be an extra loss of welfare to taxpayers. Taxpayers' incomes are expected to be significantly higher in the future, leaving people with more to consume after paying higher program costs than they do today. They may see Social Security and Medicare as guaranteeing something that they value very much for themselves, a minimum pension and basic medical care in their old age. If Social Security and Medicare are believed to be the best ways to guarantee those goods, people may be willing to pay for them.

For these and other reasons, any argument that the future costs of Social Security and Medicare would be "unaffordable" is a matter of guess and opinion. It involves guesses about the amount of that spending, the incomes from which that spending will be financed, and other government costs. It involves opinions about the value of Social Security and Medicare. I argue that there is better reason to believe the programs are worth preserving than that they should be radically "reformed."

The following pages are an attack on conventional wisdom. Conventional wisdom says there is an entitlement crisis. That definition of the policy problem presented by Social Security and Medicare threatens serious policy errors.

The more obvious risk is that poverty and lousy health care could become much greater risks for elderly persons—which potentially means each of us— without meaningfully improving the economy. The less obvious risk is that, if the public's appropriate doubts do block dramatic "fixes" to Social Security and Medicare, the United States will forgo the sensible, incremental measures that would fairly address concerns about an aging society without abandoning basic security for the elderly.

The actual costs of "savings" cannot be assumed away, and neither equity nor the economy requires a rush to make large changes in Social Security and Medicare. Modest changes as proposed in this book will do as much good as needs to be done. Future generations can be expected to take care of the rest.

"Control of entitlements" is often treated as a matter of responsibility, and suggestions that the conventional wisdom is overstated are considered a form of irresponsibility. That is simply wrong. Planning ahead is not responsible if you ignore consequences, get the facts wrong, and do unnecessary damage. Responsibility about Social Security and Medicare means the following.

We have a responsibility to maintain a decent society. Social Security and

Medicare are part of that. We have a responsibility to make changes that will work, based on the information we have. There is nothing responsible about radical reform that will do more harm than good. We have a responsibility not to confuse solving the government's problems (by cutting its expenditures) with solving society's. No matter where we started, cutting Social Security and Medicare would be good for the budget. Eliminating them would be better. But the government does not exist just for its budget. The government exists to make the country a better place to live.

Social Security and Medicare do make this a better country, and they can and should be preserved from the attack on "entitlements."

PART I

The Stakes: What Social Security and Medicare Do

TWO

Why Americans Trust Social Insurance and Distrust Entitlements

Policy choices about Social Security and Medicare might be made with reference to only those programs' specific details. Yet they are, instead, caught up in fears about entitlements. These fears define the programs as bad in principle, on the grounds that entitlement is in some way immoral.

An alternative view also puts Social Security and Medicare within a class of programs, the class of "social insurance," but in this view the programs are in principle good. Chapters 3 and 4 look more closely at the details of the individual programs; details are crucial to practical policy choice. In this chapter we look at the principles that justify the social-insurance approach to policy design, how Social Security originated in those principles, and the contrast between that view and the focus on entitlements.

Because Social Security and Medicare are government programs, their affordability ultimately depends on the fiscal capacity of the federal government, and their future rests on whether voters will want to continue them. Yet the financing of Social Security and Medicare raises issues of "bankruptcy" that seem to mean the programs are at risk. It is important to understand why Social Security and Medicare have that dedicated financing.

That brings us to the nature and reasons for social insurance. This chapter emphasizes the history of Social Security because Medicare was designed in the context of that history.

Origins and Rationale of Social Security
Security and Government

Old Age Insurance was initiated in the Social Security Act of 1935 and has been extended and modified in many steps since then. The most important modification, including the creation of survivors' benefits, occurred in 1939, after the report of the first Advisory Council on Social Security in 1938. The 1939 reforms are commonly viewed as having created, along with the original act, the basic framework that we know today (Derthick 1979: 212–38; Berkowitz 1996).

The original package put the program for elderly persons that we now think of as the core of Social Security in a context of other measures, such as unemployment compensation and Aid to Dependent Children. All of these measures responded to the same basic concern: how to protect people against the economic uncertainties that are created both by swings in the entire economy (quite obvious in the midst of the Great Depression) and by fluctuations in personal circumstances. They responded, however, in significantly different ways.

The report of President Roosevelt's Committee on Economic Security noted that "there is insecurity in every stage of life." Then, as now, people did not entirely control their own fates. Savings could be impaired and lost as a result of all sorts of bad luck: general bad times such as the Depression, an expensive family crisis, or personal unemployment. The committee noted that for the largest group of citizens, "the people in middle years who carry the burden of current production from which all must live, the hazards with which they are confronted threaten not only their own economic independence but the welfare of their dependents." Policies that protected the dependents, whether young or old, therefore would also help workers, by reducing their burdens. In the case of the elderly, the committee emphasized that

> insecurity is doubly tragic, because they are beyond the productive period. Old age comes to everyone who does not die prematurely and is a misfortune only if there is insufficient income to provide for the remaining years of life. With a rapidly increasing number of the aged, and with the impairment and loss of savings, this country faces, in the next decades, an even greater old-age security problem than that with which it is already confronted. (Committee on Economic Security 1985: 72)

Concern for an "aging society" is nothing new, as this shows. And elderly persons *are* different, because once they get into trouble, there is less they can do to get out by their own efforts.

How much protection is appropriate, and why must it be provided by government? As FDR declared in signing the Social Security Act, "we can never insure one hundred percent of the population against one hundred percent of the hazards and vicissitudes of life" (Committee on Economic Security 1985: 145). Nevertheless, government needed to guarantee some minimum, as he explained in his radio address on the third anniversary of signing the act, because in a modern economy dominated by "the often intangible forces of giant industry," a man's "individual strength and wits" cannot guarantee security. At one time people could turn to neighbors, but neighbors were not enough anymore, if they ever had been. And, Roosevelt emphasized, this was not a matter of government providing security only for the poor. Government had already been in the business of helping develop the economy for a long time, responding to the "rich and the strong." FDR asserted that "none of the sums of money paid out to individuals" under the act "will spell anything approaching abundance. But they will furnish that minimum necessary to keep a foothold, and that is the kind of protection Americans want" (147–48).

Roosevelt's explanations respond to two bases for criticism of Social Security. One is that the benefits might be excessive—more than "a foothold" and too close to "abundance." That must be a matter of collective judgment and can be addressed by altering benefit levels. The second criticism is more fundamental, more a matter of how one believes the world works. Can individuals really provide entirely for their own security? Here, supporters of a government role argue that modern libertarians and other conservatives simply misunderstand how individuals' fates are determined in the modern economy. They argue that using the government to ensure a foothold does not deny individual responsibility, but defines responsibility in a way that is reasonable and fair to people in the real world. Most individuals face too many uncertainties in both their personal lives and general economic performance to be able to guarantee their own security (Thompson and Upp 1997). None of these factors mean that government should guarantee people all they want, but they justify government guarantee of some minimum.

But should government guarantee benefits even to people who are not prudent and responsible? One of the commonest criticisms of government in-

come support programs is that they hurt the economy and even the beneficiaries by encouraging them to be irresponsible. Such criticisms, and a desire
to ensure that the public would not be exploited by people who chose welfare
rather than work, were a major factor in the repeal of the Aid to Families with
Dependent Children program in 1996—one of the few "entitlements" to be
eliminated (Weaver 2000). We do not need to discuss the dubious merits of
the 1990s attack on AFDC itself in order to recognize that this concern could
be legitimate.

The answer, in the form of Social Security and some other programs, such
as Unemployment Insurance and Medicare, is to link benefits to work through
social insurance, based on contributions made while the future beneficiary is
able to work. This approach does not fit some situations, especially those involving children. Children cannot entitle themselves by working, and in many
cases—a widowed young mother, or divorce, or no marriage—there is no parent whose work could be used as a basis for benefits.[1] That is why the original Social Security Act included a separate, means-tested, program that was
the predecessor to AFDC. But the abolition of AFDC made clear, if it was
not clear already, how important the social-insurance approach can be.

Social Insurance and "Protecting the Prudent"

In social insurance, people contribute to a program in order to receive protection against certain risks. Beneficiaries must either be contributors or be related to contributors (e.g., for survivors' benefits). Because they are entitled by
contribution, the beneficiaries cannot be suspected of being slackers or irresponsible. But social insurance differs from private insurance because participation is compulsory and may be designed to serve further social goals, such
as adequacy.

Richard A. Musgrave (1986a,b) explains the case for social pension insurance by beginning with the insurance part. Pensions involve unpredictable
needs. Some people will live longer and need more retirement income; some
will need less. If people wanted to cover the risk, it would not be in the interest of all to save for the maximum need, because some would not get to use
the money. If they pooled their money under an agreement that those who
needed it would get it, each would be protected and they would pay less. Mus-

grave imagines three individuals, Calvin, Homer, and Jack; logically, they might all buy insurance against the risk of living longer.

Now imagine that Jack is "irresponsible" and does not buy the insurance. Later on, he is poor and suffering. What then? In Musgrave's account, Calvin and Homer will end up paying for some means-tested benefit for Jack, out of humanitarian concern. A cynic might doubt that but should recognize that virtually all current critics of Social Security assert some support for such means-tested benefits.[2] One can be a humanitarian of this type without any interest in equality or any of the other values that are more politically controversial.

Under the circumstances, however, what would have been the effect of having a system like Social Security? *Jack would already have contributed.* So Social Security is in Calvin and Homer's interest. As Musgrave explains,

> Insurance could be purchased privately but becomes a matter of public concern only because Jack will not do so, while Calvin and Homer will. Given their humanitarian premise, Calvin and Homer must bail out Jack should the contingency arise. They will require therefore that Jack should insure. Social insurance is now insurance in the technical sense, but its basic function (and especially the rationale for making it mandatory) is . . . to avoid burdening the prudent."
> (1986a: 69–70)

Economist Rudolph Penner, former director of the Congressional Budget Office, makes the same point about the difference between social insurance and alternative income support approaches when he writes that "Social security must be the most popular civilian program ever invented in the United States. . . . The compulsory nature of the new system was vitally important in protecting it against freeloaders" (1994: 4).

This function was especially clear to the designers of Social Security in the political context of the time. They saw not only that existing local means-tested programs were inadequate (humanitarianism goes only so far) but also that there was a powerful political campaign for a no-strings-attached, general-revenue-financed pension for all the elderly, the Townsend Plan. Social Security's design was a middle ground between the inadequacies of previous means-tested efforts and the entitlement (as we now call it), based purely on age, of the Townsend scheme (Committee on Economic Security 1985: 45, 53–

54). The 1938 Advisory Council declared that Social Security's "method of encouragement of self-help and self-reliance in securing protection in old age is
essentially in harmony with individual incentive within a democratic society."
It emphasized that social protection was "related," in this way, "to past participation in the productive processes of the country" (185).

This early statement remains by far the primary justification for Social Security. Benefits are based on having contributed to the nation as a whole, "participation in the productive processes of the country." It was and is a social
contribution that earns social support for social security. That is different from
results in the market, advocates for which must maintain that whatever you
happen to get is "just," whether that is due to your own unusual good or bad
luck or skill, and there is no such thing as "need." Social Security relates a social judgment of need (the benefit rules) to a social demand for contribution
(the tax rules). You contribute to establish your claim on the rest of us.

Issues within the Terms of Social Insurance

If contributing is a social act, in which participants pull their weight in the
shared enterprise of guaranteeing a modicum of security by paying a fixed
share of their wage income, it is not the same as an investment or any form of
personal saving. Nor does the logic of social insurance meet some more egali-
tarian or leveling notions of "fairness."

Social Security taxes apply only to wage income and only to a portion of
that income (the first $76,200 in earnings in 2000). Egalitarians object that
higher-income Americans pay smaller proportions of their incomes than
lower-income workers do. However, this "regressive" tax follows from the program's purpose: the cap on covered income simply says that beyond some maximum, society is not especially interested in people's ability to replace their
working incomes. So the excess is counted for neither taxes nor benefits.

Four other issues about the relation of contributions to benefits were relatively easy to resolve in 1939 but may seem more difficult now. First, why is
redistribution confined to the pension formula, rather than affecting all income? If income were redistributed first, workers would be better off while
working, and Social Security pensions would look more like private investments or insurance. Yet the reasons for confining redistribution within the
pension benefit design were and remain politically and practically compelling.

Less money has to be redistributed if only pensions, not the incomes on which pensions are based, are affected. Furthermore, redistribution earlier would help lower earners not for the popular purpose of protecting them in their retirement, when they could not do more for themselves, but during their working years, when perhaps they could. Moreover, the low earner at one time may be a high earner later and may have contributed enough for a passable retirement on average; so the earlier adjustments would turn out to have been unnecessary for pension purposes. Because help will be targeted more accurately if pensions are adjusted at the end of a career, redistribution is within the benefit formula rather than on the contribution side (Musgrave 1986a: 70; 1986b: 112–13).

The effect of redistribution within the benefit formula, however, is that higher-income participants may feel they receive less for their contributions. Chapter 3 explains the mechanisms by which higher earners receive lower *replacement rates*.[3] For the first three or even four decades of the program, this was not a serious problem. The ratio of workers to retirees was high, and earnings grew quickly; thus, even high-wage retirees could receive benefits far in excess of the investment value of their contributions without workers feeling too burdened by payroll taxes. Those conditions have now changed, however, and so the balance between the goals of adequacy and relating benefits to contributions has become more politically problematic.

The second issue involves the extent to which the program should be "funded" or "pay-as-you-go." This issue also can be debated as a matter of principle, economic or otherwise, but it was answered in 1939 according to practical considerations.

In current debate, two basic arguments are made for a "funded" system. One is that a generation should pay for its own retirement, as a matter of fairness or "intergeneration neutrality." The other is that by building up the fund, the nation would increase its pool of savings and thus its eventual wealth.

The original Social Security Act contemplated paying benefits only in the future, after a fund had built up. Musgrave explains that this early intent was abandoned for two reasons: "First, it seemed unacceptable to exclude the then old generation from benefits, the more so since their plight was accentuated by the Great Depression. And second, the 1937 recession, which followed rapidly upon the introduction of the system, rendered a substantial system surplus undesirable on grounds of stabilisation policy" (1986b: 110). That is, during a major recession the government should not be taking money out of circulation; extra savings can wait for another day. At a time of high unemployment, encouraging older workers to leave the workforce, so as to provide opportunities for younger workers starting out, was also a policy goal (Committee on Economic Security 1985: 187). In reaction to these and other concerns, the 1939 legislation postponed scheduled tax increases that had been planned to build up the fund and initiated payment of some benefits immediately.

At present, when for better or worse there is more concern about savings than about maintaining demand for goods, and when future prospects make keeping people in the labor force seem more useful than encouraging them to leave it, one can imagine making a different decision. But a pay-as-you-go system is what we now have, in any case, and there are costs to changing that design. As the analysis of privatization proposals in chapter 8 shows, any transition to a funded system requires making some people "pay twice," both to fund some of their own benefits and to pay for the benefits of those who are in retirement while these people are working.

The third important issue is how the benefits and the risks of macroeconomic trends should be shared. Here the key factors are the changes in price level and in real wages.

Current Social Security law raises benefits automatically with a Cost-of-Living Adjustment equal to the previous year's increase in a version of the Consumer Price Index. Thus benefits are said to be "indexed" to inflation. Indexing of benefits to inflation was not enacted until 1972 and is controversial among the people who care most about the budget, but the basic case for it is strong. If individuals contribute now to their elders' pensions in return for a promise of adequate pensions later, those pensions cannot be allowed to be eroded by inflation. As Musgrave puts it, "an explicitly and rigidly adhered to provision for inflation adjustment, such as contained in the present law, is essential to the design of a meaningful inter-generation contract. The contract, by its nature being of a long-term character, becomes meaningless without such an adjustment" (1986b: 110).

When wages rise more quickly than prices (that is, when *real wages* are rising), the cost of benefits (other things being equal) rises more slowly than total wages, so price indexing is affordable. Some advocates for higher pensions argue that it would be more fair to index benefits to wages, so that the rising

national product would be shared among all the public (Eisner 1998). However, if real wages decline, as they did significantly from 1979 to 1980 and marginally in other years since, indexing doubles the burden on wage earners: they
must pay the cost of inflation not only in their own purchases but for the elderly as well.[4] Wage indexing would force elderly persons to share in the nation's bad times as well as good. In practice, other things are not equal; with a
growing ratio of beneficiaries to workers, and with wages normally growing,
price indexing likely strikes the best balance between adequacy and affordability.

The fourth issue is the size of payroll-tax financing. The payroll tax is the
logical basis for social insurance because work is the contribution to society.
It is especially logical for a pension program, whose point is to replace wages.
Yet payroll, and especially covered payroll, is only a portion of national income. In 1998 it was about 40.9 percent of GDP and was projected to decline
slightly over time.[5] As costs grow and payroll's share of national income declines, there might come a point at which the necessary payroll tax looks too
large. If so, is the right response to limit benefits, or find other revenues?

This issue was actually addressed by the first Advisory Council, and the answer as of 1938 may surprise readers. Arguing that "the Nation as a whole, independent of the beneficiaries of the system, will derive a benefit from the
old-age security program," the council recommended that some general revenues be used to supplement payroll taxes. Looking ahead to 1980, the council members expected that by then the cost of the program would be between
10 and 12 percent of covered payroll, and they recommended that general revenue financing be implemented as needed then (Advisory Council on Social
Security 1997a: 188, 198).

Replacement rates in 1980 were almost exactly as anticipated and the
needed contributions a little lower, because the baby boom raised the working-age population more than expected (Ball 1985: 166–67). By 1998 the payroll tax for OASI was 10.70 percent and costs were about 9.70 percent, which
yielded a surplus. Because costs as a share of payroll are expected to increase,
however, we are now at a point where the 1938 council would have recommended serious consideration of general-revenue finance.

There seem to be two reasons why general-revenue finance has not been explicitly on the table. First, at a time of great concern about budget deficits,
even many liberals wanted to use any increases in general revenues for other

purposes. Second, using general revenues would seem to violate public un-
derstandings of how people buy their benefits with their contributions. Is it
possible to maintain the argument that Social Security has the advantages of
social-insurance finance if it uses some general revenues? The 1938 Advisory
Council apparently believed so, and we might argue that, so long as benefits
were paid mainly from contributions, the basic understanding of Social Security should not change.

The questions I have posed here are central to much of the controversy
about "reforming" Social Security. Many proposals should be understood as
efforts to resolve tensions with the least possible pain. Although all of the issues regarding the terms of social insurance for pensions are worth discussion,
none suggest that social insurance per se is a bad idea. The critique of entitlements does.

How Entitlements Became an Issue

The case for social insurance is that it is the right way to conduct certain national programs, precisely because it ensures that the recipients will be "de-
serving." By contrast, entitlements could be viewed as negative on the assumption that the recipients are "undeserving."

The Legal Theory of Entitlements

As Kent Weaver explains, "the concept of entitlement is of fairly recent ori-
gin." It developed from legal theories of the 1960s, which argued that when
legislation defined social welfare benefits, the beneficiaries had "something
akin to property rights in them" (1984: 308–9). As Justice Brennan wrote in
Goldberg v. Kelly, "such benefits are a matter of statutory entitlement for persons qualified to receive them" (397 U.S. 254 [1969]). As a result, Weaver
writes, "recipients can sue if payments allotted to them by statutory formula
are not forthcoming." Even if an entitlement program does not have a dedicated funding source and must be paid for by annual appropriations, "Congress ordinarily considers itself bound to appropriate the amounts required by
law" (1984: 308–9).

Litigation and legal controversy have tended to involve welfare benefits (as in *Goldberg v. Kelly*) and so have associated the term *entitlement* with the negative connotations of welfare. For example, in a public opinion survey, the American Hospital Association asked, "Are Social Security and Medicare entitlement programs, or do people get benefits that their taxes have already paid for?" As John Gist points out, "the answer, in this case, is yes to both," yet the way the question was posed shows how the term *entitlement* commonly has a negative connotation (1996: 331).

Entitlement as a Budgetary Category

Although the legal origins of the entitlement concept helped make it controversial, budgetary politics is what made entitlements fearsome.[6]

From a budgetary perspective, entitlements are one kind of spending commitment by the federal government. The Congressional Budget Act of 1974 refers to authority "to make payments (including loans and grants), the budget authority for which is not provided for in advance by Appropriations Acts, to any person or government if, under the provisions of the law containing such authority, the United States is obligated to make such payments to persons or governments who meet the requirements established by such law" (sec. 402 c 2 C). Such "mandatory" spending can be distinguished from the majority of programs, for which law creates a bureau that then must be funded each year. The latter spending is now called "discretionary," since the law that authorizes the programs generally does not compel particular annual appropriations. For many years the annual appropriations process was viewed as the norm for federal budgeting (Wildavsky 1964; Fenno 1966).

From that perspective, any other kind of program, especially the entitlements defined in *Goldberg v. Kelly*, represents an evasion of budget control. There have always been expenses that were not controlled by annual appropriations, the most obvious being interest on the debt. Pensions for veterans are as old as the republic. Yet Social Security and Medicare are by far the largest among the hundreds of programs that fit the budgetary definitions of entitlement or mandatory spending.

Until the mid-1960s, the discretionary programs accounted for enough of the budget (67.5% in 1962) that budget totals could be adjusted basically by manipulating the annual appropriations. But as defense spending grew more slowly or declined after Vietnam, and as programs such as Medicare, Medicaid, and Social Security grew, the share of the budget consumed by the discretionary programs fell to 55.7 percent of the budget by 1972, 43.7 percent in 1982, and 33.7 percent in 1997.[7] It became impossible to control the deficit through manipulating the shrinking part of the budget. How to create better annual budget control over entitlement spending (still not routinely called by that term) therefore was one of the subjects of budget process reforms in 1974 and 1980 (Schick 1980; Gilmour 1990; White and Wildavsky 1991). But it took the politics of the Reagan deficits to make entitlements per se a major public issue.

As the deficit then became the major theme in American politics, "entitlements and other mandatory spending" became the standard term used to talk about these programs within the budget world and thus the standard term associated with most of the spending side of the federal deficit.[8] It became a commonplace for budget experts to complain that the deficit would not be controlled until Congress controlled entitlement spending. Thus "entitlements" became defined as the cause of national irresponsibility, the federal deficit. The biggest entitlements, Social Security and Medicare, from this perspective looked like threats to the nation.

The growth of entitlement spending was related to budget deficits, though the importance of that relationship must depend on one's perspective. Between 1963 and 1983, Social Security nearly doubled as a share of the economy, from 2.6 percent of GDP to 4.9 percent. It grew partly because of demographics, as a larger share of the population became elderly and was entitled to full benefits under the program, and partly because of policy choices to raise benefits, particularly in 1972 (Derthick 1979; Light 1985).[9] Medicare, which did not exist until 1966, had grown to 1.6 percent of GDP by 1983. As a matter of mathematics, then, one could argue that a deficit that reached a peak of 6.1 percent of GDP in 1983, compared to 0.8 percent in 1963, was largely due to the growth of those two entitlements. And Medicaid explained some more.

Ironically, the 1980s, during which large deficits seemed to become systematic, was not a time of especially large entitlement growth. Social Security's costs as a share of the economy fell during the 1980s, as the demographic surge ended and the economy grew more quickly. Medicare cost controls became more effective. Other entitlements, such as unemployment compensation, were cut and also declined for economic reasons. If one looked only at the immediate causes of a mismatch between spending and revenues in the

1980s, one would have to emphasize the 1981 tax cuts, the defense buildup, and the ways in which the deficit fed on itself to raise interest costs.[10]

Nevertheless, as the budget battles of the 1980s continued, a consensus that the "real problem" was entitlements grew. Medicare costs were controlled relatively well compared to health costs in the private sector, but Medicare and Medicaid did grow as a share of GDP through the 1980s.[11] By the time the Republicans took control of Congress in 1994 and then pledged to balance the budget by 2002, budget forecasts especially fit the idea that health-care entitlements were to blame for the deficit (CBO 1995: 57 and table 2–14).[12]

These budget forecasts underestimated future revenues, overstated future Medicare and Medicaid cost increases, and so proved far too pessimistic. Yet the notion that entitlements threatened massive deficits was too entrenched to be abandoned even when the deficit disappeared. And it could still seem true, if one looked far enough into the future.

In May of 1998, the Congressional Budget Office projected that rising entitlement costs would send federal deficits spiraling out of control in the 2030s. In January of 1999 it was projecting that debt would not become unmanageable until sometime after 2050 (CBO 1998b: xvi–xvii; 1999: 43–44). Chapter 5 argues that the very volatility of these estimates is reason to hesitate to base action on either optimistic or pessimistic numbers. But the salient political fact was that analysts and commentators went out of their way to look far enough ahead to find a disaster that entitlements would create.

As the largest entitlements, Social Security and Medicare thus were transformed into objects of budgetary fear. As part of the class of programs that *Goldberg v. Kelly* defined, Social Security and Medicare could be associated with some of the unpopularity of "welfare." Good "social insurance" was also bad "entitlements."

Social Insurance and Entitlement Perspectives on Future Burdens

From a social-insurance perspective, Social Security and Medicare are subjects of an intergenerational contract. Workers pay for benefits for the current retirees, in return for assurance that their own benefits will be funded by future workers' contributions. There will be some variations in costs due to demographic and economic factors, but the "burden" on any given set of workers is offset largely by the security that they receive from the continuation of the Social Security and Medicare systems. From the perspective of critics of entitlements, however, benefits at any given time are an unnecessary burden on the persons who are the workers at that time. If costs rise over time, that just means the entitlement is becoming more onerous.

Chapter 7 considers issues of intergenerational "equity" in greater detail, but here it is worth stopping to look at the different ways we might think about future costs. We will focus mainly on Social Security as the clearer example, relying on the "intermediate" projections by the Social Security Administration actuaries.

Costs as a Share of the Economy

As table 2.1 summarizes (see the "Costs as % of GDP" column), costs have been stable in recent years but are expected to rise slowly through about 2010. Then, as the baby-boom generation retires, they will rise much more quickly, before stabilizing around 2035. The total expected cost increase is about 2.6 percent of GDP over the next seventy-five years. During the period of greatest growth, from 2010 to 2030, it is about 2 percent of GDP. From the perspective of the entitlement critic, this is all unjustified extra cost.

Yet, first of all, spending for various government accounts has risen or fallen by larger shares of GDP at many points in the past. Other voters, at other times, have dealt with significantly larger "problems."

Social Security spending rose by more in the fifteen years from 1950 to 1965 than it is projected in table 2.1 to rise from 2010 to 2030. Government spending in the United States on the baby boomers themselves rose by more during the period from 1950 to 1970, to pay for their public education. The effects of military buildups have been much larger. In 1940 defense cost 1.7 percent of GDP, within a federal government budget of 9.9 percent. By 1951 it had risen to 7.5 percent of GDP, within a total budget of 14.5 percent. It is unlikely that anyone would argue that the economy was worse in 1951 than in 1940. Yet government spending had grown by 4.6 percent of GDP—becoming essentially 50 percent larger than before.

If spending is seen as entitlements, and thus inherently suspect, then we might view any increase as negative. Yet increased spending on a given gov-

TABLE 2.1
Indices of Increasing Social Security "Burden"

| Calendar Years | Costs as % of GDP | Dependency Ratios | | Workers per Beneficiary |
		Aged Only	Total	
1950	0.27	0.138	0.719	16.5
1960	2.20	0.173	0.904	5.1
1965	2.49	0.182	0.946	4.0
1970	2.94	0.185	0.898	3.7
1980	4.31	0.195	0.749	3.2
1990	4.33	0.209	0.701	3.4
2000	4.19	0.211	0.697	3.4
2005	4.30	0.207	0.673	3.3
2010	4.57	0.214	0.660	3.1
2015	5.06	0.239	0.674	2.8
2020	5.70	0.274	0.710	2.5
2025	6.26	0.319	0.760	2.3
2030	6.62	0.355	0.800	2.1
2035	6.75	0.370	0.810	2.1
2040	6.69	0.370	0.802	2.1
2045	6.62	0.369	0.796	2.0
2055	6.64	0.383	0.811	2.0
2065	6.75	0.406	0.834	1.9
2075	6.83	0.421	0.846	1.9

SOURCES: Figures for 1950–90 for Costs/GDP are author's calculations for those fiscal years from *Historical Tables: Budget of the United States Government, Fiscal Year 1999* (Washington, D.C.: GPO, 1998), tables 11.3, 15.1. All other data in the table is for calendar years, from Board of Trustees 2000a: tables II.F19, II.H1, III.C1.

ernment function, in and of itself, does not mean much. Any economic and social effects will depend, first, on what is going on in the rest of the budget and the economy. Second, opinions of the effects will depend on how we value the object of spending. When the need for military or education spending rose, the spending was accepted. In the same way as military danger and later a larger population of schoolchildren caused higher military and education spending, a larger population of retirees is expected to raise Social Security's share of the economy. If we believe the program is a good idea to start with, spending more as the need increases can seem entirely sensible.

Dependency Ratios and Other Demographic Effects

Another approach to measuring the burden of entitlements for retirees focuses on how many workers are paying to support how many elderly people. This is the major factor in creating the GDP ratio for Social Security and a major factor for Medicare, since if there are more elderly people per worker, one would expect (productivity being equal) a larger cost relative to national product. It is certainly the major influence on the payroll tax rate. Yet, when viewed in isolation, beneficiary-per-worker figures are highly deceptive.

For instance, Peter G. Peterson informs us that "in 1960 5.1 taxpaying workers supported each Social Security beneficiary. Today, there are 3.3. By 2040, there will be no more than 2—and perhaps as few as 1.6. In effect, every young working couple, in addition to their other tax burdens, will have to pay the Social Security and Medicare benefits of at least one unknown retired 'relative'" (1996: 22). The basic numbers are accurate enough, yet Peterson's interpretation is highly suspect.

His most obvious misstatement refers to that "one unknown retired 'relative.'" After all, these workers are likely to have living parents, and if they are paying for somebody else's parents, then somebody else is paying for theirs. By sleight of word processor, Peterson has defined *entitlement* as entitlement for strangers, rather than as part of how we guarantee security for our families. He has ignored the function of social insurance as providing relief *for workers* from worry about poverty for their parents.

But Peterson's measure also says little about the actual burden on workers' budgets. That depends not only on the costs of Social Security (and Medicare) but also on the other expenses workers must pay. Considering demographics alone, we would want to know not simply the ratio of workers to the elderly but also the ratio of workers to all the people they support. That is the *total dependency ratio*. If there are fewer children and more retired people, then some of the higher cost for the retired is balanced by lower costs for supporting children.

The "Aged Only" column of table 2.1 shows the ratio of people of normal working age (20–64) to those of retirement age (65 and over).[13] This "aged dependency ratio" will be twice as high in 2035 as it was in 1965 and 1970. Yet if we count all potential dependents, as in the "Total" column, the story is very different. This should be no surprise: the baby boomers were children once, and there had to be more of them as children than as eventual old folks. So we see that the total dependency ratio was actually higher in 1965 and 1970 than it is anticipated to become even in 2075.

It seems reasonable to ask why, if members of the baby-boom generation were dependents once and the United States economy survived (even thrived), the baby boom should be unaffordable when its members are over 65 instead of under 21. Or, put another way, why, if the baby boom was "entitled" to support as children, which I think even Peter G. Peterson would not doubt, could the same citizens not also be "entitled" to some security when they are elderly?

In fact, children are expensive but not as costly per capita as elderly persons; this is partly because the costs of medical care for the elderly are much higher and partly because working-age adults tend to want (or at least be willing) to share their homes with their kids but not their parents. Although education costs naturally are higher for children, the most careful attempt to adjust for these differences, based on the demographic forecasts available in 1988, concluded that support for each elderly person is substantially more expensive than for each youth (Cutler et al. 1990).

With those adjustments, the total dependency burden could be expected to pass its 1965 level in 2055.[14] Yet that conclusion still suggests that the social burden of future elderly persons has been overstated by the entitlement Cassandras who look at only one side of the demographic ledger. A slightly higher dependency burden in the distant future hardly looks like a calamity unless you believe that the economic performance of the 1960s was poor, which would be an unusual view.[15]

In spite of the fact that purveyors of panic about entitlements talk about horrible demographic burdens, the demographic figures simply are not that bad. What, then, is the problem? The problem is that Social Security and Medicare benefits are paid from the government budget. Most expenses for children (though by no means all, given the costs of public education) are paid through family budgets. So if you see government programs as inherently suspect, increased costs for Social Security and Medicare will look worse.

Yet if you believe that Social Security and Medicare are the best ways to guarantee a basic pension and medical insurance to the elderly—meaning, hopefully, yourself and your parents—then effects on government spending totals should not seem relevant. Some things might be better done by the government (such as insuring against financial risks); some are better done in families (such as raising children). In short, the debate is not really about the "burden" on future workers. It is about the role of government.

Within that debate, Medicaid is getting relatively little attention. That is both strange and strangely appropriate. In concluding this discussion of social insurance and entitlements, we turn to a program that is not quite social insurance yet technically an entitlement.

Medicaid and Values

From a purely budgetary perspective, one might expect Medicaid to be joined with Medicare and Social Security in discussions of the entitlement crisis of an aging society.

Although Medicaid's public face may be mainly poor mothers and children, in 1996 about a third of its individual benefits were paid to elderly persons and about a third to the blind and disabled.[16] An aging society will raise Medicaid costs, especially since the program is the major source of long-term nursing home finance, and the need for that service should grow substantially.

Sometimes Medicaid is lumped together with Medicare and Social Security in entitlement discussions, and sometimes it is not. This book emphasizes Social Security and Medicare because they are larger expenses for the federal government, because the absence of trust-fund financing means the question of "bankruptcy" cannot be raised for Medicaid, and because the objections to hasty action on Medicare would apply to Medicaid as well. In its 1997 and 1998 reports about long-term budget choices, the Congressional Budget Office made the same decision. But Medicaid also has an ambivalent relationship to the policy debate about entitlements because it represents different values than Social Security and Medicare do.

Medicaid and Universalism
Unpredictability

Medicaid is neither as reliable an entitlement nor as predictable a cost as Social Security and Medicare.

Medicaid is a federal-state program, in which some eligibility standards are uniform and some depend on state options. States are not required to participate, and they extend eligibility both formally (by law) and informally (through the extent of their outreach efforts) to very different populations. State governments may do little to inform inhabitants that the state could be spending money on them. Medicaid is means-tested, so as people's incomes change, they go back and forth between being eligible and not; Social Security and Medicare beneficiaries are eligible once and for all.

For all these reasons, participation in Medicaid is much less predictable than enrollment in Social Security and Medicare. So are costs per capita. States have substantial control of the costs of their programs and thus of the federal spending that those programs generate. There is a politics of cost-shifting between the levels, and any attempt to forecast costs systemwide must depend on assumptions about a wide range of state policies and their success.

The Politics of Means-Testing

Perhaps more important politically, the means-tested nature of Medicaid gives it a different politics than Social Security and Medicare have. As a program for the poor, Medicaid's constituency seems much weaker and the program more easily endangered. For defenders of Social Security and Medicare, one of the greatest dangers is that they might be turned into something more like Medicaid—a program for poor people, whose right to benefits is always in question.

That is exactly what critics of Social Security and Medicare recommend: that those programs target the poor and cease being "middle-class entitlements" paid to people who do not need the help. Thus, Peter G. Peterson calls Social Security "a massive and indiscriminate middle-class welfare program," part of an "entitlement ethic" in which "a very broad spectrum of America's middle-class" think of themselves as "victims." "We thus came to accept a nonsensical notion: universal entitlements" (1996: 95–97).

If a program pays only for people who cannot help themselves, following the logic of a means-tested program like Medicaid, how can we be sure that the beneficiaries deserve the help? Is poverty a sign of virtue? Most Americans do not seem to think so and are suspicious of programs for the poor (Burtless, Weaver, and Wiener 1997: 118). Indeed, the main cash benefit for children, AFDC, was abolished in 1996, largely because of a belief that parents who were not working did not deserve help. That means-tested benefits threaten work effort is an argument made by economists of all political stripes.

In contrast, Peterson's "nonsensical notion" of "universal entitlements" is one of the most common policy measures in the world, since it describes the "social security" systems of all advanced industrial countries. Taken to its logical conclusion, Peterson's critique suggests that middle-class people should not receive benefits from government, which would raise some interesting questions. Why is there public education? Why not tolls on every road? What is so different about retirement income and health care? If anything, the contributory basis of social insurance seeks to avoid the practical and moral hazards of a means-tested program like Medicaid.

That does not mean that I would like to see Medicaid cut. But the program's actual future costs depend on far too many factors, it is not part of the discussion about trust-fund shortfalls, and its character is too different from that of Social Security and Medicare to justify inclusion in this book.[17]

"Unproductive" Elderly Persons versus Children

Behind its facade of concern for equity and the economy, much of the objection to "middle-class entitlements" for the elderly is based on a notion of society that mixes harsh economics and antigovernment values. Consider the reply of Peterson and the Concord Coalition that he helps fund to arguments that he has overstated the future demographic burdens. Responding to an article by Richard C. Leone, a Concord report declared:

> Yes, families spend a lot of their own money on their kids, and if we took this into account it would narrow (but not eliminate) the gap in dependency costs. But why should we? In our economy, there's an obvious difference between personal spending and public spending (for one thing, only the latter runs up the public debt). And in our political system, there's an obvious difference between compulsory transfers and voluntary giving. Some might argue that personal spending on a dependent is not really voluntary. But this doesn't wash. Perhaps some people may regard helping out grandma as an other-than-voluntary burden. But this is not ordinarily the case with children, since the decision to raise a family is usually a matter of choice. (Peterson 1996: 26–27)

Concord's response ignored a few things. One is public education, for which people are compelled to pay taxes even though they are not compelled to receive benefits (which hardly seems fairer than Social Security). Concord also ignored the ways in which Social Security and Medicare may be the surest means for a worker to guarantee a minimum standard of retirement and health care for her parents. After all, these programs pay even if the parent or the worker hit a bad patch and have few resources of their own. And the extent to which extremely popular government programs are not a "choice" could also be debated. Individual preferences, through votes, tend to constitute political choices.[18]

Still, whatever you may think of the Concord Coalition's argument, it is clearly about values—the government's role, and whether children are some sort of consumption good. But the "most profound" (in their words) issue follows: "Leone is perplexed that Americans look forward to the senior boom with anxiety but didn't consider the 1960s an era of 'deprivation,' even though the total demographic dependency ratio was higher in 1960 than it will be in 2030. The difference is that thirty-five years ago adults were sacrificing to *build the future* while thirty-five years hence they will be sacrificing to *reward the past*" (Peterson 1996: 26–27; emphasis in original text). In other words, the real problem with spending on programs for elderly persons is that they are not productive. It is a waste of money: pure consumption, not investment. You cannot invest in retirees: because they are retired, there can be no "return" to society.

The difference between support for social insurance and fear of entitlements could hardly be expressed more starkly. Unlike the antientitlement activists, many people might argue that there is nothing wrong with "rewarding the past." After all, what other than the past can ever be rewarded? The past is all that we ever know. And most Americans look to a decent retirement as a well-deserved reward for years of hard labor. Supporters of Social Security and Medicare believe all human beings are worthwhile; all should be able to live with some dignity and minimum competence; and the standard of a good society is one in which a decent life is possible throughout one's days. From this perspective, saving for economic growth and guaranteeing a minimum income to the elderly are not values that must contradict each other but part of the same goal. Indeed, if people know that they will be secure in their old age and that their parents are also protected against economic ill luck, that may have value to them even when they are younger, and they may believe they live in a better society.

Readers can make their own choice between visions. But nobody should believe that the argument made by advocates like Pete Peterson and the Concord Coalition against entitlements is value-neutral. It is based on a vision of society that emphasizes what its believers would call "self-reliance" and what its critics would call exposing individuals too greatly to random risks that have little to do with personal virtue (Kosterlitz 1996).

The debate about Social Security and Medicare is rarely about technical "affordability." I consider cost issues carefully in the rest of this book. But the basis of much of the conflict is the contrast between two visions, one in which Social Security and Medicare are examples of something good, social insurance, and one in which they are examples of something bad, entitlements.

The more liberal budget "hawks," whose commentary has fed the hysteria about entitlements, see the value of social insurance and believe they are merely recommending prudent planning for the future. I attempt to show in succeeding chapters why their fears for the future are exaggerated. As a political matter, the attempt by well-meaning centrists to scare the public into "responsible" action mainly has served the interests of Mr. Peterson and many far more conservative advocates, whose real purpose is to attack social insurance out of a belief that such entitlements are fundamentally immoral.

The basic original arguments for Social Security as a form of social insurance remain the reasons for the program. If you believe people can and should fend entirely for themselves, you should not support Social Security or Medicare. But if you have doubts about that, even only of a "humanitarian" sort, then the case for social insurance should look a lot stronger.

THREE

Social Security

There are many possible versions of social insurance, and the details matter. Confusion about aspects of both Social Security and Medicare can distort the debate about reform. This chapter highlights the details relevant to the Social Security debate.

Social Security includes two programs: Old-Age and Survivors Insurance (OASI) and Disability Insurance (DI).[1] Old Age Insurance was created in the original Social Security Act of 1935; benefits for dependents and survivors were added in the major amendments of 1939; and DI was created in 1956. Grouped together, these are Old Age, Survivors, and Disability Insurance (OASDI).

Almost all workers and their employers are required by law to contribute to OASDI through taxes on wage income (*payroll taxes*). Based on these contributions, OASDI pays pensions to retired individuals, disabled persons, and their spouses or survivors. The major exceptions at present are some state and local government workers, students, and some federal civilian employees hired before 1984 (U.S. House, Committee on Ways and Means 1996: 10).

Social Security is designed as insurance against some of life's risks, such as becoming disabled or losing a family's breadwinner (survivor's coverage, similar to life insurance) or, most fundamentally, if hardest to remember, outliving other retirement resources. As with any insurance, the value of the package depends not just on average benefits paid but also on the value of the protection against risk.

Contributions

Employees and their employers contribute equally to the system. In 2000 each paid 5.30 percent of covered payroll for OASI and 0.90 percent for DI, that is, 6.2 percent each and 12.4 percent in total. Taxes are paid, however, only on earnings up to a limit. No tax is assessed on individuals and employers for wages above that limit ($76,200 in 2000), and such higher earnings also are not reflected in eventual benefits. If a person is self-employed, she pays the employer portion as well, up to the same limit.[2]

These payroll taxes are by far the largest source of income for Social Security: about $406 billion in 1997. But the program also is credited with the taxes paid by certain beneficiaries of Social Security on their benefits. In essence, all individual beneficiaries with incomes below $25,000 per year, and couples with incomes below $32,000, receive Social Security benefits tax free. Above those thresholds they pay tax on a portion of the value of their benefits. The income thresholds are high enough that in 1997 less than a quarter of OASDI beneficiaries paid tax on their benefits.[3] This benefits tax leads to all sorts of theological or purely posturing arguments—is it really a tax, or a backhanded benefit reduction?—in budget politics.[4]

Benefit Rules and Principles

The formula for benefits begins with individuals' contributions. In order to collect any benefits, a person must have contributed payroll taxes for earnings above a very low minimum during forty quarters (that is, ten years, but the years do not have to be full or consecutive).[5] Then the formula looks at earnings over a working life: for old-age pensions, it considers the average of a retiree's thirty-five highest-earning years. Each year's earnings are indexed to account for changes in average wages over time (so an income of $7,000 in 1969 is treated as much higher than an income of $7,000 in 1999). Once a person begins to receive benefits, the amount is adjusted each year to compensate for inflation (a Cost of Living Adjustment, or COLA). These adjustments are used to calculate each individual's Average Indexed Monthly Earnings (AIME).

Benefits are related to earnings because every dollar of extra AIME increases

TABLE 3.1
Illustrative Primary Insurance Amount Calculations

	Lower Income	Moderate Income	High Income
AIME[a]	$900.00	$2,000.00	$3,500.00
PIA[a]	$551.90	$903.90	$1,254.87
PIA as % AIME	61.3	45.2	35.9

[a]PIAs and AIMEs are based on 1997 bend points. AIME = Average Indexed Monthly Earnings

NOTE: The figures here generate pensions for people who retired in the mid-1990s with full benefits (i.e., at age 65). The average pension in Social Security is lower than the "moderate" figure here for many reasons. The characterizations of how these AIMEs compare to average and maximum earners are based on U.S. House, Committee on Ways and Means 1996: 24, table 1-12.

TABLE 3.2
Illustrative Replacement Rates
(Using Standard SSA Earnings Examples)

Year of Retirement	Low Earners	Average	Maximum
1990	58.2%	43.2%	24.5%
2032	56.0%	41.8%	27.7%

SOURCE: U.S. House, Committee on Ways and Means 1996: 27, table 1-14.

NOTE: Retirement in 1990 is at age 65; retirement in 2032 is at age 67 (see text for explanation).

one's benefit. Yet the formula favors individuals with lower incomes, through the calculation of individuals' Primary Insurance Amount (PIA). The PIA is essentially the monthly benefit one would receive, absent all other adjustments, upon retirement at age 65 as a single individual. The formula pays lower percentages of earnings as earnings rise. As table 3.1 shows, a lower earner (assuming there are no further adjustments) receives a far larger share of his or her earnings, but a higher earner still gets a significantly higher pension.

Because most people do not think of their pension in terms of its relation to their adjusted average lifetime income (who knows that figure in advance?), the Social Security Administration summarizes benefits in terms of *replacement rates:* nominally, benefits expressed as a percent of earnings in the year before retirement. The standard calculation is unrealistic in some ways but sufficient to show the program's distributional impact and trends.[6] Table 3.2 shows both the better rates for lower earners and that, because of legislative changes in 1983, the replacement rates will change marginally in the future.

Adequate Protection

The benefit formula and results reflect a tension between two principles: that benefits should be related to contributions and thus income (so in that sense earned) and that benefits should be adequate. Adequacy would be impossible if everyone received the same replacement rate, for a rate that would be affordable for the program as a whole would leave low earners with extremely low pensions. Even with the favoritism in the formula, the pension for a low-income worker is still quite low.

Adequacy is also pursued by other aspects of the OASDI benefit formulas, which are too often overlooked. Most fundamentally, benefits are paid as long as the beneficiaries live. Thus, old-age benefits are really insurance: *Social Security protects against the risk of a longer-than-normal life*. In Social Security, if two people retire with the same pension and one lives twice as long, that person receives twice as much.

This is very different from private savings, which would create a fixed "nest egg" upon retirement that could be used up. In private markets an individual may seek to guarantee payment as long as she lives by purchasing an annuity. But then, for any given purchase price, the seller of the annuity will provide a lower monthly check if it expects the annuitant to live longer.

The principle of adequacy is embedded in Social Security in another way that is both basic and easily forgotten. *Social Security is not a return on an individual's investment but a payment to a family unit*. Larger families need higher incomes, so the benefit based on a given PIA is higher for wage earners with more dependents. Dependents may include children and even parents of the retired or disabled beneficiary, but the most significant category is spouses. Social Security provides a spousal benefit of 50 percent of the wage earner's benefit, so if two workers have the same earnings histories, but one is single and the other part of a couple, the latter will receive 50 percent more.

Another aspect of adequacy is what the benefits will actually buy. When a person saves privately, the value of investments and their earnings can easily be eroded by inflation, as occurred for many people during the 1970s. The automatic inflation adjustment of benefits offers beneficiaries another degree of protection that simply does not exist for private savings.

Any pension program requires rules about when enrollees can begin collecting benefits. Under current law, people can receive "full benefits" if they begin collecting at age 65 (the *normal retirement age*). They may retire as early as age 62; but if they do, their benefits are *actuarially adjusted*. Their monthly check is reduced by an amount intended to ensure that on average they will collect the same total value of benefits as the people who retire at the standard retirement age. In 1997 that meant a 20 percent reduction to the checks for people who retired at age 62 rather than age 65.[7]

As life expectancies increase, any given normal retirement age must become more expensive, because people on average will collect benefits for a longer time. In order to reduce costs, therefore, Congress in 1983 adopted legislation that will raise the normal retirement age to 67 by 2022. The increase is phased in over two periods, 2000–2004 and 2017–22. A person like myself, born in June of 1952, will not be able to take full retirement at age 65 in June of 2017. Instead, I will have to wait until June of 2018, when I hope to be 66 years old (U.S. House, Committee on Ways and Means 1996: 19).

The benefit formulas for Social Security have many modifications beyond the basics mentioned here. Disability Insurance involves many complexities, especially determining who is disabled and therefore eligible to receive benefits. The key point, though, is that Social Security benefits are based on collectively set standards of need and contribution, not on returns on investments in markets.

How well does Social Security balance the demands for adequacy and a "fair" return on contributions? That is both a political question and a matter of personal values; for issues of adequacy, see chapter 7, and for returns, see chapter 8.

The Trust Funds

The money from OASDI contributions flows into, and benefits are paid out of, the widely misunderstood Social Security trust funds.

The trust funds are a form of federal budget accounting. For most programs, Congress creates "budget authority," the right to spend an amount of money, in annual appropriations acts. Social Security works differently. The money raised by each payroll tax is deposited into a separate trust fund account within the Treasury, and the trust-fund balances, by law, automatically constitute budget authority. Whatever is in the funds can be spent without further legislative action. The funds offer legal certainty that contributions will be turned into benefits and therefore greater political certainty than would exist if the programs depended on annual appropriations.[8]

Because there are two separate accounts, DI and OASI, common references to "the trust fund" are a technical error. Nevertheless, Congress over the years has shown a sufficient willingness to move money between the funds while maintaining the same total tax rate that the two can be considered together. More serious confusions involve how the Social Security trust funds compare with private trust funds or investments.

The trust-fund device does not keep Social Security from being mostly a "pay-as-you-go" program. Although my taxes establish my legal and political claim to later benefits, they go into the pool that pays my mother's and aunt's and other current elderly or disabled people's benefits. My money does not pay for my benefits in the same way as my private investments eventually pay (if they go well) for my personal consumption.

Even in such a program, there is reason to accumulate a surplus in the trust funds. The surplus should be large enough that unexpected bad news does not run a fund to zero, eliminating authority to pay benefits, before Congress and the president can agree on a response. On various occasions, funds have neared the zero point, most notably in early 1983, and then Social Security "rescues" have been necessary (Light 1985; White and Wildavsky 1991).

Given the capacity for gridlock within the American constitutional design, the target of policy might, therefore, be to maintain a balance of a year or more's expenses. Yet legislation in 1983 created an annual surplus that has been accumulating for many years; this accumulation has encouraged arguments about whether that surplus is or is not being used to finance Social Security in the future.

Unlike private parties, the federal government has not had the option of putting extra funds into private investments such as stocks, bonds, or even savings accounts. In the past, policymakers have feared either the power that would give "big government" or possible corruption. Fortunately (depending on one's view), there has always been a simpler thing to do with the money: reduce federal government borrowing or debt.

If the Social Security surplus is $40 billion with a federal deficit of $200 billion, having the government sell $200 billion in bonds to the public seems silly. The $40 billion could be used to reduce the federal government's need to sell bonds to $160 billion, saving, in each subsequent year, the interest on $40 billion. Similarly, if the budget were in balance and Social Security had a $40 billion surplus, it would make sense to retire $40 billion of the federal government's existing debt. That too would save the interest on $40 billion in each succeeding year.

Each year's Social Security surplus, then, is used to reduce federal debt. It is recorded as a special kind of Treasury bond. These bonds then accumulate within the trust funds and are credited with interest, which is recorded as more bonds. *The balance in the funds and the interest accrued on that balance are ways of expressing the amount of money that Social Security surpluses have allowed the Treasury to save by not borrowing on the financial markets.* If the surplus had not existed, other things being equal, the federal government would have sold that much more debt and would have been obligated to repay that much more principal and interest.

Claims That the Surpluses Were "Wasted"

During the 1980s a wide range of commentators declared that Social Security surpluses did not, in fact, reduce national debt. They reasoned that, without those surpluses, the government's deficit would have seemed larger. If the deficit seemed larger, politicians would have done more about it. So Social Security surpluses "masked" the true size of the deficit, allowing politicians to "waste" them by financing other spending.[9]

As a political analysis, this was nonsense. The political question, properly phrased, is whether, in the absence of the Social Security surpluses, Congress and the president would have agreed on larger reductions in spending on other programs or higher increases in other taxes (Penner 1994). Those who assume a positive answer are saying politicians would have done more if the problem seemed bigger. Their logic, essentially, is that politicians have to be scared into recognizing problems and doing what is right. Although this fits public views of politicians, it does not fit the facts of budget politics in the 1980s and 1990s.

The budget deficit dominated national politics from 1981 through 1997. A raft of books provide accounts of various years' battles.[10] The deficit persisted not because it was ignored but because there was no consensus on a package of spending cuts and revenue increases big enough to eliminate it. Majorities at any given time felt that the consequences of such a package would be worse than the deficit itself.

Since there was no agreement on measures large enough to balance the budget, *every deficit-reduction package from 1982 on was created by defining the problem as something smaller, not larger, than how to balance the budget* (White 1998a). The Tax Equity and Fiscal Responsibility Act of 1982 and the Deficit Reduction Act of 1984 were both described as down payments on deficit reduction. In 1990 President Bush and the Democratic Congress first had to settle on the proper target. The Democrats insisted on $500 billion in deficit reduction over five years, and they prevailed. Nobody talked in terms of balancing the budget (White and Wildavsky 1991). President Clinton promised in his 1992 campaign to cut the deficit in half by 1996. When that seemed too difficult (given the unduly pessimistic projections at the time), his economic advisers settled on a $140 billion reduction in the deficit projected for 1997, on the grounds that a reduction of that size would satisfy the financial markets (Woodward 1994). In 1995 congressional Republicans did set a balanced budget as their target, but they promised balance not until seven years in the future, in order to reduce the needed policy change to what they hoped would be a politically manageable level. Even that seemed a stretch at the time (Maraniss and Weiskopf 1996).

By making the deficit-reduction target smaller, politicians set goals that they could meet. That enabled them to get at least some credit (for making progress on the deficit) to balance the political pain of spending cuts and tax increases. Making the problem seem bigger would have made it harder, not easier, for them to claim that they had accomplished anything. A senior senator expressed the logic nicely in a confidential interview back in 1986. "Once the deficits got as big as they did," he explained, "no one thing would make a perceptible difference. If abolishing the Marine Corps would end the deficit, then Congress would abolish the Marine Corps. But if you abolished the Marines you'd have $210 billion left to go and all the Marines mad at you."

In everyday life we do not assume that making a task harder causes people to do more. Sometimes they will quit, instead. In short, there is at least as much reason to believe that deficit reduction was facilitated by making the problem seem smaller as to conclude that deficit reduction could have been helped by making the problem seem bigger.[11] The argument that Social Security surpluses caused less action on the deficit does not stand up to investigation. Its supporters need to explain in what year, in what way, Congress and the president would have done more.

Throughout the period of high deficits, therefore, it seems fair to say that Social Security surpluses reduced total federal deficits by about the amount of the surpluses.

Debt Reduction and Fiscal Capacity

When surplus OASDI contributions save future taxpayers interest costs on the forgone debt, these savings improve what in public-finance terms is called the federal government's *fiscal capacity* (White 2000). A government's fiscal capacity is its ability to finance spending through taxes or borrowing. Fiscal capacity depends, among other things, on the existing level of government spending. Lower spending on some programs must make it easier to finance others. Surpluses in the OASDI trust funds should improve the federal government's future fiscal capacity, by reducing its future interest costs. Voters in 2020 will be willing to pay more for pensions if they are paying less for interest.

The argument made here about what the trust funds do may seem unfamiliar, yet it is the position reached by the first Advisory Council on Social Security in 1938. While considering significant changes to the program, the council debated the program's financing. It recognized that "there are other ways of financing the old-age insurance system which upon further study may prove to have greater advantages than the present system" but declared that the subject was extremely complex and no final judgment seemed possible at the time. "Upon one aspect of the general problem," however, the council deemed "it advisable at this time to allay unwarranted fears . . . the method of handling the funds collected for old-age insurance purposes." The Advisory Council then explained that

the United States Treasury uses the moneys realized from the issueance of these special securities by the old-age reserve account in the same manner as it does moneys realized from the sale of other Government securities. As long as the budget is not balanced, the net result is to reduce the amounts which the Government has to borrow from banks, insurance companies and other private parties. When the budget is balanced, these moneys will be available for the reduction of the national debt held by the public. The members of the Advisory Council are in agreement that the fulfillment of the promises made to the wage earners included in the old-age insurance system depends upon, more than anything else, the financial integrity of the Government. The members of the council, regardless of differing views on other aspects of the financing of old-age insurance, are of the opinion that the present provisions regarding the investment of the moneys in the old-age reserve account do not involve any misuse of these moneys or endanger the safety of these funds.[12]

Ignoring the first council's focus on federal fiscal capacity (or "financial integrity"), standard discussion of the trust funds now makes either of two mistakes: saying the funds do less or more than the truth.

On one side, critics of Social Security call the trust funds some kind of fake or Ponzi scheme. The Concord Coalition, for instance, refers to "the charade of trust-fund accounting." It reasons this way: when the Social Security Administration goes to the Treasury to cash in some trust-fund securities, so as to pay benefits, what will the Treasury do? It will tax or borrow to get the money. If there were no surplus, what would the Treasury do to pay benefits? It would tax or borrow. So from this perspective, the funds are "mythical."[13] Yet this argument is equivalent to saying that reducing your own debt does not improve your fiscal position, because you will still have to earn money to cover future spending. In fact, you would still rather have less debt, so you would owe less interest.

On the other side, the standard analyses of Social Security's long-term prospects are expressed in terms of the amount that payroll taxes would need to be raised now in order to pay for the program over a period of seventy-five years. Thus, the *Report of the 1994–1996 Advisory Council on Social Security* indicated that the deficit over seventy-five years was 2.17 percent of taxable payroll, meaning that "if payroll rates had been increased in 1995 by just over 1 percentage point each on employers and employees . . . the system would be in balance over this 75-year period" (Advisory Council on Social Security 1997a: 11). Such analyses assume that surpluses built up in the early years would help pay for the program by being run down in the future. But although you can sell off the assets in your personal portfolio without making any claim on the rest of your earnings, such as your wage earnings, the federal government cannot sell the assets in Social Security's portfolio without digging into its other earnings, namely general revenue. If the advantage of building up the trust fund is that federal fiscal capacity is increased by avoiding interest costs, then the assets in the fund cannot be run down without forfeiting the advantage gained by building them up.

On balance, of course, it is better to borrow later than sooner. Money not borrowed now may instead be used for investment, which may create a larger economy in the future. That larger economy may make paying Social Security benefits easier. But *the most basic value of the Social Security surplus for financing the program in the future is represented not by the accumulation in the trust funds but by the interest on those balances.* To the extent that they reduced federal debt obligations, past surpluses have not been wasted, and future surpluses' positive effects should be understood and preserved.

Financing Social Security's Future Shortfalls

The alternative perspectives on the trust funds presented in the preceding section have different implications for assessment of Social Security's financial position. Chapter 2 described trends in terms of Social Security's share of GDP. That expresses spending in terms of the economy's ability to pay. Another common approach is to compare revenues and costs in any year to taxable payroll in that year. This comparison shows the adequacy of financing under the current basic funding arrangement. Either way, our view of the function of the trust funds will determine our assessment of Social Security's financial condition. We can use table 3.3 to illustrate the different views.

If we view the program entirely on a pay-as-you-go basis, then the relevant question will be the difference between the program's *income rate*, its earnings from taxation (including taxation of benefits); and its *cost rate*, which includes all expenditures. By this standard, as of the 2000 projections, OASDI would be in trouble beginning in 2015, the first year in which costs exceed tax revenues, causing the pay-as-you-go balance to become negative.

Following the standard analysis, however, the goal should be to maintain a cost rate and income rate that leave some trust-fund balance intact until the end of the estimation period, in 2075. On the one hand, that means action must be taken by 2036, the last year when there is any balance on which to earn interest (see the "Interest/Payroll" column). On the other, as estimated

TABLE 3.3
Projected OASDI Income and Costs as Share of Taxable Payroll

	Income Rate	Cost Rate	Pay-Go Balance	Interest/ Payroll	Balance with Interest
2000	12.65	10.34	2.31	1.73	3.92
2005	12.68	10.74	1.95	2.39	4.32
2010	12.74	11.55	1.18	3.04	4.19
2015	12.81	12.91	−0.10	3.46	3.33
2020	12.91	14.66	−1.75	3.46	1.68
2025	13.00	16.24	−3.24	2.96	−0.31
2030	13.08	17.35	−4.26	1.99	−2.31
2035	13.14	17.86	−4.72	0.68	−4.07
2036	13.14	17.88	−4.74	0.40	−4.38
2040	13.16	17.87	−4.71		
2045	13.18	17.85	−4.67		
2050	13.21	17.96	−4.76		
2055	13.24	18.27	−5.03		
2060	13.27	18.63	−5.36		
2065	13.30	18.95	−5.65		
2070	13.32	19.24	−5.92		
2075	13.34	19.53	−6.18		

SOURCES: Long-term tables available as a supplement to Board of Trustees 2000a, posted at ⟨www.ssa.gov/OACT/TR/TR00⟩, tables II.F13, III.B1, III.B3; plus author's calculations.

in 2000, an immediate increase in payroll taxes of 1.89 percent total would have covered the shortfall through the entire period (Board of Trustees 2000b).

Critics of the trust funds would object that the standard analysis is wrong because increasing payroll taxes by 1.89 percent total would still leave a shortfall in pay-as-you-go terms in, say, 2030 (1.89 − 2.31 = −0.42). The implication of my argument about the trust funds, however, is that it would be legitimate to use general revenues to fund Social Security up to the amount of interest that the funds are said to earn in a given year, because that interest is in fact savings to the general fund. By that standard, although the critics would see a shortfall of 1.75 percent of payroll in 2020, for example, I am arguing that general revenues up to 3.46 percent of payroll ("Interest/Payroll" column) could appropriately be used, more than covering the shortfall. However, though the standard calculation shows the program still in balance in 2030, I would argue that the available interest savings in 2030, and thus the appropriate financing from general revenues, are much less than the pay-as-you-go deficit. Even raising taxes by 1.89 percent of payroll would leave a small gap (1.89 − 2.31 = −0.42).

To put this another way, the standard calculation identifies 2036 as the crucial year. The pay-as-you-go critique emphasizes 2015. The fiscal-capacity perspective sees 2025 as the year by which, if the estimates were correct, some reform would be needed, because in that year the appropriate spending from general revenues becomes less than the program's shortfalls from dedicated taxes.

If we interpret Social Security surpluses in terms of their effect on federal fiscal capacity, then the goal of policy could be to stabilize the trust-fund balances in the early 2020s. Then the amount of interest at that point would represent (other things being equal) a fixed payment that could be made from general revenues to help cover Social Security benefits from that year forward, because it would be the amount of interest that would, if there had been no surpluses, be being paid to other parties.

Such a fixed dollar payment would become a smaller and smaller share of taxable payroll over time. Eventually, therefore, savings from programmatic revenue increases or benefit adjustments would need to approach (though never equal) the pay-as-you-go figures. But counting the accumulated interest as a legitimate use of general revenues would allow the chosen measures to be introduced more slowly than under a strict pay-as-you-go regimen, thereby stretching some of the cost increase in the 2010–35 period over subsequent decades. In that sense, current surpluses would indeed help finance Social Security during the baby-boom generation's retirement.

Any analysis other than in pure pay-as-you-go terms assumes that some general revenues will be used to finance benefits for some period of time. My argument here presents the questions that must be asked about that use of general revenues. First, What amount of general revenue finance is justified by earlier surpluses? I am arguing that the appropriate amount would be based on the interest on the trust fund balance; the traditional accounting implies use of general revenues to cover both interest and cashing in the principal.

Second, on what schedule should those general revenues be spent? That choice depends on how we would want to use general revenue finance to reduce the need for other measures. If policymakers chose to stabilize the trust fund balance as of 2024, that would produce general revenue financing equal to each year's earnings on the fund. That amount would decline as a share of GDP as GDP itself grew. Alternatively, they could try to stabilize the balance as a share of GDP, so that the interest earnings figure as a share of GDP also was (relatively) stable. That would require larger reforms early, but smaller changes over the long run.

Last, how much general revenue finance would we want to provide? If we want to do more, yet not reduce future federal fiscal capacity, we would want to run larger surpluses than if we wanted to use less general revenue.

Although I believe the standard analysis of Social Security's financing in terms of long-run actuarial balance is too optimistic, that method is much more useful for evaluating specific reform proposals. Any given policy could be measured in terms of its effects in each of seventy-five years, but then comparing measures would be very difficult. Measuring in terms of long-term actuarial balance provides a way to compare very different measures. Therefore I use the standard methodology in order to discuss individual proposals later in this book. But I assess packages in terms of their annual effects on federal fiscal capacity.

We have delved into only a small portion of Social Security's complexities, in order to highlight the points that, for political and policy purposes, are most important. Two are crucial.

First, the benefits of the program are much different from returns on a private investment. They are related to personal contributions but not nearly proportionally so. They are adjusted to ensure adequacy in many ways, including protection against market risks, a subject considered at more length in chapter 8, where I analyze privatization plans. Social Security is insurance, not a standard investment.

Second, Social Security's intergenerational character and the fact that trust funds are not invested in private securities raise all sorts of confusions about what surpluses at any given time could possibly accomplish. We have seen here why both the standard justifications and critiques of Social Security surpluses and their uses are misleading.

FOUR

Medicare's Structure, Benefits, and Financing

"If Social Security is an 800 pound gorilla," a highly experienced political analyst once commented, "Medicare weighs in at about 750" (Burke 1997: 258).[1] The likely reason is simple. The prospect of elderly persons doing without health insurance is about as frightening, for them and their children, as the thought of their doing without Social Security (Bowman 1997).

If a retired couple who were both eligible for Medicare had to buy comparable coverage in 1997, the bill could easily have been over eleven thousand dollars per year—not much less than the median Social Security benefit for a couple.[2] The point of health insurance, of course, is that without it bills in any given year could be much, much higher—far beyond what the average person could hope to pay. Whereas an elderly couple's children might be able to supplement a more meager pension, they could be financially ruined by the medical bills they might face without Medicare. Before Medicare was created, only 38 percent of the nonworking aged had any insurance. Elderly persons in poor health were particularly likely to be uninsured, and the insurance that existed covered only a small part of hospital bills (Marmor 1971: 18–19).

Medicare's Origins and Their Consequences

Medicare was designed as an addition to the framework of social protection that Social Security initiated (Marmor 1971; Derthick 1979; Ball 1997; NASI 1999). The two programs remain linked in the public mind as different from other government programs and peculiarly important.[3] Yet, because of the political maneuvering that created Medicare, the program is also a most peculiar mix of methods and rationales.

President Roosevelt did not even attempt to include health insurance in the Social Security Act because it was far more controversial than pensions, especially in light of fervent opposition from the American Medical Association. President Truman's efforts to create a national health-insurance program were routed in Congress (Marmor 1971: 7–14). In 1951 advocates of social insurance, based in the Federal Security Administration (which oversaw Social Security), switched to an incremental strategy in which hospital insurance for the elderly was to be the first step.

As Theodore R. Marmor (1971: 13–18) explains, the elderly-first strategy for hospital insurance was designed to blunt the most popular objections to a government health-insurance program. It could be defended against charges of being a "give-away" to the undeserving because the aged, "through no fault of their own . . . had lower earning capacity and higher medical expenses than any other adult age group." The program would not need a divisive means-test because aged people as a group especially needed coverage, and entitlement would be based on having contributed to OASI. Covering only hospitalization was expected to limit the potential increase in services and, more politically important, blunt charges that the program would involve federal control of physicians.

Medicare's advocates were blocked by President Eisenhower and by the congressional "conservative coalition" of Republicans with southern Democrats. Wilbur Mills, an Arkansas Democrat, who as chair of the House Ways and Means Committee had jurisdiction over all taxes and thus OASDI, promoted means-tested help for elderly poor people. His Kerr-Mills plan passed in 1960 (Marmor 1971: 35–38; Derthick 1979: 327–28). Kerr-Mills did not lead to much coverage for the elderly, and President Kennedy's assassination and the subsequent Democratic sweep in the 1964 elections changed the political balance radically in favor of passage of further health-insurance legislation for elderly persons.

In order to preempt the hospital insurance proposal, both the American Medical Association and John W. Byrnes, the Republican leader on the Ways and Means Committee, proposed plans that in fact covered more, but on terms that their sponsors believed were less of a threat. The current form of Medicare was established when Chairman Mills, to general surprise, proposed merging the HI and Byrnes proposals. Ways and Means then devised a bill that created two separate insurance packages, Hospital Insurance (HI), and Supplementary Medical Insurance (SMI). HI would be Part A and SMI would be Part B of this compromise version of Medicare. HI would be compulsory and financed, like Social Security, from a payroll tax. SMI would be a voluntary program in which individuals paid premiums, but those premiums would be subsidized by the federal government (which originally was to pay 50% of the costs), from general revenues.

Mills's maneuver, Martha Derthick has explained, was meant to preempt later pressures to cover physician services within the Social Security framework. It "was much more acceptable to conservative interests" because "it was voluntary in principle, placed most of the responsibility for administration in the hands of 'carriers' (that is, private organizations under contract to the government) rather than the SSA, and promised to pay physicians 'reasonable' charges with few and vague tests of what was 'reasonable'" (1979: 331–32). Mills also believed that health-care costs were too unpredictable to be safely financed by the payroll tax.

In a further step, Mills adapted the AMA's proposal to expand the means-tested Kerr-Mills program, applying it to poor people of all ages. This would become Medicaid, Title XIX of the Social Security Act. In essence, Medicaid was designed to do for the general population what Kerr-Mills failed to do for the aged: blunt any campaign for social insurance by providing a means-tested alternative.

Mills's synthesis and the HI proposal to which he was responding established the basic outlines of Medicare, with a series of consequences. First, the enrollees in HI are not contributing during the time they are enrolled. Although they have contributed earlier, and although they contribute to SMI, one might argue that they should pay some amount while actually receiving HI benefits.

Second, a program of health insurance mainly for the elderly makes the effects of demographic change on costs seem more significant than they would if everybody was insured in the same system. When a person turns 65, his entire Medicare cost is suddenly a new expense and burden on the government's budget. In other countries, with the elderly in the same plans as almost everyone else, a person's sixty-fifth birthday does not create comparable transfers of costs.

Third, the set of provisions to mollify physician and other provider opposition guaranteed that costs would explode. It is asking for trouble to pay providers their "usual and customary" fees and reimburse them based on whatever "costs" they incur. Medicare's advocates saw that that could happen, Robert Ball reports, but "had a naive faith that when we had more experience with the program, we could get reasonable changes made in the law" (1997: 34). They did, but it took a long while. In the meantime Medicare became identified among policymakers not as a program that successfully served a vital national goal but primarily as a continual cost problem (Oberlander 1995).

Fourth, Mills's strategy probably did help block expansion of social insurance for health care. Medicare eligibility was expanded only by adding disabled individuals (who belonged there logically, since they were part of Social Security) and victims of End Stage Renal Disease (ESRD), meaning kidney failure. ESRD victims were comparable to elderly persons in that insurance coverage for ESRD care, meaning dialysis or kidney transplant, was quite rare in the early 1970s and the uninsured, unless extremely rich, would die from lack of care (Nissenson and Rettig 1999; U.S. House, Committee on Ways and Means 1996: 196–99).

Fifth, Medicare's benefits were designed for the medical system of the 1960s. Subsequent increases in the importance of pharmaceutical treatment and outpatient surgery have made the benefit package less adequate. Nothing about the design prevents adding new benefits, but that of course costs money.

Sixth, although Medicare is now managed by the Health Care Financing Administration (HCFA), much of the day-to-day business is still performed by the private carriers and intermediaries, adding an extra layer of confusion and blame-passing to the program's administration (GAO 1999).

Finally, SMI has a different rationale than HI does, and it is not as insulated from arguments that it should be means-tested as HI and OASDI are. Senate support in 1997 for proposals to means-test the SMI premium showed that SMI's design allows some policymakers to view Part B not as social insurance but as a "government subsidy program."

Eligibility and Benefits

Although both beneficiaries and public discussion normally refer to Medicare as a whole, HI and SMI are separate insurance plans. About a sixth of

Medicare beneficiaries do have coverage that merges the two programs (Igle-hart 1999: 144). The federal government pays managed-care organizations a premium to provide individuals with both Part A and Part B benefits. For lack of a better term, we'll call this minority but growing form of Medicare "Com-bination Plans."

Part A (HI) covers inpatient hospital care (except for physician services), skilled nursing facility (SNF) care if related to a hospital stay, hospice care, and some home health care. Individuals are entitled to benefits by age (given sufficient contribution to OASDI), by disability status under DI (after a two-year waiting period), or by qualifying under the ESRD program.[4]

SMI covers not only physician services (in and outside hospitals) but also outpatient surgery, laboratory and other diagnostic tests, radiation therapy, home dialysis, and many other services. Until 1997 it covered home health care only for people who did not have HI coverage. As of mid-2000, it provided no reimbursement for the costs of prescription drugs, save a few special cases.[5]

Any person eligible for Part A, plus all other persons age 65 or older, may enroll in Part B voluntarily. In the early 1970s Congress responded to rapid increases in Part B costs, and so of the premium, by limiting the annual pre-mium increase to no more than the annual cost-of-living adjustment for So-cial Security. Since medical costs continued to grow more quickly than gen-eral prices, the Part B premium fell from the original 50 percent to below 25 percent of Part B costs. Congress in various years amended the law to keep the premium close to 25 percent and in 1997 set the premium permanently at that level, which came to $45.50 per month in 2000. Since 25 percent of costs is quite a discount, virtually any eligible person who does not have some other party (normally an employer or a spouse's employer) paying for her health in-surance enrolls in SMI. As one consumer's guide put it, "Make no mistake: Part B insurance is the bargain of the century" (Mason and Nohlgren 1989: 3–4). In 1999 SMI was expected to have about 37 million enrollees and HI about 39.2 million.[6]

Although it is an excellent deal for its enrollees, Medicare does not come close to providing full coverage for medical costs. It appears to provide less financial protection than 85 percent of private employer-sponsored plans.[7] The most prominent excluded services are prescription drugs and long-term care. Medicare does cover nursing home services if incident to a hospital stay but not if a person simply has reached the point where she is unable to manage the tasks of daily living. The latter group of Americans must rely on private resources or Medicaid.

Medicare also requires substantial beneficiary contributions (cost-sharing) for the services that it covers. These provisions are summarized in table 4.1. The deductible for HI is unusually high, and benefits can be used up, leaving a patient with no further protection. So a Medicare beneficiary's potential expenses are unlimited.[8] Congress and the president tried to fix that in 1988, with the Medicare Catastrophic Coverage Act, but that legislation was repealed in 1989 (Rovner 1995).

For the bulk of its covered benefits, Part B establishes an approved payment amount and pays only 80 percent of the cost. Either the patient or supplemental insurance (described below) must pay the "balance." One area of political controversy involves the desire of providers, especially physicians, to charge more than Medicare's fee schedule, in which case patients have to pay more than 20 percent of the Medicare fee.[9]

A series of measures have given physicians strong incentives to accept Medicare's fee levels. Because of these provisions, in 1996 the standard 20 percent cost-sharing applied to 96 percent of claims for physician services. Extra-billing can be far more significant for other services, such as durable medical equipment and especially outpatient surgery that is performed in a hospital. Hospital charges may greatly exceed the Medicare rate, and the Medicare Payment Advisory Commission reported in 1998 that, as a result, beneficiaries or their supplemental insurers on average paid close to half of the Medicare schedule amount (MedPAC 1998a: 59; Moon 1996: 4). In addition, nonhospital HI services generally require an initial hospitalization, so a person who needs admission to a skilled nursing facility, for instance, but not hospitalization, is not covered (ProPAC 1997b: 104–5; U.S. House, Committee on Ways and Means 1996: 166–68).

Exceptions to the rule of significant cost-sharing include hospice and home health care. When legislation in 1980 loosened the link between home health benefits and hospitalization, that ultimately led to skyrocketing costs (Med-PAC 1998b: 108–9; ProPAC 1997b: 110–14). For both substantive and political reasons, those cost increases also raised doubt about why home health benefits were part of HI at all. In 1997 the law was changed so that only home health benefits that were clearly related to hospitalization would be main-

TABLE 4.1
Medicare Cost-Sharing Requirements (and Probabilities)

Service Category	Deductible in 1999	Other Patient Charges	Coverage Expires?
Hospital Insurance (Part A)	($768.00)		
Hospitalization	$768.00 (first day)	$192.00/day for days 61–90; then 60-day "lifetime reserve" at $384.00/day.	No coverage after 150 days, or 90 days if lifetime reserve previously consumed
Skilled Nursing Facility (SNF)		No charge days 1–20; $96.00/day days 21–100	No benefits after 100th day associated with a given hospital stay.
Hospice		Very limited, for certain drugs and respite care	
Home Health		None	
Supplementary Medical Insurance (Part B)	($100.00)		
Physician Services		20% of Medicare Schedule Fee for "participating" physicians; Up to 29.25% of the schedule for physicians who do not accept assignment	
Outpatient Surgery/ Procedures		20% of charges; In ambulatory surgical centers this is 20% of the set fee, but in hospital facilities, this averages almost 50% of the Medicare fee.	
Durable Medical Equipment		Varies greatly. Medicare pays 80% of its schedule or of the amount charged, whichever is lower. Patient pays the rest.	
Physical Therapy and Speech Therapy (combined)		20% coinsurance	Benefits expire after Medicare pays $1,500
Occupational Therapy		20% coinsurance	Benefits expire after Medicare pays $1,500
Home Health Services		None	
Clinical Lab Services		None	

SOURCES: Board of Trustees 1999c, table III.C1; ProPAC 1997b: 105–14; MedPAC 1998b: 59–75, 85.

tained as part of Part A, and the rest is being transferred to Part B over the six years from 1998 through 2003 (O'Sullivan et al. 1997: 44).

Finances
Revenues

HI revenues are much the same as OASDI's, save that any projected medium-term surpluses are more fortuitous than based on plans to "save for the future." Employers and employees each pay a 1.45 percent payroll tax. Self-employed persons therefore pay 2.9 percent. Unlike OASDI, there is no cap on pay subject to the HI tax, so higher-income people pay on all their wages. HI also receives some revenue from taxation of OASDI benefits, and interest is credited on the fund's balance.

As with OASDI, HI revenues are expected to become inadequate at some point in the future. The basic problems are that medical costs per person normally rise more quickly than per capita GDP, and enrollment will in the future increase more quickly than population.

The HI trust fund has frequently been projected to go broke within a decade. That has not occurred, because of either legislative action or helpful events. In 1997 the HI fund was projected to run out of money by 2002 (Board of Trustees 1997a: 34–35). Both the provisions of the Balanced Budget Act of 1997 and some surprising good news caused projections of HI's financing to improve dramatically by 2000. As this book was being edited, the Medicare trustees were projecting that tax income would exceed costs through 2009, taxes plus interest would exceed costs through 2015, and trust-fund assets would not be exhausted until 2023. There remains plenty of reason for concern, for those projections may be optimistic, and in the long run there is little doubt that the financing base of HI, as for OASDI, will not cover all current commitments (Board of Trustees 2000b).

SMI also has a trust fund, but no taxes are separately dedicated to it. The only dedicated funding consists of beneficiaries' premiums, which are only supposed to pay 25 percent of costs. The balance of SMI's funding comes from general revenues, which have to be appropriated by Congress each year, preferably in the annual Departments of Labor, Health and Human Services, and

Related Agencies appropriations act.[10] Thus, SMI is an "appropriated entitle-ment."

What would happen if Congress did not appropriate the money—as, af-ter all, happened during the government shutdowns at the end of 1995? In the long run, the courts can be expected to order it to do so. But Congress keeps the balance in the SMI fund above the level that is likely to be needed in a given year, so as to guard against running out of cash because of (a) spending being higher than expected or (b) gridlock such as occurred in 1995.

So the SMI trust fund is not quite meaningless but also does not have the same effect as the OASDI trust funds. And ironically, because there is no ded-icated funding stream, there is no basis for saying that funding would ever be inadequate. Because it is based on general revenues, the estimates always pre-sume that SMI will be funded. It could not "go bankrupt" unless the whole federal government did so. In short, "Medicare" cannot go bankrupt; only HI can. When politicians use projections of HI insolvency to argue that they must cut Medicare to "save" it, and then propose cuts in SMI, they are being dis-honest. The honest argument would be that Medicare, including SMI, is sim-ply too expensive. But that would be awkward for politicians who claim to be "saving" it.

Costs

Medical services in general have been moving out of the hospitals in recent years, the two programs are subject to the same demographic pressures, and home health costs are now being shifted to SMI; therefore, SMI costs, which have grown more quickly than HI's over the past two decades, should con-tinue to do so (U.S. House, Committee on Ways and Means 1996: 137; CBO 1997a: 123).

In fiscal year 1999, Medicare spent a total of about $213 billion (Board of Trustees 2000c: 29; 2000d: 28). That was actually less than in fiscal year 1998, a shocking development. But it is still a lot of money. We look at cost trends in more detail in chapters 5 and 7, but two points are related to Medicare's function as social insurance.

First, compared to other American health insurers, HI and SMI both pay larger shares for benefits and smaller shares (less than 2% of spending) for administration. That is not because the federal government is wonderfully competent but because compulsory government programs have no marketing costs, no profits, no underwriting, and no separate expenses for collecting the money (the tax system is already in place).

Second, the value of insurance to its enrollees is not its average cost but the value of protection against the risk of much higher costs. This is especially true of HI: in 1997 it spent about $3,640 per enrollee, but barely a fifth of enrollees received covered services. Therefore the value of HI benefits to those who used them averaged over $16,500.[11]

Medicare's Other Purposes

The debate about both Social Security and Medicare involves the contrasting positive view of social insurance and negative view of entitlements. Yet Medicare has collected a series of functions that are not really part of social insurance logic. Reforms cannot help affecting Medicare's "other" roles (NASI 1999).

One is support for capital investment in hospitals. Medicare got into this business on the grounds that capital investment was a cost that, like other costs, should be reimbursed. But guaranteeing payment for at least some of the costs of any investment fueled the "medical arms race" that is widely believed to be one cause of rising costs systemwide.[12] Now Medicare's capital payments are being revised so that hospitals will receive funds according to a formula, but paying capital costs even when hospitals do not invest seems no more reasonable (ProPAC 1997b: 70–72; 1997a: 22–26). The basic problem here is that Medicare is not set up, and the relevant interests do not want it to be set up, in a way that would enable HCFA to make decisions about what hospitals will be funded to build what.

Medicare plays an even more significant role in funding graduate medical education. "Direct" graduate medical education (GME) payments provide an amount per resident (trainee) physician per hospital, prorated by Medicare's share of the hospital's inpatient days. These payments totaled $2.2 billion in fiscal year 1997.[13] Indirect Medical Education (IME) payments support extra costs besides the salaries of residents. For instance, as part of training the doctors, patients may be given more diagnostic tests. So hospitals get an IME payment based on the intensity of their teaching activities, as measured by the ratio of interns and residents per bed. IME payments totaled about $4.6 billion in fiscal year 1997. This funding support is widely criticized on the grounds that hospitals, which benefit from cheap resident labor, end up training more physicians, especially specialists, than the nation needs. Reform initiatives have even included paying hospitals not to train doctors (somewhat like paying farmers not to plant wheat) (Commonwealth Fund 1997; Iglehart 1998; MedPAC 1999b).

Medicare also provides support for the nation's health-care "safety net." The rationale is that hospitals with an unusually high share of low-income patients incur extra costs because poor people are sicker on average when they enter the hospital; they tend to be in neighborhoods that create extra costs; and they tend to have more uninsured patients, who cannot pay. Therefore both Medicaid and Medicare include provisions to subsidize "disproportionate share hospitals" (DSH payments). Medicare DSH was expected to cost $4.5 billion in fiscal year 1997 (MedPAC 1998d: 61–69). The only policy reason to include this financing in Medicare is that it was possible this way and might have been more difficult politically through any other means.

Medicare's payment rates are also adjusted in other ways to support health-care provision in areas, such as rural communities, that would otherwise be "underserved." Each of these extra functions has some rationale. They create obstacles, however, to reforms that would seek to make Medicare more like private insurance that does not have those extra goals. The extra functions also increase the "eyes-glaze-over" factor in policy debate—I fear I am losing my readers already and that if I say more about DSH or IME, you will be gone. So I won't.

Covering the Gaps

Medicare's gaps produce the strange phenomenon that even advocates of radical reform as part of the need to control entitlements often claim that they also want to expand benefits. Coverage for prescription drugs in particular became a hot issue as this book was being completed. The merits of specific drug-coverage proposals are outside the scope of a book whose purpose is to defuse the campaign to reduce Medicare's function as social insurance. But the gaps mean there is some truth to the argument that Medicare is only part of a broader system of health insurance for the elderly, and policy choices should address both it and other, supplemental, coverage.[14]

Supplemental Insurance

Supplemental coverage can be obtained through a Medicare combination plan, individually purchased "Medigap" policies, employer-sponsored "wraparound" policies for retirees, and public programs such as Medicaid or veterans' benefits.[15]

Medigap plans normally cover most or almost all coinsurance, but few of their enrollees receive much coverage for prescription drugs. Benefits are limited in part because, as an individually purchased form of insurance, the plans are subject to serious adverse selection. Insurers expect the people who need the benefit most to purchase the pharmaceutical coverage, and so they both limit benefits and charge high premiums.[16]

Employers provide wraparound coverage for a variety of reasons, ranging from employees' demanding it in union contracts, to the usefulness of such coverage in persuading employees to retire. Employer-sponsored coverage tends to be significantly more comprehensive than individual Medigap insurance. It is also a much better deal, because even if employers make no contribution to the costs of the plan, employees may still benefit from being charged less for insurance marketing and underwriting than they would if they purchased coverage individually. The average retiree from a large firm nevertheless paid $948 for his employer-sponsored wraparound in 1996. In addition, fewer employers are providing benefits than in the early 1990s, and many are restricting benefits and modifying eligibility requirements (PPRC 1997: 321–26).

The third major source of supplemental coverage is Medicaid. Persons who otherwise qualify for Medicaid because of poverty will have their Part B premiums and cost-sharing paid and will receive Medicaid's further benefits. The Qualified Medicare Beneficiary (QMB) and Specified Low-Income Medicare Beneficiary (SLMB) programs use Medicaid to reduce the burdens of Medicare's cost-sharing (for QMB only) and premiums for elders who would not otherwise be eligible for Medicaid. As is common for means-tested, state-administered programs, however, participation is both significantly lower than eligibility and varies greatly by state. Therefore, about 78 percent of persons eligible for QMB assistance and 16 percent of those eligible for SLMB actually were covered in 1998 (Rosenbach and Lamphere 1999).

In general, then, supplemental coverage is either pricey or, in the case of Medicaid, nominally free but often unavailable. In addition to these weaknesses, supplemental insurance is often criticized by economists on the grounds that, by paying for cost-sharing for services that Medicare does cover, supplemental insurance raises the program's spending. Many economists favor cost-sharing on the grounds that it provides an incentive for beneficiaries to forgo care that is likely to be of little value (assuming they can identify the value of medical care, a big assumption). Yet the holes in Medicare's benefit package also mean that even strong advocates of cost-sharing argue that some further coverage is desirable (Wilensky and Newhouse 1999: 94–95). And the fact that a portion of the elderly population does not have this coverage means that medical care for the elderly is less equal than Medicare's universality might seem to promise. Individuals with no drug coverage fill substantially fewer prescriptions per year than those with extra coverage. Over 20 percent of enrollees without supplemental coverage reported, in 1996, that they had delayed care because of its cost, compared to about 6 percent of those who were in combination plans or had private supplemental insurance (MedPAC 1998b: 124, 130–32; Davis et al. 1999: 237).

Combination Plans

Other things being equal, combination plans should be a better way to buy extra benefits, for two reasons. First, the economic effects of eliminating cost-sharing would not be the federal government's problem. The government pays fixed amounts to combination plans, and if their enrollees then consume more services, that is the plans' problem. Second, if combination plans can provide the HI and SMI benefits at lower cost, the government and the plans' enrollees can split the savings, the government reducing its outlays for HI and SMI and the enrollees reducing their outlays for supplemental coverage.

These hopes or arguments are one reason why transforming Medicare into a system of competing combination plans, as discussed in later chapters, is the most prominent radical structural reform proposal. Yet experience with combination plans to date has been mixed at best.

Extent and Distribution of Combination Plans

This experience consists almost entirely of Health Maintenance Organizations operating as Medicare Risk Plans through 1997. Enrollment in Medicare Risk Plans expanded dramatically in the 1990s but remained extremely geographically uneven. In March of 1998, 28 percent of Medicare enrollees lived in areas where no risk plan was available, whereas 39 percent lived in areas where they could choose among five or more plans (MedPAC 1998c: 39). Risk plans enrolled over a third of Medicare beneficiaries in Arizona and California in 1997 but none in nine other states (ProPAC 1997b: 29–39; also U.S. House, Committee on Ways and Means 1998: 174–75; PPRC 1997: 35–38).

One reason for this variation is that HMOs themselves are more common, and more popular, in some parts of the country than in others. At least equally important, however, is that Medicare would pay an HMO much more, per enrollee, in some areas than in others. Where the payments have been higher, HMOs have seen better opportunities to make profits and have been able to offer more extensive extra benefits without charging any extra premium.

Here is not the place to delve into the details of the system of paying HMOs 95 percent of the Adjusted Average Per Capita Cost (AAPCC) amount in each county. Clearly the AAPCC rate affected HMO availability. In 1999 plans were available in 97 percent of counties with an AAPCC of over $550.00 per month but in only 23 percent of counties where the AAPCC was under $379.84 (MedPAC 1999a: 41). Equally clearly, one of the few things on which virtually all analysts of Medicare agree is the need for some better method of paying for combination plans.[17] Some of the variation is appropriate: some areas have higher basic costs and sicker enrollees. But the AAPCC system also has rewarded plans in areas where historic price levels were higher than normal or where medical caregivers are prone to provide a lot more than the national average amount of services for a given type of patient, a pattern that, in the literature, is generally associated with higher costs but no better outcomes.[18] Hence, HMOs gave extra benefits to Medicare enrollees in areas where medical care was least efficient (U.S. House, Committee on Ways and Means 1996: 207; PPRC 1997: 69). In addition, plans were paid as if they contracted with hospitals that received large DSH or medical education payments, even if they did not (PPRC 1997: 64, 364–65; ProPAC 1997a: 27); and plans tended to avoid counties with small numbers of enrollees and, thus, average costs that varied significantly from year to year (PPRC 1997: 69; ProPAC 1997b: 36–37).

Who Joins Combination Plans?

Combination plans have tended not only to be most prevalent in areas that are more expensive than the norm but also to have members who are less expensive to treat. Plans seek less risky members through tactics ranging from sending mailings to certain zip codes but not others, to situating their office on the second floor of a building without an elevator. As Marilyn Moon asks, rhetorically, "How many health plan advertisements feature seniors in wheelchairs or hospital beds instead of playing golf or tennis?" (1999: 110). Plans might even choose to avoid getting a reputation for being too "good" at treating expensive conditions, not wanting to attract those patients. But even without the plans' efforts, sicker people may be less likely to choose to switch to the HMOs, because sicker people tend to want to stick with the medical providers whom they know. In short, beneficiaries appear to have been more likely to enroll in combination plans if they have needed little care and more likely to cancel their enrollment in those plans if they expected to need care.[19] Policymakers have long recommended that payments be adjusted for patients' risk of expenses, but that is much, much easier said than done. Medicare Risk Plan enrollees at least through 1995 appeared to have had expected costs 12 to 14 percent below average, so paying premiums only 5 percent less than the average meant that Medicare overpaid (PPRC 1997: 81; 1996; Newhouse, Buntin, and Chapman 1997; Lee and Rogal 1997).

In short, combination plans in the past have cost Medicare money, not saved money. They also have improved benefits significantly for some people, particularly those in high-expense areas. The 1997 report by the Physician Payment Review Commission estimated that the average Medicare Risk Plan enrollee "received about $69 per month in net benefits ($87 in benefits for an $18 premium)" (PPRC 1997: 46–51, quote on 49).[20] The exceptions are areas with high usage of Medicare HMOs (because HMOs are deeply ingrained in local medical practice) but low AAPCC levels (because costs are relatively low), such as Portland, Oregon, and Minneapolis (49–51).

Favoring recipients in high-cost areas is not all bad; after all, without combination plans, the extra costs would have been income for providers instead of benefits to seniors and the disabled. Yet a payment system that has the effect of making Medicare a more generous program for beneficiaries in some markets than others is rather hard to justify in principle.

Quality of and Satisfaction with Risk Plans

As with all "managed care," there is also extensive controversy about the quality of care in Medicare HMOs. The only safe conclusion is that some managed-care plans are better than others.

Surveys of self-reported access to care show slightly worse access in Medicare HMOs than for individuals with other supplementary coverage, but better access than for enrollees with no supplement at all (MedPAC 1998b: 130–33; see also PPRC 1997: 138–43; Gold et al. 1997). Many studies attempt to measure quality of medical care more directly. Unfortunately, measuring quality is hard. Since most people at any given time are not sick, they are not likely to have negative experience with their HMOs. When studies involve short periods of time, they may understate differences that evolve over longer periods.[21] There are lags in the data, so the HMOs in most studies are very different from those available in many areas, and even the studied HMOs' performance may be different now than at the time of the study.[22] Moreover, evidence about quality in traditional fee-for-service medicine, Medicare or otherwise, is hard to come by, making comparisons especially difficult.[23]

Much of the available evidence reports no difference between HMO and fee-for-service settings on particular health outcomes. Some studies report a better process of care in HMOs (Oberlander 1998). Unfortunately, the data limitations leave plenty of room for caution. Moreover, the few studies on which HMOs did significantly worse tend to be particularly relevant to Medicare. On three particularly well-conceived studies, Medicare enrollees with chronic conditions and diseases had significantly worse outcomes (Miller and Luft 1997). The fact that people who cancel their enrollment in HMOs and return to traditional Medicare tend to be "much less healthy" than those who switch from one HMO to another also suggests that quality measures for HMOs may be skewed favorably by selection. Disenrollment might itself indicate quality problems, at least for specific plans with high turnover (Riley, Ingber, and Tudor 1997).

If combination plans did not seem a good deal to some Medicare beneficiaries, the plans' enrollment would not have grown through 1997. Yet Medicare has lost money on the combination-plan enrollees, the plans' record on quality of care is mixed, and they offer extra benefits in part by cream-skimming in high cost areas. Both the successes and the difficulties explain why the Balanced Budget Act of 1997 transformed the Medicare Risk Program into "Medicare + Choice." When we consider proposals to transform Medicare into a voucher system, we will look at both the problems identified when Medicare + Choice was designed and the difficulties that arose in its first two years of implementation.

A Flawed but Vital Program

Medicare is much more complicated than Social Security, because Medicare includes an entire extra level of issues. We do not worry about the "quality" of pensions, or about controlling the costs of "pension providers," about beneficiaries being induced to consume extra pensions, about the political battles among different providers of pensions, or about non-social-insurance functions of Social Security.

Medicare also provides a meager benefit package, compared to the norms for both American private insurance and the coverage guaranteed to all citizens in most advanced industrialized countries.[24] Combining the Part B premium, cost-sharing for covered services, and expenses for uncovered services, the average Medicare enrollee appears to spend a great deal of money for medical benefits in a year. Urban Institute scholar and Medicare public trustee Marilyn Moon projected that in 1996 the average Medicare beneficiary incurred $2,605 in costs, not counting nursing home expenses (1996: 5–11). A study for the American Association of Retired Persons by the Lewin Group estimated that aged Medicare beneficiaries paid an average of $2,149 per person in 1997, not including costs for home health care or nursing facilities (AARP 1997). Moon's figure translates into 21 percent of average household income for the noninstitutionalized elderly person, and the AARP-Lewin figure is 19 percent. Some beneficiaries, of course, would pay much higher costs.

In spite of its failings, however, Medicare offers its beneficiaries a far more reliable guarantee of care than is available to all other Americans. At any given time, over one-sixth of the rest of the population has no insurance at all. Comparing themselves to their fellow citizens, seniors have very good reason to fear that without Medicare their lives would be much less secure.

PART II

Challenges That Are Not Crises

FIVE

Why All the Fuss? The Story behind the Savings Crusade

Much of the political controversy over entitlements is related to ideas about how commitments for Social Security and Medicare will affect the federal budget and therefore the economy. Thus, Peter G. Peterson wrote,

> A momentous question now looms over America's economic future. The way we face this question will likely have vast bottom-line consequences for your personal retirement. It may also determine whether your children will participate in the American Dream of rising affluence or whether our nation's wealth-producing engines will fail within your lifetime.
>
> The question is this: How will America prepare and pay for the growing dependency of our rapidly aging population? (1996: 3)

He went on to explain that the issue was not how to balance the federal budget then but "how to control the projected explosion in entitlement costs *after* 2002" (4). Why was this a problem? "The risk we now run is that unless we begin again to save for the future, we will leave our economy without the savings we all need in order to prosper" (6).

In the 1980s, Peterson saw the Reagan era's deficits as part of a "national consumption addiction" that, by lowering national savings, endangered future prosperity. He concluded that "the crux of America's undersaving, or, if you like, overconsumption, is the addiction to universal entitlements—welfare for all, in effect." If entitlements were slashed, he argued, workers' wages would be higher because the government would not have engaged in deficits, "negative saving by government" that "cancels out private saving and investment dollar for dollar." Moreover, if retirees could not count on receiving Social Security and Medicare, they would choose to save more, further increasing investment (1996: 6, 8, 10, 11).

This notion that the eventual costs of entitlements threaten to sink the economy remains the basis for much of the campaign to slash Social Security and Medicare. It has become part of the conventional wisdom of Wall Street and Washington, D.C., as witnessed by endorsements on the jacket of Peterson's book by former Federal Reserve Board chairman Paul Volcker, famed investor Warren Buffett, and television anchor Diane Sawyer—and by the quotations by David Broder and others in the introduction of this book.

Yet the claim that cutting entitlements is the key to whether "your children will participate in the American dream" is fundamentally false. Mainstream econometric estimates do not confirm the argument that changes in government savings rates of any plausible size would have the kinds of effects on the economy that Peterson implies. So it is perfectly reasonable to conclude that the evils of slashing entitlements are worse than the evils of the very slightly smaller economy that would, in the standard models, result from not slashing them.

The merits of the case in favor of higher savings, and its relevance to decisions about Social Security and Medicare, have been obscured by the strange politics of federal deficits. The politics of surpluses shows signs of being equally confusing. In order to clarify those issues, I emphasize the following points in this chapter:

1. Peterson's exaggerations seem plausible to David Broder, Diane Sawyer, and other elite commentators because many of the nation's most eminent policy economists, associated with both political parties, have shared Peterson's concern about savings and have made arguments that in significant ways parallel his own.[1] These mainstream economists fully understood the difference between social insurance and means-tested benefits but, as Peter Passell of the *New York Times* put it at the end of 1996, saw "the need to increase the nation's anemic savings rate as the paramount issue" (1996). This chapter explains the origins and logic of economists' emphasis on savings, in order to show why the linkage with Social Security and Medicare was as much a misguided political tactic as an economic analysis.

2. There are actually two separate arguments about savings, the budget and the economy, and they tend to get confused. One asserts that, under nor-

mal economic circumstances, greater savings will enhance economic growth. The direction of this economic argument is likely right; but the implications for policy are more limited than its sponsors have claimed, both because the effects are modest and because the political arguments about those effects were badly flawed.

3. The second argument emphasizes that deficits could feed on themselves until they became so large that they could not be financed and would swamp the economy. These doomsday scenarios do have numbers that fit their conclusions. But doomsday scenarios are highly sensitive to economic assumptions and events, and during the 1990s doomsday kept receding into the future even though the government took only modest steps to reduce deficits. It just is not sensible to premise major policy change on such extremely volatile forecasts of events three or more decades into the future.

4. By 1999 the arguments about savings had a new twist: surpluses. Much of the formulation had switched from how to get higher savings to the case for preserving savings that were anticipated in the Congressional Budget Office's forecasts. There is a better case for preserving anticipated surpluses than for increasing savings through larger surpluses (or lower deficits). But efforts to "lock in" those savings were wrongheaded because the forecasts were based on highly unreasonable assumptions and because the "lockbox" provisions would require counterproductive economic policies.

How Fiscal Policy Became Savings Policy

Current rhetoric about the economic effects of entitlements originated in the battles of the budget during the 1980s.[2]

The Devaluation of Keynesian Demand Management

In the 1960s and 1970s, the Keynesian (then-mainstream) economic analyses emphasized how budget policy could be used for "stabilization": directing the economy to more or less inflation or employment by manipulating aggregate demand. If the government spent more relative to its income, that would increase demand and so raise both employment and inflation. If it spent less relative to its income, lower demand would reduce employment and inflation.

Policy choice, then, would depend on whether you believed unemployment or inflation was the bigger problem at the time. By the 1980s, however, many economists who once had been proponents of Keynesian analysis had decided to downplay or even abandon attention to demand-side effects. They argued instead that deficits are normally bad, because they reduce national savings.[3]

This switch had many causes. Keynesian analysis did not seem to offer an answer to the stagflation of the 1970s (though that in itself shows not that the Keynesian analysis is wrong but only that it was not comprehensive). The most activist version of Keynesianism, "fine-tuning" the economy, turned out to be extremely hard to implement. Then, although panic about the short-term effects of deficits proved unfounded in the 1980s, the very failure to link the deficit to short-term evils also suggested that its short-term effects on demand should not be the focus of attention.

This conclusion that deficits did not matter so much for short-term trends was reinforced by a growing belief that monetary policy mattered more. The current cult of Alan Greenspan began with the credit given Federal Reserve chair Paul Volcker for breaking inflation in the 1980s. It is not so easy to disentangle monetary from fiscal effects in the events of the early 1980s, since they moved at the same time in the same direction (White and Wildavsky 1991). Yet monetary policy could seem a better instrument on practical grounds alone: it seemed more likely to move in the direction its master at least claimed to intend, and if political officials wanted to pursue certain economic goals, and the Fed disagreed, the Fed could block them.[4]

Reasons for Emphasizing Savings

Savings first became an issue as a result of the "productivity crisis" of the 1970s. After 1973 America's rate of economic growth declined significantly from the pleasantly high rates of the previous two decades (Levy 1987). Thus, from 1963 to 1973 real disposable personal income per capita rose by 46 percent, whereas from 1973 to 1983 it rose by only 13 percent. The major factor in income growth should be an increase in workers' productivity. In fact, from 1963 to 1973 the productivity of labor in the business sector had risen by about 36 percent, whereas from 1973 to 1983 it rose by only 13 percent. What, then, could economists recommend, and the government do, to increase the growth of productivity? Reaganomics did offer an answer: tax cuts to spur the "supply side."

But it did not work: productivity grew by only 14 percent from 1983 to 1993, virtually the same performance as from 1973 to 1983.[5]

Within the framework of mainstream economics, the clear alternative way to increase productivity was to increase investment by increasing the amount of savings available to be invested. National savings is the amount of money not consumed in a given year. The effect of the government's budget on national savings is an accounting identity:

National Savings = Personal Savings + Corporate Savings + Government Savings

Any of the numbers on the right side of this equation can be negative, reducing the total. The federal government could increase national savings by either reducing its deficit or adding to a surplus. In the mid-1980s, as Barry Bosworth (1986) and other economists argued, the available data did suggest that government dissaving was driving down the national savings rate.

This argument had one evident flaw: productivity growth fell before the savings rate did. The sequence of events suggests that other factors could be more important than savings; therefore, policies to increase savings might not have large effects. But economists viewed government savings as a variable that could be manipulated much more easily than anything else in the economy, simply by changing the budget (changing the budget seems simpler to economists than to the people who have to enact those changes, perhaps because many economists have tenure and legislators do not). And even if lower savings did not cause the productivity slump, who would want to make the productivity problem even worse?

By 1988 Charles L. Schultze, who as a former budget director and chairman of the Council of Economic Advisers had been a major figure in attempting to implement the old economic understanding, was arguing that the primary economic function of the budget should be "as a device for making inter-temporal transfers, by increasing or decreasing the nation's savings rate . . . the influence of the budget on national saving should be a principal determinant of the targets we set for overall budget policy" (1990: 15). Neither Schultze nor others who adopted this analysis would argue that stabilization effects were irrelevant; the econometric models that provide the estimates used below do include such effects. But they believed savings and their long-term benefits should be the normal priority.

Making Economic Policy for the Long Run

This understanding was synthesized in 1983 by Edward M. Gramlich, future chair of the 1994–96 Advisory Council on Social Security, in a paper in which he provided an unusually careful answer to the question "How bad are the large deficits?" Reviewing arguments and evidence about short-term effects, he concluded that they were much less convincing than the "primary reason" why deficits would be bad: namely, that "higher deficits represent increased 'dissaving' by the government. Unless offset by a corresponding increase in private saving, this increased governmental dissaving will lead to a large reduction in the share of total output devoted to capital formation in the United States in the long run" (1984: 44). By increasing demand, however, deficits might even increase consumption for a long time—in Gramlich's model, "for close to a quarter century" (61–62). He concluded that "deficits look undesirable only when thought about from a very long-term perspective, and we should probably begin thinking about (and worrying about) them from just such a standpoint" (65). Gramlich's analysis was quickly endorsed by other mainstream economists and incorporated into the Congressional Budget Office's description of why the deficit should be reduced (CBO 1985: 93–104; Minarik and Penner 1990). Schultze provided the pithiest summary of this analysis, describing deficits as like "termites in the basement" (1990: 15).

Critics from both the left and the right offered alternative policies to increase economic growth. But the analysts who emphasized savings could quite plausibly argue that options such as greater public investment, tax cuts, and deregulation did not offer larger benefits.[6] Another alternative, a policy to increase individual savings and investment, requires changing the behavior of individuals or firms, and the generalization that government is bad at changing personal behavior is true in many contexts (Wildavsky 1979). For example, those Reagan tax cuts that were marketed as ways to increase personal savings did not seem to have done so (Bosworth 1986).

Limiting recessions does tend to require some attention to demand, and both politicians and economists often show that they believe this in practice even if they critique the idea in principle (Stein 1996). Yet the deficit-reduction legislation of 1990 and 1993 did not slam the economy. One reason may be that reduced domestic demand becomes less important as trade and international financial flows become a more important aspect of economic performance (Bryant 1994). The balance of evidence and inference suggests that, other things being equal, greater government savings would lead to greater national savings and thus to a stronger economy. But would that increase be large enough to justify either substantial cuts to government programs or higher taxes, as Peter G. Peterson promised?

The Return on Savings
Economic Return

Peterson's claims are highly exaggerated.[7] The basic flaw in his argument is that new government savings do not translate directly into new domestic investment and thus new productivity. Only part of the new savings becomes new investment, for three reasons:

Offsets: In response to their reduced ability to consume because of higher taxes or lower benefits, some people will reduce their personal savings. Therefore, not all of any increase in government savings will turn into national savings. CBO (1997a) estimated that this offset could range, depending on the method of deficit reduction, from 20 to 50 percent of the total.[8]

Displacement: Some of the extra savings that occurs then displaces foreign investment in the United States, rather than creating new investment. In 1993 CBO (1993: 75) estimated that between 32 percent and 47 percent of net deficit reduction would be devoted to reducing net capital inflows. Americans would get the profits from investment that previously flowed to foreigners, but when Americans invest in place of foreigners, there is no increase in productivity.

Depreciation: As new capital stock is created by new investment, the amount of depreciation increases (for there is more to depreciate). More investment is needed just to replace what depreciates, and eventually any increase in the savings rate should generate enough new capital stock that the higher savings are needed just to pay for the higher level of depreciation (Aaron, Bosworth, and Burtless 1989: 73). So, within standard models, eventually the extra investment stops creating extra growth.

Estimates of the benefits of savings vary from model to model, depending on both other parameters and how they account for these three effects.[9] At the low end, using a model developed in the International Monetary Fund, Ralph Bryant (1994) estimated that reducing the U.S. federal deficit by half a percent of GDP for six successive years—3 percent overall—would eventually increase GDP by 1 percent. At the high end, adapting a model developed by the Federal Reserve Bank of New York, the General Accounting Office estimated that a permanently balanced budget would, after thirty years, produce an economy 6.6 percent bigger than it would be with a permanent deficit of 3 percent of GDP (1995: 9). The Congressional Budget Office in 1993 concluded that "for each percentage point of permanent increase in the ratio of national saving to GDP, consumption will eventually be permanently raised by about 1 percent above what it would have been without the saving increase" (1993: 74–75).

If we adopt CBO's figure, we should remember that the federal government's savings position would have to alter by a larger amount. For instance, to get a 5-percent-of-GDP increase in national savings, even with the minimal offset of 20 percent, the budget position would have to improve by 6.25 percent of GDP.

Political and Policy Returns

What do these figures really mean? They mean that a 3-percent-of-GDP change in federal budget policy—equivalent to about a $275 billion combined cut in spending and increase in taxes for fiscal year 2000—would increase consumption by about 2.5 percent sometime around 2030. To pose that as a policy choice, if Congress and the president in the year 2000 had virtually eliminated the entire military, or had cut Social Security and Medicare by nearly half, citizens in 2030 could consume 2.5 percent more.[10]

Peter G. Peterson might think cutting Social Security and Medicare so much would be worthwhile because he does not like universal entitlements anyway. There may be people who would be willing to sacrifice the military for a meager amount of extra economic growth. But few believers in either Social Security and Medicare on one hand, or the military on the other, would think the macroeconomic benefits were worth the pain.

By normal, simple, political logic, then, one might expect defenders of Social Security and Medicare to be leery of campaigns to cut deficits or increase surpluses. Instead, many of the economists who were campaigning for increased national savings argued that their policy would actually help save Social Security.

Savings and "Saving" Social Security (and Medicare)

Growing concern in the 1980s about national savings occurred at the same time as the Social Security rescue package of 1983. That package was designed to build up a reserve in the trust funds that, by the standard accounting, would help finance future costs. Critics, as I explain in chapter 3, claimed that this reserve was fake. Economists who believed that increasing national savings would create a larger economy had an answer.

The Hole and the Doughnut

Lawrence H. Thompson (1990), Schultze (1990), and others connected increased national savings and paying for Social Security's long-term cost increases by arguing that higher taxes paid by the baby-boom generation would translate into increased capital formation, and thus into a larger economy that would pay for the boomers' benefits.[11] Neither Thompson nor Schultze meant what many people might assume, namely, that adding surpluses to the trust funds would make higher payroll taxes unnecessary. Instead, as Thompson and Henry Aaron explained, worrying about the taxes themselves would be to "focus on the hole instead of the doughnut" (1987: 93). What matters to workers, they claimed, should be how much income they had left over after taxes (the doughnut), rather than the taxes themselves (the hole). If the economy grew more, the metaphorical circle of dough (pretax income) would be bigger. So even if the hole (the percentage taken for payroll tax) was bigger, they would be better off because there would be more doughnut remaining. Future workers when they paid higher taxes then would essentially be giving back some of the higher incomes that the baby boomers provided for them by increasing national savings by running the Social Security surplus.

This argument was barely visible (if it existed at all) in 1983. Robert Ball, one of the two main negotiators for the Democrats, claimed that if it was adopted, "it was when I was out of the room." Nevertheless, by 1988 it was widely accepted among policymakers and mainstream economists.

Social Security as a Means to the End of Savings

The National Economic Commission, created after the 1987 stock market crash to recommend what to do about the deficit (after the 1988 election!), was unable to agree on concrete antideficit measures. But its Democratic members, led by Senator Daniel Patrick Moynihan (D-N.Y.), who was the other principal Democratic negotiator of the 1983 Social Security package, issued a ringing declaration in favor of the savings-and-Social-Security link:

> There already exists an *immense* revenue stream that will flow into the federal fisc for the next thirty years, which if properly used, which is to say saved, would raise our savings rates significantly, and thereby, at least presumably, perk up all the indices that follow from savings. We refer of course to the accumulations of surpluses in the trust funds of the Social Security retirement and disability system. (1989: 51)[12]

This emphasis on savings remains central to mainstream discussion of Social Security's future. In the most recent authoritative collection of essays on the subject, *Social Security in the Twenty-first Century,* the chapter titled "What Economic Role for the Trust Funds?" refers to how the program can be "a vehicle for raising national saving" (Bosworth 1997: 168). In the same volume Gramlich writes that "the United States Social Security system could even provide a convenient way to mobilize new national saving and provide for higher living standards" (1997: 150).

Language like "opportunity," "convenient way," and "vehicle" suggests that Social Security is subordinate to the quest to increase national savings. But advocates of the conventional wisdom claimed that national savings was necessary for Social Security as well. As the *New York Times* paraphrased Robert Reischauer, "only with high rates of savings and investment will the economy be big enough to support the retiring baby boomers in the style to which they have grown accustomed. With low rates, the debate over Social Security, he contends, will deteriorate into a battle between generations in which aging parents and their children end up squabbling over who will make the greater sacrifice" (Passell 1996). Neither the economic benefits nor reasonable political calculations, however, support such claims.

Weaknesses in the Savings Argument

The economic benefits of extra savings, as projected in mainstream estimates, are far too small to prevent jealousies among generations. Even without extra savings, if productivity per worker grows, in Robert Eisner's words, at "a modest 1 percent per year, total output per worker will come to more than 40 percent" in about thirty-five years (1996). If a very large budget surplus made the economy 5 percent larger, compounding on Eisner's underlying 40 percent growth, the economy would be 47 percent larger instead. It is hard to believe that the difference between 40 percent larger and 47 percent larger would be recognized or credited by future workers—never mind enough to make the difference between program acceptance and "generational warfare."

Even the advocates of the savings-to-save-Social-Security argument recognize its political implausibility when they think through its implications (Schultze 1990: 8; Aaron and Bosworth 1997: 299–300). In Thompson's words,

> although higher savings today can compensate future workers for higher Social Security burdens, the future workers will probably never recognize that they have been compensated. Suppose that a far-sighted nineteenth century Congress recognized that citizens of the twentieth century would have to bear increased burdens to finance national defense and decided to promote capital formation—say by awarding land grants to encourage the building of railroads. Such an action might have accelerated the growth of national income enough to offset the higher defense burden. Even if such a scenario could be demonstrated, would it change our attitudes today about the fraction of our national income we want to devote to defense spending? I doubt it. . . . If I am correct, this form of "advance funding" of the Social Security burden is an analytical exercise with essentially no political meaning. (1990: 45–46)

The effects as estimated by the argument's own advocates are both too small to be politically noticeable and likely to be swamped by other economic factors over a period of decades. Eugene Steuerle, though himself an advocate of both savings and cutting entitlements, nicely summarized the problem when he wrote that "it takes several leaps of faith to accept that extra gross deposits translate to increases in net investment translate to substantial increases in economic income translate to such increases being available for retirement and health policy programs" (1997).

The estimated economic benefits of any plausible change in the government's budget position are far smaller than the uncertainty about our underlying economic future. They are much smaller than the differences among the Social Security Administration's three long-term economic forecasts.[13] They are even smaller than the effects of technical changes in the Bureau of Labor Statistics calculation of the Consumer Price Index that were made in the late 1990s.[14] The standard estimates of the importance of savings to economic growth simply do not justify radical changes in either the federal budget or entitlements for elderly persons.

That does not mean that lower deficits or even surpluses are a bad thing for Social Security. Other things being equal, a slightly larger economy can only help. More important, the basic argument for a better budget situation, in terms of lowering federal interest costs and thereby improving the government's fiscal capacity, is independent of the economic arguments. But the linkage of the campaign for greater national savings to "saving" Social Security was and is misguided.

The argument in favor of savings, however, is only one kind of long-term argument about the budget and entitlements and the need for major reform. During the 1990s a second argument, which can be called the doomsday scenario, became prominent.

The Doomsday Scenarios
Doomsday Logic

Assume that the government's budget deficit as a share of the economy was trending upward, as was normally true from about 1980 until late 1997. If nothing was done at all, each deficit would raise borrowing and interest costs, creating a larger deficit the next year, and they would compound on each other. Eventually deficits would pass 2 percent of GDP and 4 percent, and 6, and 10, and on upward—so long as nothing at all was ever done after the deficits appeared. Federal borrowing would soak up a larger and larger share of the combined pool of Americans' savings and foreigners' investment in the United States, until eventually the funds available for investment would be less than each year's depreciation. As the nation's capital stock began to decline, production would fall, the economy would enter a permanent recession or depression, deficits would rise even more, and so on. Whether the economy would totally crash first or the government would have to default when foreigners stopped buying its bonds is hard to say.

This doomsday scenario is very different from the standard argument about the benefits of increased savings. *Doomsday scenarios depend not on the economics of savings but on the logic of compound interest.*

Following this logic, there were a series of estimates beginning in 1992 showing how, if there was no action at all, the budget and the economy would eventually crash. These estimates produced different charts of the road to perdition because they started from different situations and made somewhat different assumptions (CBO 1997b: 16–18). In spite of these differences, there is a clear pattern over time: doomsday has steadily receded.

Doomsday Forecasts

Table 5.1 displays long-term budget forecasts made by the president's Office of Management and Budget (OMB) and two congressional agencies, the General Accounting Office (GAO) and the Congressional Budget Office (CBO). Our real concern should be not the level of deficit at which the economy im-

TABLE 5.1
Changes during the 1990s in Estimates of Long-Term Budget Shortfalls

	Estimated Surplus or (Deficit) as % of GDP					
	2000	2010	2020	2030	2040	2050
GAO June 1992 (a)	(−5)	(−8)	(−20)			
GAO April 1995 (b)	(−3)	(−7)	(−15)	>(−23)		
CBO March 1997 (c)	(−2)	(−3)	(−7)	(−17)		
GAO October 1997 (d)	0	0	(−2)	(−7)	(−13)	(−20)
OMB January 1998 (e)	0	2	2	2	1	1
GAO February 1998 (f)	0	1	(−1)	(−5)	(−10)	(−16)
CBO May 1998 (g)	0	1	(−1)	(−5)	(−10)	(−23)
CBO January 1999 (h)	1	3	1	(−1)	(−3)	(−6)
OMB January 1999 (i)	1	3	3	2	2	1
GAO May 1999 (j)	1	3	2	(−1)	(−2)	(−4)

SOURCES: (a), (d) both estimated from U.S. General Accounting Office, "Budget Issues: Analysis of Long-Term Fiscal Outlook" GAO/AIMD/OCE-98-19 (October 1997), fig. 2; (b) estimated from GAO 1995, fig. 2; (f) and (j) from spreadsheets kindly supplied by Office of the Chief Economist, U.S. GAO; (c) CBO 1997b: table 5, with economic feedbacks and discretionary spending growing with the economy after 2007; (g) CBO 1998b: summary table 2; (h) CBO 1999: table 2-1, summary table 3; (e) *Analytical Perspectives* 1998: table 2-2; (i) *Analytical Perspectives* 1999: table 2-2.

plodes (in these tables, around 30% of GDP) but the level at which it would become quite difficult to stop the accumulation of interest toward doomsday. In wartime even deficits of 20 percent of GDP can be (and have been) lived with. But it seems fair to say that, absent war, 20 percent is too big: it inevitably involves massive interest costs and is very hard to reverse.

Table 5.1 shows that, starting from the deficit and health-care-cost forecasts of 1992, GAO predicted extremely dangerous deficits by 2020. The end of the recession and the budget package of 1993 improved the situation, but the 1995 forecast, with its deficit of 15 percent of GDP in 2020, still might seem to have required action.

Yet, even without new legislation, the forecast deficit in 2020 was cut in half by CBO's March 1997 projection. The Clinton administration in 1997 even projected that its policies would essentially solve the long-term problem, but that was based on a highly unrealistic assumption about the long-term trend of discretionary spending, an issue that became particularly significant by 1999.[15]

Six months later, in October of 1997, the situation had again improved significantly. The Balanced Budget Act of 1997 (BBA) was, by most accounts, a smaller deficit-reduction package than those of 1982, 1990, and 1993. But the BBA was supplemented by greater economic growth than expected and surprisingly large revenue growth relative to the economy; and as GAO and CBO redid their forecasts, deficits were projected not to begin to verge out of control until around 2040. By 1999, even though there had been no further deficit-reduction legislation, more good news on spending, revenues, and the economy left CBO projecting that the deficit would not rise to Reagan-era levels for another fifty years. Doomsday, if it occurred, was further in the future than D-Day was in the past.

In short, during the Clinton administration, in spite of the absence of dramatic "reform" of entitlements for the elderly, doomsday receded, according to mainstream forecasts, by more than a generation. This happened because small differences in assumptions and beginning conditions lead to big differences in results when the logic of compound interest is spread over decades.

The volatility of estimates caused by changes in the beginning economic conditions and budgetary assumptions, which is implicit in table 5.1, was shown by another set of figures produced by the Congressional Budget Office. CBO reported what immediate change in budget position would be necessary to eliminate the problem for the foreseeable future. They defined that as keeping the federal debt at its 1997 share of GDP through 2070. In May 1996 CBO estimated that a 5.4-percent-of-GDP immediate increase in revenues (or reduction in outlays) would be necessary. By March of 1997, the estimate had fallen to 4.1 percent of GDP. This alteration in the space of ten months was due to a very small amount of policy change, economic improvements, new Medicare and Medicaid estimates, and technical changes in CBO's models (1997a: 16–17). In the same report, CBO projected that if the budget were balanced in 2002, then "long-term imbalances in the budget would be reduced from 4.1 percent of GDP to 2.3 percent" (22–23). By August of 1998, even though the BBA was somewhat less stringent than the legislation CBO was assuming in its earlier projection, the shortfall was down to 1.2 percent, and by January of 1999 it was 0.6 percent of GDP (CBO 1999: 43).

It is important to note that none of these analyses say that balancing the budget per se is crucial. The important step is to hold the deficit at a given level and not let it grow. In 1997 CBO estimated the economic effects of two scenarios: balancing the budget by 2002 and maintaining balance thereafter, or simply maintaining the deficit at the 1996 level, 1.7 percent of GDP. The simulation predicted that the economy would be 21 percent larger if the deficit was maintained at 1.7 percent of GDP, as opposed to 23 percent larger with a balanced budget. This estimate is basically what one would expect from the discussion of the economic benefits of extra savings earlier in this chapter: the economy would be roughly 1.7 percent larger if the government saved an additional 1.7 percent of GDP.

Lessons of the Doomsday Forecasts

The doomsday forecasts and how they changed reveal some important points. First, earlier action does have serious benefits. Second, *anything* that reduces interest costs is good for the future budget, whether that is tax increases, spending cuts in social insurance, or other spending cuts.

Third, these analyses have very little to do with the argument for national savings, whether it is made by the mainstream economists or by people like Peter G. Peterson who claim to offer a return to the growth of the 1950s. The relatively low return on national savings in the standard estimates is based, as one CBO analyst told me, on "changes among sustainable policies." The doomsday projections involve unsustainable policies: at some point, regardless of your macroeconomic theory, debt can run beyond the ability to pay for it, and then there are big benefits from moving to *any* sustainable policy. The relationship between the budget and the economy is different when one is talking about avoiding huge interest costs, rather than simply enhancing national savings.

But, fourth, one should take only so seriously projections of doomsday that extend decades into the future. Relatively small changes in policy or even estimating techniques can alter the projections quite significantly. It makes no sense to say such changeable estimates of reality many decades in the future should force major policy change in the present.

What, then, would be a prudent approach to doomsday scenarios? I suggest that a responsible approach would be to have at any given time, given reasonable assumptions, a budget policy that does not threaten serious movement toward the doomsday spiral within two decades. Serious movement can be defined as projections that deficits would be heading toward 10 percent of GDP and accelerating. By this standard, CBO's estimates in 1997 suggested that the budget at least required close watching, if not immediate action, because the deficit looked likely to spiral upward sometime around 2020. But estimates are too volatile to justify significant changes in policy at any time when the estimated benefits, if they exist at all, will not occur for more than two decades in the future. In the standard projections as of 1999, doomsday was so distant that any claim that politicians "must" slash entitlements to save the economy should not be taken seriously.

An Embarrassment of Riches: Budget Surpluses

The arguments that Social Security and Medicare must be cut so as to save the national economy are seriously flawed. Yet those arguments were originally made during a period of large, immediate deficits. This book appears in an era of projected budget surpluses, of all things. How does that change either the substance or politics of the campaigns to "save" Social Security, Medicare, and the economy?

The basic economic and fiscal relationships that I have described in this chapter are unaffected by current surpluses. Surpluses, whether in Social Security or the rest of the budget, can increase federal fiscal capacity by reducing future interest costs. The new forecasts merely change the data: there is less reason to worry about doomsday scenarios than there was in the past, and federal fiscal capacity looks adequate for a longer period.

But the advent of current, and projected future, budget surpluses has led to some rather misleading political maneuvers and even creates some legitimate policy dilemmas. The major policy question is whether the budget's move into overall surplus will mean that the argument I made in chapter 3, that Social Security surpluses from about 1983 on did not reduce budgetary discipline in other accounts, will apply in the future. There was good reason to believe that, with deficits already large, Social Security surpluses did not reduce them to a level that caused politicians to think they did not have to act. But if the normal goal of policy is to balance the overall budget, and if Social Security surpluses put the overall budget in surplus, then policymakers might feel they have extra money to spend on tax cuts or program increases.

From this perspective, the debate that erupted in 1999 about "preserving" surpluses to dedicate toward Social Security (in particular) was not totally senseless. Unfortunately, it included a whole series of new misunderstandings and distortions. Congressional Republicans and President Clinton accused each other of wanting to misuse (that is, eliminate) part of the surpluses in order to finance pet spending or tax cuts. The perhaps temporary result of this competition to blame each other for threatening Social Security was to produce a new informal norm: that the budget should be balanced not counting the Social Security surplus. This norm was easier to follow since forecasts were projecting surpluses even excluding Social Security. Still, it represented a dramatic, humongous, and unprecedented change in budget policies (Taylor 1999a,b,c,d; Broder 1999b; Hager 1999b; Penner 1999; Horney 1999; Samuelson 1999).

The political pressures behind this new norm were powerful, but they still might be overcome by spending or tax-cut pressures—especially if the 2000 election unites Congress and the presidency under the same party's control. So it is reasonable to ask how, if desirable, the projected surpluses might best be protected. But one should first ask whether the surpluses being projected as this book was written were credible and desirable.

Why Most Surplus Estimates Have Been Excessive
Hidden and Drastic Spending Cuts

Virtually all projections assumed major cuts in the share of the economy dedicated to federal discretionary spending—everything except entitlements and interest costs. CBO in 1999, for instance, assumed these accounts would decline from 6.6 percent of GDP in fiscal year 1999 to 5.0 percent in fiscal year 2009. That meant almost a 25 percent cut relative to the economy, over ten years, in the accounts that pay for the national defense, health research, federal law enforcement, NASA, the EPA, veterans' medical care, diplomacy, collecting taxes, patrolling borders, job training—in short, most of what the federal government does.

There were two reasons for the assumed constraints on discretionary spending. First, the Balanced Budget Act of 1997 established caps on total discretionary spending through fiscal year 2002. Since those caps were set in law, CBO assumed that discretionary spending would decline accordingly, thereby falling to 5.7 percent of GDP by 2002. Because budget estimates are supposed to project spending under existing law, CBO could hardly make different projections.[16] After 2002, however, there was no existing law from which to make projections. Discretionary spending depends on annual appropriations, for which the laws are passed each year. CBO adapted a common assumption used for "current services" baselines and projected that total discretionary spending would be increased each year by the amount of inflation. Since GDP grows each year not only with inflation but with productivity and population, increasing discretionary spending only with inflation meant that it would continue to shrink relative to the economy.

Spending caps enacted in 1990 and 1993 were basically followed. Total discretionary spending declined from 8.7 percent of GDP in fiscal year 1990 to 6.4 percent in fiscal year 1998, greatly contributing to the elimination of federal deficits (CBO 2000: 145). But that was made much easier by the military build-down of the 1990s, and by 1997 there was little support for further declines in the military share of GDP. Nor was there evidence of majority support for slashing nondefense programs (Reischauer 1997c). So, even though Congress and the president agreed to further declines in the 1997 Balanced Budget Act, in 1998 and 1999 appropriations exceeded the caps by about $30 billion per year (CBO 2000: 11).

By the beginning of 2000, the *Congressional Quarterly* was reporting that "Even GOP's Toughest Budget Hawks Perceive Fiscal Caps' Time Has Passed." "The caps are not very realistic anymore," declared House Budget Committee chair John R. Kasich (R-Ohio). "It kills me to say that, but it's true" (Parks 2000a). Neither the House nor the Senate adhered to the caps in its Budget Resolution for fiscal years 2001–5. Even the spending constraint that they did assume was widely viewed as unrealistic. Among the strongest critics were Republican legislators on the congressional appropriations committees (Parks 2000b).

Given that spending enacted in both 1998 and 1999 exceeded the caps substantially, the minimum reasonable projection for discretionary spending trends from 2000 on is not the baseline that was used in most previous forecasts but an alternative presented by CBO in its budget overview document at the beginning of the year. This baseline assumed that discretionary spending would grow with inflation beginning with the appropriations made in the year 2000. That difference alone would reduce projected surpluses over the following ten years by $1 trillion (Parks 2000a).

Even the inflation-adjusted baseline, however, may be unrealistic. An inflation adjustment would not help a program keep up with growing population nor allow wages to keep up with private-sector wages. Some savings might be possible from higher productivity, and some programmatic needs, such as the amount of weather to be forecast or the size of external military threats, are not related to population growth. Even those programs, however, could justify inflation adjustments (absent dramatic decreases in need); if other programs need more, spending overall would need to grow by more than inflation in order to maintain even existing service expectations.[17] Predictions that Congress and the president will reduce the value of government programs during a time of massive budget surpluses do not seem plausible.

What Would Be Done with the Money?

Surplus forecasts also beg the question of what happens when there is no more debt to be retired. CBO in 1999 was projecting that the debt would disappear in 2012 and the federal government would begin to accumulate, and earn interest on, assets. These interest earnings would be one reason that surpluses could be maintained for another decade. But how, exactly, would the federal government do that?

In what would the federal government invest its money? As chapter 8 discusses, allowing the government to invest Social Security surpluses in the stock market, on the trust funds' behalf, is controversial enough. But it must be easier to justify investment to finance Social Security than investment merely because the federal government has more cash than it knows what to do with.

Moreover, eliminating the federal debt would abolish the main means by which the Federal Reserve manages the money supply, which is by buying and selling that debt. As Paul Samuelson summarized in his textbook, "by selling or buying government bonds in the open market (mostly in New York City), the Fed authorities can tighten member bank Reserves or loosen them. These so-called 'open-market operations' are a central bank's most important stabilizing weapon" (1970: 297). If there were no federal debt to buy and sell, the Federal Reserve's task would be much more difficult. Before the government committed to eliminating its debt, it would be nice if someone would explain how monetary policy then would work.

In its budget outlook report at the beginning of 2000, CBO noted that "it might be more plausible to assume that the Congress and the President would decide to cut taxes and increase spending" than do something else with extra cash. But the forecasts assume that surpluses instead will be invested in some way because "CBO makes no assumptions about future policy actions" (CBO 2000: 19).[18] Fair enough for CBO, but not good enough for policy.

Excessive Optimism about the Economy

The final reason for skepticism about forecast surpluses is that the run of economic and budgetary good news that began in 1997 can be expected to reverse eventually. That does not mean that the CBO estimates in 2000 were irresponsible. It does mean that careful budget analysts and policymakers might choose to make somewhat more conservative assumptions.

As an example, I did some rough estimates of budget trends using the General Accounting Office's model as of early 1999 but with more realistic policy assumptions. Using the GAO 1999 figures made both the economic baseline and the assumptions more conservative than those used in CBO's projections during 2000. My discretionary spending assumptions also included modestly more spending than in CBO's inflation-adjusted baseline.[19] I also made

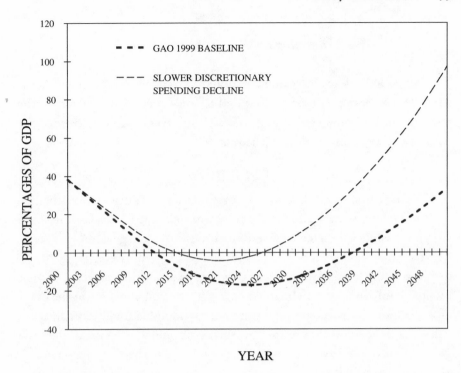

Fig. 5.1. National debt owed to the public under two budget scenarios

slightly less optimistic assumptions about Medicare spending than GAO had included in its model.

Under this projection the federal government's positive balance would top out at just over 4 percent of GDP in 2020, and the national debt would reappear in 2026 (figure 5.1). The deficit in 2030 would be about 2.5 percent of GDP. It would reach 5.5 percent of GDP in 2040 and begin spiralling upward. In this scenario, there would be reason to consider further action in the late 2020s.

Even with these more conservative assumptions, at the time of the 2000 election doomsday was not close enough to be considered a serious prospect. But the more cautious forecast does give some basis for being a bit more cautious than the standard estimates used in policy debate and electioneering at the time.

Protecting the Rest of the Surpluses

This brings us back to the vexing question of how to ensure that Social Security surpluses have the most positive and reasonable effect on the rest of the government budget, so that lower interest costs eventually help finance the costs of entitlements for elderly persons.

Doing It Wrong

The first thing to do is to get the baselines right. Policy choices that diminish the long-term decline in discretionary spending that is built into the current baselines would not be diverting surpluses to other government spending at all; they would simply be a correction to a flawed baseline.

Second, any legislation that set budgetary goals in stone as if the current economic forecasts were right could have perverse consequences in the event of a recession. In a recession, government spending naturally rises and revenues fall; if the law requires that predicted surpluses be attained, then the government would have to cut spending or raise taxes, thereby making the recession worse.

For both of these reasons, virtually all the plans promoted by congressional Republicans as ways to "protect" or "preserve" social security surpluses in 1999 were irresponsible demagoguery. These versions of a "lockbox" would have forced on-budget surpluses to match the CBO baseline forecast at the beginning of 1999 and so would have mandated the long-term decline in discretionary spending, even though that was not debated and even though Congress was unable to meet the legislated target for fiscal year 2000. They would have required spending cuts if the economy did worse (even if the budget were still in surplus, and even if that would hurt the economy further). In addition, experience with such targets in the Gramm-Rudman-Hollings act was less than successful. As Allen Schick put it, "one of the lessons Congress derived from the failure of GRH is that it is futile to set fixed-dollar limits on annual deficits" (1995: 39). There is no reason to believe that fixed targets for surpluses would work any better.

President Clinton added to the confusion when, in his 1999 State of the Union address, he proposed to "save" federal budget surpluses to help pay for Social Security. He suggested taking $2.7 trillion out of the projected budget

surpluses. A small share of that total would have been used for private investments to diversify the trust funds' portfolio (as explained in chapter 8). The
rest would have been used to buy Treasury bills and notes from the public.
These bills and notes would then have been added to the Social Security trust
funds. The extra budget authority in the funds, regardless of its economic
value, would have given SSA the legal right to pay full benefits for about another fifteen years, without any further action by Congress ("The Text"
1999).[20]

The difficulty with this proposal, naturally immediately pointed out by the
president's critics, was that the share of the budget surplus that he proposed
to dedicate to Social Security was suspiciously similar to the Social Security
surpluses themselves. In essence, the same funds would be credited to the trust
funds twice: once as Social Security surplus and once as budget surplus (Feldstein 1999).

The administration's defenders asserted that if the surpluses were not used
to buy bonds from the public, the administration's opponents would cut the
surpluses by slashing taxes or increasing spending. "All they would change,"
asserted Gene Sperling, the president's chief economic adviser, "is the use to
which the surplus would be put" (Weinstein 1999a; see also Hitt 1999; Kuttner 1999; Davidson and Galbraith 1999). The administration's defenders were
right about their opponents. As described in chapter 8, privatizers such as Feldstein indeed meant to divert federal surpluses to private accounts, and they
even claimed that doing so would increase national savings because, otherwise,
the government would have spent the money. But the Clinton administration's position did not meet the right test of a policy, which should be to ensure that the first deposit of surpluses into Social Security trust funds accurately reflects an improvement in the federal government's long-term fiscal
capacity. In fact, it presumed that the first deposit did not do so.

Doing It Right

Fortunately, sensible budget policy is not so hard as the debates about
"lockboxes" and the like may suggest. There is no need to establish specific
surplus targets. Instead, restrictions should target existing spending and revenue law. That is how the Budget Enforcement Act of 1990 (BEA) fixed
Gramm-Rudman-Hollings (Schick 1995; White and Wildavsky 1991).

BEA created two basic enforcement mechanisms. One requires that sixty senators support violations of points of order that enforce the rules. The second establishes that if legislation passed by the end of a fiscal year is determined to have violated the limits, then either discretionary spending accounts (if the caps were violated) or selected entitlement spending accounts are subject to "sequesters," automatic spending cuts.[21] These could be updated by applying them to any legislation that increased entitlement or other spending or decreased taxes, rather than being based on budget totals.

These measures are not airtight. The programs subject to the entitlement sequester are so limited that a large violation could not be offset. Caps can be exceeded by agreeing that spending is an "emergency" or through accounting games. But the real lesson of 1998 and 1999 is that implausible discretionary spending targets will not be enforced. If the targets are plausible, then, as from 1990 to 1997, the enforcement measures seem to be adequate.

Once legislation established a more reasonable current law baseline for discretionary spending, "protecting" the surpluses then would mean preventing non–Social Security legislation that would violate the baseline.[22] Any legislation that increased discretionary appropriations over the targets would be out of order unless it was offset by cuts in other programs or by revenue increases or declared to be an emergency. The current sequester process also could be continued. Any legislation that increased entitlement spending or decreased revenues would be subject to points of order based on the expected effect on spending or revenues, rather than on the deficit or the surplus.

These measures would not provide absolute protection against the "diversion" of Social Security surpluses to other uses. But absolute protection would inevitably be inflexibly dangerous. Indeed, the proposal I make here is fiscally conservative enough to make me uneasy. It means that, for instance, legislation to create national health insurance would face the same kind of procedural obstacles that it faced in 1994, even though the budget would be in surplus. My personal belief is that the benefits of national health insurance would justify spending some extra money. However, as part of a package to reduce fears about Social Security and Medicare, I am willing to subject future national health insurance efforts to those constraints.

No measure could or should absolutely bind future Congresses and presidents. Therefore the rules, and targets, should be set for only five to seven years at a time. What we need is not absolute guarantees but methods that will work for the moment and could work in the future; they need to be flexible enough to allow change if needs change. The measures that I am proposing would certainly assure that Social Security surpluses did not "mask" the underlying fiscal situation. Surpluses then would not mislead the public into allowing politicians to spend more money than they would otherwise have been able to spend.

All of the economic analysis about the budget and savings presumes that economists have a reasonably good idea about the nature and size of the relationships involved. In fact, more is unknown than known. The decline in productivity growth after 1973 was not caused by changes in savings but, if anything, caused that later decline. In the 1980s economists who were worried about savings were talking about termites in the basement; but by 1997 the economy was still growing nicely. One has to suspect that because other factors intervene, the relationship between savings as it is usually measured and economic growth is not so strong.[23]

Over the past two decades, the notion of an "entitlements crisis" has been promoted and oversold as part of a campaign to increase national savings. Other things being equal, increasing savings is a fine idea. But one does have to consider the other things, such as the consequences of budget cuts. And one has to be realistic about the potential benefits. They are much smaller than political propaganda commonly suggests.

The 1990s analyses of the federal government's own financial position did raise a relevant concern. The federal government should avoid conditions in which debt and interest costs grow so quickly that they will feed on themselves, pushing the government toward bankruptcy. The question is how realistic it is to worry about the budget how far into the future. I proposed in this chapter a moderate standard that policymakers could use to judge when long-term forecasts justified immediate action. The budget situation in 2000 was far better than that.

With the budget situation having improved to a point where virtually all of the Social Security surpluses for many years might be available to reduce the federal debt, there are good reasons to try to ensure that the funds are used in that way. But that would not be a good idea if other needs seemed more pressing or if the favorable budget forecasts were based on undebated, poorly understood, large cuts in the ability of other programs to perform their tasks. Nor is it really sensible to plan to eliminate the federal debt entirely; at a minimum, some thought has to be given to how subsequent federal assets would be managed and how monetary policy would operate in that strange (and unlikely) world.

Part 4 of this book suggests measures that would allow the federal government's finances to match the projections made by the major estimating agencies at the beginning of 1999, without the risks and unwise policies that were built into those estimates as hidden assumptions. I think the policies I suggest would improve future budget circumstances in a prudent manner. But any change should be evaluated in terms of both its costs and benefits, not out of panic in response to a mythical economic or budgetary crisis.

SIX

___

Can Americans Afford to Grow
Old and Sick?

___

Even aside from the debate about entitlements' effects on the budget and national savings, some analysts have argued that health-care costs for the elderly, in the words of the eminent economist Victor Fuchs, "could plunge the nation into a severe economic and social crisis within two decades" (1999: 11). Such arguments are based on extrapolations of trends of Medicare spending at some times in the past and on a theory about the causes of health-care spending growth. This theory says that costs increase mainly because the diffusion of new technology raises the norms of medical care, so that many more services are offered over time. Are we, then, facing impoverishment-by-medication?

Mainstream budget forecasts suggest otherwise (see chapter 5). The difference between these budget forecasts and the doomsday projections of Fuchs and others is, essentially, the extent to which one believes that policy can control costs. I argue in this chapter that the variation in spending over time for Medicare, cost trends in other countries, and the differences among periods of cost growth in the American private sector all show that whether medical cost growth is held to tolerable levels is a matter of choice.

Medicare spending can be expected to grow, both for demographic reasons and because some increase in spending per enrollee will probably be both desirable and desired. If people spend a larger share of their growing incomes for medical care that allows less painful, more active, and longer lives, they may consider that a very good use of the money. If many of those people are elderly, because better medicine helps people live longer, that could seem to be an achievement, not a crisis.

There is good reason to believe that Americans spend more for health care, both within and outside of Medicare, than they need to. So we will need strong policies to control costs. Calls for radical reform of Medicare, however, both are based on and threaten serious errors. For example, there is little substantive reason to view only potential Medicare costs as threatening, and ignore the costs of private-sector health insurance. And there is something more than a little ludicrous about pretending that health-care costs can be controlled decades from now, whether that is desirable or not. Yet many analyses are structured in a way that makes radical reform seem desirable in principle, even though they offer no assurance that those reforms would do more good than harm.[1]

Estimating Medicare's Spending Far into the Future

As in other long-term spending analyses, it is best to think about Medicare's costs in terms of its share of the Gross Domestic Product. Medicare's projected spending as a share of GDP depends mainly on two things. One is Medicare enrollees' expected share of the population. The other is the relationship between the growth of medical care costs per enrollee and the growth of the economy per capita.

The number of workers paying payroll and other taxes, the proportion of Medicare beneficiaries in the population, and the age of the beneficiaries depend above all on forecasts of birthrates and death rates. Estimates of such effects on Medicare for the next twenty years should be close to reality, since lower or higher birthrates would not affect the working-age population by then. Longer-term forecasts could involve larger errors. The best one can say for demographic estimates is that the procedures used by the Social Security Administration, whose estimates are also used by the Health Care Financing Administration (HCFA), are widely believed to be unbiased. Moreover, the basic trend toward longer life spans seems clear (Advisory Council on Social Security 1997b: 141–59).

The relationship between increases in health-care costs per enrollee and economic growth per capita is harder to predict than the demographic trends and, in some forecasts, is at least as large a cause of projected spending growth. As we will see, medical costs per capita have grown at very different rates relative to per capita GDP at different times, and they have grown unpredictably from year to year.

Long-term forecasts can differ substantially both between sources and from year to year. Small differences among estimating assumptions can compound to large differences in results over decades. Even small differences in starting points can develop into substantial differences eventually.

Table 6.1 displays some of this variation, using forecasts both by the trustees of the HI and SMI trust funds and by the Congressional Budget Office. All these estimates show substantial cost increases as the baby-boom cohort becomes eligible for Medicare and as life expectancies subsequently continue to increase. All show a slowdown during the 2040s as the baby boom dies off (lowering the average age of Medicare beneficiaries). Yet even the same organization's forecast can change significantly in a short period of time. For example, HCFA's estimate of spending in 2040 declined from 7.74 percent of GDP in 1997 to 5.25 percent in 1999, eliminating half of the originally expected increase.

What happened? One factor was the Balanced Budget Act, which was designed to reduce spending and, according to the estimates, did so. But estimated effects of the BBA were already in the projections made in 1998. Projected spending shrunk further in the following year partly because the lower-than-expected spending in 1998 reduced the baseline from which further growth would occur. But estimation is also a continual process, and as

TABLE 6.1
CBO and HCFA Estimates of Long-Term Medicare Spending Trends
(in Percentage of GDP, Calendar Years)

	2000	2010	2020	2030	2040	2050	2060	2070
CBO 1997	(3)	(4)	(6)	(7)	(8)	(8)		
CBO 1998	2.68	3.67	5.01	6.29	6.89	7.02	7.34	7.76
CBO 1999	2.54	3.38	4.60	5.76	6.28	6.34	6.62	6.96
HCFA 1997	3.03	4.23	5.72	7.14	7.74	7.80	8.03	8.38
HCFA 1998	2.68	3.46	4.70	5.85	6.29	6.29	6.47	6.71
HCFA 1999	2.61	3.04	3.92	4.88	5.25	5.26	5.42	5.67
HCFA 2000	2.33	2.75	3.50	4.36	4.76	4.79	4.93	5.19

SOURCES: CBO: CBO 1997b: xv, summary table 2. Note that this table was reported only in whole numbers; it did not extend beyond 2050 because, for reasons explained in chap. 5, CBO had the economy collapsing afterward. 1998 figures are from backup material provided by CBO staff in June 1998, from which I performed the calculations; they are consistent with the whole-number figures in CBO 1998b: 48, table 4-2. 1999 figures are from backup material provided by CBO staff in March of 1999 and are consistent with CBO 1999: 43, table 2-5.

HCFA: 1997 estimate is from Board of Trustees 1997c: 70, table III.B1. 1998 estimate is from Board of Trustees 1998c: 78, table III.B1. 1999 estimate is from Board of Trustees 1999c: 76, table III.B1. 2000 estimate is from Board of Trustees 2000c: 82, table III.B1.

the trends in specific costs changed in 1998, HCFA (and, to a lesser extent, CBO) analysts reduced their estimates of the cost growth that was likely in the future.

Thus good news in the short run compounds into large differences in long-term estimates (as does bad news). Much of the proportional change in the HCFA 2040 and 2070 numbers is already evident in the difference between the 1999 and 1997 figures for 2010. One point to remember here is that legislated savings in early years can be very useful in later years. But even unexpected good news in one year can have substantial effects in later years.

Table 6.1 also shows that different, equally reputable, estimators can have significantly different estimates. Even in the 1998 forecasts, HCFA's estimate for spending in 2070 was a full percent of GDP less than CBO's. This difference is not exactly small—the equivalent of $85 billion in 1997. Yet it resulted from quite small and mainly technical underlying differences between the two agencies' methods.[2] When such small differences in estimating procedures produce differences of tens of billions of dollars, we should take all estimates with a shaker or two of salt.

The gap between HCFA and CBO estimates widened in 1999 because the HCFA actuaries reduced their shorter-term cost estimates more severely than CBO's analysts did. Who was right? No one could be sure.

Demographic Factors

Table 6.2 breaks down the 1998 forecasts by the Congressional Budget Office of Medicare costs for selected years through 2070. The final two columns show the effect of enrollment trends alone. That depends on whether our concern is total Medicare spending or net spending (the government's expense minus its revenue from the Part B premium). The latter figure, which is the budgetary effect, is shown in the last column. If costs increased only in line with demographic pressures, then net spending was projected to rise from 2.3 percent of GDP in 1995 to 4.3 percent in 2070, or a total of 2 percent of GDP.

This increase was proportionately greater than forecast increases in Social Security spending, because Social Security benefits are, in the forecasts, expected to decline relative to per capita GDP.[3] We would add the forecast So-

TABLE 6.2

Demographic Trends as a Factor in Projections of Long-Term Medicare Spending Trends

(Congressional Budget Office Estimates, May 1998)

Calendar Year	Enroll. as % of Pop.	Spending Shares as % of GDP			
		Total Medicare	Medicare Net of Premiums	Total If Spending Grew Only with Enroll.	Net Amount If Spending Grew Only with Enroll.
1995	13.6	2.6	2.3[a]	2.6[b]	2.3
2010	14.8	3.7	3.2	3.0	2.6
2030	22.0	6.3	5.5	4.4	3.9
2050	23.1	7.0	6.2	4.5	4.0
2070	24.7	7.8	6.8	4.8	4.3

SOURCE: CBO 1998b: table 4-2 for cols. 2-4, table 4-5 for cols. 5 and 6.

NOTES: The Part B premium is expected to grow more quickly than overall program costs, both because of the move of some home health benefits to Part B, and the estimates that Part B will grow more quickly than Part A. Therefore, premiums as a share of spending grow faster than spending, creating the slower growth of net spending (col. 4) than of total spending (col. 3).

The estimates here are taken from an option of allowing spending per enrollee to grow only at 4% per year as part of a defined-contribution approach. The report describes this as an increase "equal to the average annual rate of growth projected for GDP per capita" (CBO 1998b: 57). Background materials supplied to me by CBO, however, show estimates for given years as being slightly higher or lower than 4%. So the estimates here for given years, such as those for 2010, will be slightly different from the estimated GDP trend.

cial Security spending increase to this 2 percent of GDP to get the total expected increase in future budget expenses on elderly persons, other things being equal, from demographic effects in Social Security and Medicare.

Medicare's Peculiar Demographic Problem

From an international perspective, however, the demographic effects on Medicare are quite unusual. America is not aging as severely as many other countries, but the effects on Medicare are worse than those on other nations' insurance systems. The reason is that only the United States has (and therefore budgets for) a health-insurance guarantee only for the elderly and a portion of the disabled. When the average person turns 65, most of her or his medical costs suddenly become part of Medicare; so Medicare costs increase significantly as a larger share of the population ages into the program. In other countries, where elderly people are in the same plan(s) as everyone else, the effect of a person turning 65 is only the difference between his or her costs at ages 64 and 65. That is why many studies show that the effect of aging on health-care costs in other countries will be smaller than the projected effect on Medicare (OECD 1996:52; 1994: 64). The demographic side of Medicare's cost "crisis," therefore, is in part an artifact of the choice not to guarantee health insurance to all Americans. If the United States had national health insurance, the effects of an aging population on the budget would be smaller.

Since the nation has decided to guarantee health insurance to (and only to) the elderly and certain disabled persons, however, what does that imply about the effects of having more eligible beneficiaries? If we thought of Medicare as being like other government programs, we would say the need for it was expected to increase. All ideology aside, one would expect the government to be better at some things and worse at others; we would decide what we wanted government to do and then have it do as much of that as was needed. If we are to have public education, it should consume a larger or smaller share of national resources as the school-age population becomes a larger or smaller proportion of the total. Military spending should depend on the extent of the military threat rather than being set at some arbitrary share of the economy. Roads should be built according to need. So what is wrong with spending more on Medicare as its beneficiaries' share of the population grows? Does having more elderly people make their health care less important?

If you agree with Peter G. Peterson and the Concord Coalition that the elderly are unproductive, a waste of national resources, and therefore undeserving, then their health care should be of little concern. But if that logic were taken to its logical conclusion, there should be no Medicare now. If you believe Medicare should exist now, then paying for the portion of future higher costs that would be due to greater need should not seem such a bad thing.

Aging within Medicare

Peterson and other antientitlement campaigners make another argument that sounds more plausible than it is. They point out, correctly, that older people on average incur greater medical expenses. As the population ages, not only will a larger share be in Medicare, but a larger portion of that group will be the "old old," for example, people age 85 or older. So aging within Medicare itself could drive the program's burdens higher. In Peterson's typically extreme formulation, "longer life spans add to health costs at an exponential, not just a linear rate" (1996: 25).

Most estimates have assumed that aging within the Medicare population will increase costs (CBO 1998a: 124–25). In essence, they project that increases in the age of the Medicare population in the future will have the same proportional effect on costs as is observed between age groups in the Medicare population now. But that assumption is badly flawed. The major reason older people tend to cost more than younger ones is that people who are dying cost more than people who are not. An 85-year-old is more likely to die soon than a 75-year-old. But if there are more 85-year-olds in the future, that will be in part because people are living longer. Which means that at each age level, they are dying less. So they cost less.

Which effect, more "old old" or lower death rates, should matter more? On balance, lower death rates should cancel out much of the effect of having more "old old" people. In their analysis of Medicare enrollees from 1974 to 1990, James Lubitz and his colleagues not only identified the effect of lower death rates, but they also found, contrary to a great deal of rhetoric about how American doctors treat the very old as intensively as younger patients, that "the costs of medical care treatment near death decrease with increasing age of death" (1995: 1001). They therefore projected that increased longevity while enrolled in Medicare should have only a small effect on total Medicare costs in the future.[4] A study of Swiss data by one of the world's most eminent health economists, and two OECD studies of costs in many countries, showed similar results (Zweifel, Feleder, and Meier 1995; OECD 1994, 1996). Scare stories about higher Medicare costs because of having many more "old old" people are not justified.

The purely demographic impact on eventual costs could be modified either by changes in population trends—such as faster or slower declines in mortality rates or greater or smaller numbers of immigrants—or by policy choices, such as raising the age of eligibility for Medicare. Raising the age of eligibility is easy to support if one does not care about whether people have health insurance. If one does care, it becomes necessary to show that, say, 66-year-olds would obtain health insurance in other ways. If you believe that is unlikely (which, for many elderly individuals, it is), then the population age 65 and over or disabled represents the "need" for Medicare, and a 2-percent-of-GDP increase in costs is, other things being equal, an estimate of the eventual required extra spending.

Spending per Enrollee

All forecasts show costs increasing more than could be explained by demographics alone, because all forecasts assume that costs per enrollee will grow more quickly than per capita GDP. The key policy questions are whether any such further increases are necessary; whether they could be prevented; and, if some increase is necessary and acceptable, whether even that level of restraint can be achieved without radical measures.

Forecasting the Unforeseeable

In order to assess both trends and possible reforms, forecasters need to make some assumptions about the trend of costs per enrollee. But, as table 6.1 shows, it is hard to predict costs per enrollee even two years into the future, never mind thirty or fifty or seventy.

Consider the conundrum presented to the National Bipartisan Commission on the Future of Medicare. When the commission met, most of its members, its leaders, and its staff argued that the seemingly most likely starting point, the Medicare trustees' 1998 baseline, was inappropriate. The basic reason given was that the trustees' baseline presumed that after 2020, costs per enrollee would grow quite slowly, by historical standards: according to the stated assumptions, at the rate of average hourly earnings for HI and of per capita GDP for SMI. Among other critics, CBO reported that the trustees had not explained what "policies designed to achieve that result" would reduce the trend to the post-2020 forecast (1998b: xix). As his colleagues pledged to provide a more "realistic" (or pessimistic) starting point, however, Commissioner Bruce Vladeck, former administrator of HCFA, denounced the whole enterprise of forecasting costs beyond a ten-year horizon as "an enterprise in comparative fantasy" (Pear 1998).

Vladeck was essentially right. Neither HCFA, nor CBO, nor the commission in fact prepared forecasts of long-term costs based on detailed analyses of trends; all forecasts beyond the next ten years are based on general assumptions; thus, they are rather arbitrary if not "comparative fantasy."

Moreover, forecasts for the next ten years are always made, for reasons that make good sense within budget processes, by assuming that there will be no change in the law governing spending. That is highly implausible even for ten years, however (Medicare spending control legislation has been much more frequent), and absurd over a longer period.[5]

In fact, the underlying trend of Medicare spending per enrollee is exceedingly unclear. If the trustees' forecast in 1999 was right, then costs per enrollee would grow by about half a percent per year in addition to the growth of per capita GDP, for the next thirty years.[6] The previous forecasts, however, showed much faster growth of costs per enrollee, especially through 2012, though not with much justification. It is simply impossible to say what will happen, for two reasons. Spending per enrollee depends in part on what medical caregivers and patients do, which is unknown. And it depends on legislation and administration of Medicare that has not occurred.

So the right question would be, What are reasonable goals for legislation to control the trend of costs per enrollee, without radically changing the existing program?

Indicators of Potential Cost Control

One way to answer that question is to look at the performance of systems other than Medicare, such as those in other countries. Other countries provide a good comparison in part because the standard methods of cost control in their systems are similar to those that can be applied (and to some extent have been applied) in traditional Medicare.

Table 6.3 provides rates of growth of total health-care spending per capita for sixteen countries. Before the mid-1970s most countries did not really try very hard to control costs, and they did not find strong methods of doing so until the 1980s. Therefore, in order to judge potential control, I used the most recent full decade for which data was fully available, 1984–1994. For Germany I used the period 1980–90 (just West Germany) because reunification was a large negative shock to Germany's per capita GDP.

The second column of figures shows the annual rate of growth of per capita health-care spending on top of the effect of the annual increase in per capita GDP. The international norm is 1.15 percent, and if the United States were excluded it would be 1.02 percent. The column also shows that national rates of growth have varied substantially, with Sweden actually reducing costs per capita.[7]

TABLE 6.3
Trends in Total Health Care Spending Per Capita
1984–1994 (Germany, 1980–1990)

	Growth in Annual Spending Per Capita	
	In Real Local Currency (%)	Relative to Per Capita GDP (%)
Australia	2.60	1.04
Belgium	2.81	1.02
Canada	2.87	1.73
Denmark	2.03	0.33
France	2.84	1.35
Germany	2.08	0.18
Italy	3.90	1.95
Japan	3.24	0.47
Luxembourg	5.61	0.72
Netherlands	3.00	0.93
New Zealand	2.83	2.20
Norway	4.13	1.78
Sweden	−1.37	−2.01
Switzerland	2.95	2.10
United Kingdom	3.58	1.54
United States	4.78	3.13
AVERAGES		
All countries		1.15
All except U.S.		1.02

SOURCES: *OECD Health Data 97: A Software for the Comparative Analysis of 29 Health Systems* (Paris: OECD/CREDES, 1997), and author's calculations.

How does this international norm compare with Medicare's potential as revealed by experience or in some of the forecasts of future trends? Table 6.4 presents calculations of Medicare experience. It shows that sometimes, as during the periods 1985–90 and 1995–2002, Medicare has matched or even improved on the international norms. At other times it has not, but it hardly seems reasonable to assume that traditional Medicare cannot. The table also shows that the assumptions made by CBO (and the Medicare trustees until 1999) about Medicare spending for the decade after 2002 were quite pessimistic compared to both the international evidence and Medicare's seeming potential.

By the same standard, however, the Medicare trustees' projections in 1999 seem a bit optimistic. Americans, having driven costs to unmatched levels, may be able to restrain costs more severely, with less impact on quality of care, than could countries that already spend less. Sweden's exceptional cost-control performance, for instance, might be related to the fact that it trailed only

TABLE 6.4
Estimated Increases in Medicare Spending per Enrollee
(Annual Rates of Change)

	Medicare $ per Enrollee (%)	GDP per Capita (%)	Medicare over GDP Trend (%)
1985–1990	6.77	5.56	1.15
1990–1995	8.36	3.75	4.44
1995–2000	4.15	3.88	0.26
(1995–2002)	(4.25)	(3.80)	(0.43)
2000–2005	5.92	3.73	2.11
2005–2010	5.71	3.71	1.92
(2002–2012)	(5.86)	(3.72)	(2.06)
2010–2020	4.62	3.56	1.03
2020–2030	4.06	3.48	0.56
2030–2040	4.16	3.63	0.51
2040–2050	3.61	3.65	−0.04
2050–2060	3.59	3.61	0.02
2060–2070	3.59	3.84	0.24
(2002–2030)	(4.81)	(3.58)	(1.19)

SOURCES: Author's calculations from the following sources. All figures are for calendar years.

1. All Medicare enrollment figures are actually HI enrollment, from a spreadsheet supplied by the Office of the Actuary, Health Care Financing Administration, June 4, 1998.

2. GDP through 1995 was taken from CEA 1998: 280, table B-1.

3. Population figures for calculating the change in GDP per capita from 1985–90 and 1990–95 were taken from Bureau of the Census data on the Web at ⟨http://www/census/gov/statab/freq/98s0002.txt⟩.

4. Population figures for calculating GDP per capita in all comparisons from 1995 on were taken from the Social Security Administration's figures, which tend to be about 10 million people higher than the Census Bureau's in part because SSA corrects for the Census' likely undercount. The SSA figure for 1995 was taken from "Population in the Social Security Area," a table available at ⟨http://www/ssa/gov/OACT/STATS/table4c5.html⟩. But I used an interpolation of the 1994 and 1995 figures in that table to create a 1995 July 1 estimate that is consistent with the population figures that I used for all subsequent dates. Those figures are in table II.HI, "Social Security Area Population as of July 1 and Dependency Ratios. . . Intermediate Assumptions," at ⟨http://www/ssa/gov/OACT/TR/TR98/Ir2H1-2.html⟩.

5. Medicare spending for the first two rows is based on CBO 1999: 136, table F-12. Medicare spending for the third and fourth rows is based on projections in table 4.4, p. 70, in the same volume. In both cases I have converted fiscal year figures into calendar year numbers by interpolation.

6. Medicare spending figures for all rows after the first four were taken from a background spreedsheet provided to the author by CBO in March of 1999. This spreedsheet is on a national-income-and-products-account basis and includes only the transfer costs, not the administrative expenses for Medicare, in each year's total. That should not, however, materially affect calculated changes over time.

7. GDP figures after 1995 are taken from the same CBO spreadsheet.

As these explanations of sources suggest, the comparative figures involving some of the same years (e.g., 1995) are not necessarily based on the same numbers. Moreover, these figures may seem falsely precise, as there is a lot of rounding in the original data. Different data sources and choices may yield slightly different numbers. For example, using total Medicare enrollment (either HI or SMI) would give slightly different results than using only HI enrollment as the base. I used HI because CBO staff have used it in their own analyses and because HI is the larger program at present. Using 1999 enrollment estimates might yield slightly different figures (though presumably it would change CBO's spending projections as well, since they are based on 1998 enrollment).

the United States in health-care spending as a share of GDP beforehand. Put differently, the United States could do better than average in the future because it did so much worse in the past. Yet that is a bit speculative for standard-setting.

Projecting versus Planning

It would be reasonable, then, to say that Medicare costs will increase in the future by the demographic effects on enrollment plus about 1 percent per year above the growth rate of per capita GDP. That estimate could be used to guess about future budget conditions.

But it would be a very different thing to promise to hit some particular target for growth per enrollee. Supporters of "regulation," "privatization," or any other characterizations of cost-control methods cannot promise that their methods will work—except in a most limited sense.

After all, the federal government could definitely control its Medicare costs by abolishing the program. Cost control is easy so long as you do not worry about whether Medicare beneficiaries will be able to get medical care. In a less drastic way, as in some voucher plans, Congress could just legislate a contribution amount per person. Then, if coverage costs more, people would have to pay the difference or do without insurance.

The standard estimates of cost control from a voucher plan make this kind of assumption. When performed carefully, as by the Congressional Budget Office, they are accompanied by warnings that the consequences for Medicare beneficiaries may be much more negative than for the government. Less neutral analyses, such as those of the Medicare Commission staff, let that point slide (White 1999c).

It is also possible to project savings from eliminating some part of the entitlement to Medicare. Raising the retirement age and means-testing benefits are reforms that medical providers could not do so much to counter (though they might find ways to raise costs for the remaining beneficiaries). Yet controlling costs by reducing the entitlement, either with direct rule changes or by setting caps on government contributions, would not be controlling medical costs, or "saving" Medicare.

If we actually worry about availability of care, then there are two strong reasons not to expect any spending-control method to be good for decades, or even desirable for decades.

The Dynamic Challenge of Medicare Cost Control

The cynical objection is that health care provides the incomes of a large number of very smart people. Give them a decade or two or three, and they are very likely to invent either ways around cost control or ways to create great public dissatisfaction with any set of cost-control methods. It is no more reasonable to imagine that one can know how to control medical care costs in 2030 than to imagine that one can decide on a military force structure for that year. In both cases, we do not know what the challenge will look like, and any potential challengers, by adapting to our strategy, may make it fail.

We see this pattern in periods much shorter than decades. As soon as Medicare's Prospective Payment System began to reduce payments to hospitals, administrators began looking for ways to game the system: for example, through "upcoding" diagnoses. In the mid-1990s, expenses for skilled nursing facilities (SNFs) began to soar, in part because hospitals began discharging patients into SNFs that they owned, thereby collecting, for a given diagnosis, both the standard prospective payment plus some SNF fees. As the Balanced Budget Act's spending constraints began to bite, hospital and other interests mounted a powerful lobbying campaign for relief. Health-care providers will continue to innovate and politic for higher incomes.

At the same time, the cost-control successes of the mid-1990s within the private sector have begun to recede. Measures that restrained hospital or physician costs, for example, are of little help with burgeoning pharmaceutical expenses. In short, just as we have never in the past found measures that would control costs forever, we will not find such measures in the future.

Value Choices about Future Medicare Spending

The idealistic objection is that medical care is a dynamic field, in which one cannot predict the capabilities that will be offered; thus, one also cannot predict the choices that people might want to make. Innovations could even lower costs or at least be clearly of such value that most people would consider them worth paying for (Cutler, McClellan, and Newhouse 1997).

If costs per enrollee for Medicare grow more quickly than per capita GDP, then each taxpayer will pay more for health care over his lifetime. Yet most people (all except those who die before becoming eligible for Medicare) will also receive more.

So the question is whether, over a lifetime, people would choose to devote more of both their lifetime income and consumption to medical care, particularly to extend life and capability in retirement. If they would, then Medicare's financing allows people to spread out some of the cost of insurance for their care when elderly (a period when health costs compared to income will be particularly high) over their working lives. A longer and less painful or more active life seems to be something most people would want to buy, and spreading the costs over time will make it easier to finance. Therefore, to simply assume that future voters and citizens will not want to pay more for Medicare is at best presumptuous.

If people might want to spend a larger part of GDP on Medicare (and we have no idea whether they will or will not), on what basis can we decide on their behalf to view such spending as a terrible thing? In order to assume that there would be a crisis, you need to make either of two other assumptions. The first is that the growth of any government program is bad. That is clearly an ideological judgment, not an objective fact. The second assumption is that people will expect the services but not be willing to pay for them, creating a budget crisis that destroys the economy. Yet in spite of the scorn that was visited upon both politicians and the public for their supposed irresponsibility during the nearly two-decade-long battle over budget deficits that began in 1980, the budget is balanced now, and the deficits do not seem to have destroyed the economy. There is no reason to assume that future voters will not make sensible decisions.

As a matter of values, then, the reasons why action must be taken now to "fix" Medicare in 2070, or even 2030, can hardly be taken for granted. If you think Medicare is a bad idea, you should believe in the crisis; but if you think it is a good idea, you should ignore the crisis talk. The demographic component of the projected increases might seem desirable, once understood, to both present and future voters. And after the next decade or two, the component that involves estimated increases in costs per enrollee seems like something that later voters could decide for themselves. It is hardly clear that they will not want to consume ever more medical care. After all, both we and past generations have chosen to do just that.

Medicare and the Wider American Health Finance System

The whole idea of a medical cost crisis is, for these reasons, questionable in principle. Whatever the effects of future medical costs may be, we also need to distinguish a Medicare problem from a general societal problem.

Government Burdens and the Nation's Costs

As we have seen, the demographic effects on Medicare overstate society's difficulties. Many of the dollars that will go onto public budgets as individuals attain age 65 will, at the same time, go off private budgets. So private burdens will diminish as public expenses rise. Money that had been going to private insurance could go to Medicare, without the payers being any worse off. But increases in medical utilization, for instance, would have similar impacts on both Medicare and private budgets. So is the supposed problem Medicare, or the overall costs of health care, or the overall system of health care in the United States?

Workers pay a larger share of their income for their own and their immediate families' coverage than for Medicare. That will be true even as Medicare covers a larger portion of the population and workers therefore pay more for its costs.[8] Imagine even that fairly optimistic private-sector insurance cost forecasts are true. As we discuss in connection with voucher reforms, one reasonable forecast is that private health-insurance premiums will grow 1 percent per year faster than average individual income. Then, at the end of seventy years, the cost of private insurance would have doubled relative to income. Family health-insurance coverage would cost, by these assumptions, about a quarter of the median pretax family income.[9] Surely many employers would pay a much smaller share of the premiums if they paid at all, and many more workers would go without insurance.

By the same kind of logic as in long-term Medicare estimates, therefore, the current private insurance system is "unsustainable." Health-care costs for non-Medicare enrollees would seem to be as much of a problem as for Medicare enrollees. If anything, one might argue that the private sector, with its high rates of uninsurance and the growing shift of costs from employers to beneficiaries (Gabel, Hunt, and Kim 1998), poses greater policy problems.

Policy Choices

Medicare already includes policies involving the non-Medicare population, such as medical education, capital finance of hospitals, and compensation for hospitals with disproportionate shares of uninsured patients. If developments in the private marketplace endanger the survival of facilities that are believed essential for the Medicare, Medicaid, or other populations, the federal government will surely be challenged to take special steps to maintain those hospitals and other providers (as it does with the DSH payments now). So the link between Medicare and non-Medicare concerns is recognized in practice if not in theory ("Symposium on the 'Safety Net'" 1997).

Moreover, cost trends in the two sectors must be linked even without an explicit decision to do so. Medicare's administrators have long feared that if the program paid too much less than the private sector, providers would begin to avoid serving Medicare patients. If that were to occur in the future, Congress would likely slow the cost control. But if the private sector had clearly superior cost-control methods, there would be strong pressure for Medicare to follow—why should the government subsidize the private sector? It is surely no accident that the long-run trends of costs per enrollee for Medicare and private insurance have been similar.

So the real policy question is whether and how Medicare and other health-insurance policy should be explicitly coordinated. There are two very different visions of how that might be done.

One version emerges in most of the arguments for radical reform of Medicare. It begins with a vision for the entire health-care system and then treats Medicare as one version of that picture. Sometimes the proposed reform, such as medical savings accounts, barely exists in the private sector and so is proposed as the fix for both. Other times, advocates claim they want to make Medicare go in the same direction the private sector is already taking. Thus, for example, the Democratic Leadership Council promotes an approach in which enrollees would choose plans using vouchers in a way that would give them the supposed benefits of current competition within the private insurance markets (Kendall 1995).

Skeptics of radical Medicare reform prefer to believe that dissatisfaction with events in the private sector will cause politicians and voters to rethink the role of government in health care beyond Medicare. They believe that some sort of national health-insurance arrangement is morally and practically right. In 1964 no one could seriously deny that government compulsion was needed to ensure health insurance for elderly persons; both American and international experience should establish, by now, that without government action there will always be a large proportion of uninsured Americans under age 65.[10] Supporters of universal health insurance also argue that it would make cost control easier rather than harder (Goldberg, Marmor, and White 1995). Robert Kuttner explains that

> With a universal system, there is no private insurance industry spending billions of dollars trying to target the well and avoid the sick, because everyone is in the same system. . . . All national health insurance systems are facing cost squeezes, because people are living longer and costly new medical technologies keep being invented. But no national health system rewards doctors for denying care. It took the U.S. private sector to come up with that one.[11] (1998)

If something like the current Medicare program insured everyone, there would be no need for the costs associated with competing insurers' efforts to assess risk (underwriting) and avoid it (much of their marketing). Average citizens might even know what was covered and which providers they could go to and still get reimbursed.

Neither the creation of universal health insurance nor even meaningful private-sector market reform is likely in the near future. But that does not mean that it would be good policy to make Medicare more like current American private insurance. We consider that issue further in chapter 9.

Medicare is debated as a separate problem because it is a separate program for which the federal government has already taken responsibility; even conservatives cannot simply ignore it, as they might prefer to ignore or play down the problems of uninsured Americans.

It is at least half crazy to try to make Medicare policy today for 2030, never mind 2070. We do not have the facts to do it, and we do not even have the right to assume that we know what is "right."

Neither of those objections applies to efforts to reduce costs in the short run, if those efforts represent a reduction that is acceptable to the public today. Long-term estimates also are useful because they remind us that in the future, financing Medicare and Social Security will be enough of a problem that we should be prudent now. The federal budget's prospects in 2000 seemed so favorable, for such a long time, that without those long-term estimates it might be impossible to resist irresponsible pressures to loosen current cost controls.

Yet the available data and estimates provide no basis for concluding that Medicare faces any cost-control "crisis" different from that of private insurance. If Medicare's overall costs are expected to grow more quickly, that is because its potential population is growing more quickly, and Medicare, unlike American private insurance, is not set up in a way that allows (or encourages) elimination of coverage. In fact the Medicare long-term cost "crisis" is partly an artifact of a political choice not to guarantee care to other Americans, so that an aging society raises public spending more in the United States than in other countries.

The basic goal of health policy should be to provide beneficial health care where needed. As medical capabilities improve, that may justify spending a larger share of the national product on health care. Since people presumably care about their entire lives, and since they need more health care when they are older, that goal could reasonably justify spending more on health care when people are age 65 and over. But people under age 65 may also suffer and even die if they are uninsured. A policy debate that focuses only on forecasts of Medicare costs does not serve any American well.

SEVEN

Exploiting Our Grandchildren?

Medicare and Social Security cannot credibly be argued to threaten to destroy the national economy, and genuine concerns about the growth of medical costs do not justify radical reform of Medicare. But what about the third common argument asserting that Social Security and Medicare require major change: that they are unfair to future generations?

Nothing in this life is "fair" from all perspectives. The operations of both Social Security and Medicare present many specific issues that might be debated in terms of fairness or equity. Good examples include the ways Social Security favors single-earner couples over dual earners, whether spousal benefits are too high and survivors' benefits too low, and whether it is fair for Medicare beneficiaries in high-cost areas to have better access to supplemental benefits, through combination plans, than do enrollees in low-cost areas. Such issues do require debate and consideration, and that debate might justify some programmatic reforms. They do not justify notions of crisis or drastic change.

Instead, the accusation of "generational inequity" challenges social insurance itself, and especially pay-as-you-go financing of Social Security and Medicare.

Setting up Social Security and Medicare as pay-as-you-go programs may seem to have unfairly benefited the earliest recipients, who contributed far less than they collected, on average.[1] Yet collecting taxes for twenty or thirty years without paying benefits did not seem practical for many reasons; the alternative would have been to have no Social Security and Medicare at all. Then many elderly people would have had little or no pension benefits or health care. Would that be more fair?

Setting up Social Security and Medicare as pay-as-you-go social insurance programs looked fairer than the alternatives at the time the programs were adopted—which is why they were set up that way. The question now is whether the future increase in the ratio of beneficiaries to workers should change that conclusion.

Two Demographic Issues

There will be more beneficiaries in the future, relative to workers, for two different reasons, with very different implications. The first is that people are expected to live longer. But this will not, in itself, make pay-as-you-go social insurance unfair to those born later. To see why, imagine that all pensions were financed from personal savings.

If all pensions depended on savings, then as life expectancy increased, and the portion of life spent in retirement increased, each person would have to save a larger portion of her working income in order to pay for her own retirement. The "burden" of funding retirement would rise, without any exploitation at all. Pay-as-you-go social insurance has the same effect, but the money is handled differently. If life expectancies are continually increasing, then one set of workers' payments will increase through their careers as the life span of people who then are retired rises. Then, as these workers retire, their successors will pay more. In short, as the ratio of beneficiaries to workers rises because of increased life expectancy, each succeeding cohort of workers will pay more in either a funded or a pay-as-you-go system. Yet each will receive more, also. There is no inequity. More of total income goes to retirement and less to working years, because there is more retirement—for each "generation."

But there is a second demographic effect: not longer life spans, but varying birthrates. If birthrates are higher or lower for a period of time (a baby boom or bust), then there will be larger and smaller cohorts of taxpayers, and beneficiaries, in the population over time. In a pay-as-you-go system, larger cohorts' contribution rates will rise less, relative to their own benefits, as they pay for preceding smaller cohorts. Contributions by the following smaller cohorts will have to rise relatively more, as they pay for the larger groups. In a funded system, cohort size would not matter; each cohort would save only for itself. So there is a stronger argument in principle that the baby-boom bulge in particular threatens the equity of Social Security and Medicare than that the "graying of America" causes inequity.

Nevertheless, assertions that paying for the baby boom's Social Security and Medicare would be highly inequitable to future generations are themselves greatly exaggerated. There is a case for requiring modestly higher contributions from the boomers than in a pure pay-as-you-go system. But the claim of unfairness is flawed in many ways:

> The phrasing in terms of particular "generations," especially boomers versus others, is wrong.

> Cohort sizes should affect far more than Social Security and Medicare benefits and burdens, and the other effects should favor smaller cohorts.

> Fairness should be considered not only in terms of payments over time but in terms of the relative incomes of workers and seniors at any given time. It cannot be "fair" to leave the retired people much worse off than the workers. And when we look at current and future Social Security and Medicare benefits, it is hard to see how cutting benefits could, in this sense, make the world more equitable.

> The supposed inequities from pay-as-you-go financing of Social Security and Medicare pale in comparison to other trends in the economy, which are much more deserving of "crisis" talk. Measures to reduce "intergenerational inequity" are likely to make these other trends worse, not better.

Cohorts and Generations

The first point is the least significant substantively, but it is necessary for further analysis. We have to be careful when discussing "the baby boom" versus "Generation X," or ourselves versus "our children" or "our grandchildren." The baby-boom period, births from 1946 through 1964, is too small for normal definitions of a generation. Children born from 1966 to 1970 are not very likely to be the baby boomers' children, nor is someone born from 1941 to 1945 likely to be a boomer's parent. Nor does one "generation" pay for another's Social Security and Medicare. Who, for example, will pay benefits during the period when the baby boomers are between ages 65 and 85? That will be from 2011 through 2049. If we assume that workers begin to contribute at age 22 and stop at age 64, contributions will be made by people born at any time from 1947 through 2027. Only workers born between 1985 and 1989 will contribute for the whole period. Moreover, the amount paid will vary as the baby boomers move through retirement toward eternity, and at any point some of the contributions will go to nonboomers. It is obviously absurd, then, to speak as if any group of people born over a relatively long period of time share equal burdens in paying for another group's Social Security and Medicare.

In the analysis that follows, therefore, we will discuss differences among people born at different times largely in terms of smaller *cohorts*. We can speak, for instance, of the cohort of people born from 1946 to 1950 or from 1936 to 1940. When we refer to the "baby-boom cohorts," that will mean the 1946–50, 1951–55, 1956–60, and 1961–65 groups.[2]

A Balanced View of Life Chances

If cohort size varies, some groups must get a better deal from pay-as-you-go pensions than others. Serious assessments of life chances, however, should include far more than entitlement benefits and burdens.

In all the standard forecasts, the fact that workers will pay larger shares of GDP (or of their incomes) is more than balanced by the fact that a larger GDP means larger incomes. For instance, in 1998 the SSA actuaries were projecting that real wages would be about 42 percent higher in 2035 than in 1998.[3] Even after paying higher Social Security taxes, workers' net wages would be 30 percent higher.[4]

Hence spending for Social Security alone (and even increased spending for Medicare) are very unlikely to deprive future workers of all the benefits of economic growth, giving those to "greedy geezers," even though the baby boom will create an unusually large number of such geezers. The question of fairness, then, is really one of balance. Out of a growing national product, what portion should go to future workers and what portion to the people who, under current law, will be eligible for OASDI and Medicare benefits?

One factor in the answer to that question should be how cohort size alone affects incomes and living standards, aside from the effects of Social Security

and Medicare. Compared to the baby boomers, members of later, smaller cohorts should have advantages within families, in the housing and labor markets, and possibly in asset markets.

The Family Economy

Consider the following question, which I have asked in speeches to current
college students: "How many of you believe your parents have deprived you
by not giving you more brothers and sisters?"

If these students had more siblings—that is, if the baby boomers had more
children—the demographic reason for "inequity" would not exist. Should
they believe they would be better off with more siblings?

It's unlikely. If there are fewer children, more money can be spent on each
child. The child from a small family is more likely to have her own room, perhaps a car, and parents available to chauffeur her to various activities. Indeed
(I remind students at high-priced colleges), if your family is smaller, you are
more likely to be able to attend the high-priced college. Some families might
not be able to afford college at all for multiple offspring. On the whole, within
the family economy, it is better to be part of a small generation. To the extent
that these advantages translate into better training or opportunities, they
should also lead to higher incomes after leaving the family.

Cohort Sizes and Markets

Within the wider economy also, other things being equal, being part of a
smaller cohort should be a good thing.

Housing

Housing-market conditions for larger cohorts when they are forming their
households and are buyers can be expected to drive prices up, as members of
large cohorts bid against each other. But as they retire and likely want to sell
their housing, they will be a relatively large number of sellers, selling to a relatively small set of buyers (the succeeding cohorts). Following this logic, the
baby boomers, both buying and selling into unfavorable demographics, on average should experience less appreciation of housing values than either previous or successive cohorts.

Local market conditions will vary, and the earliest boomer cohorts in particular might have done better, buying from the previous cohorts and then seeing prices appreciate as other boomers formed households. But Mankiw and Weil's widely cited analysis of the housing market (1988) found that demographic trends alone predicted the housing price run-ups of the 1970s and 1980s quite well—and that demographic factors alone would predict not only stagnation but even decline of future real housing prices. Thus, whereas their parents received "unexpected capital gains in housing," the boomers are not likely to be so lucky (Sabelhaus and Manchester 1995: 802). Judging by demographics alone, post-baby-boom cohorts should do better.

Labor Markets

The reasons why labor market conditions for larger cohorts are generally less favorable than for smaller ones are clear enough: more workers in the former case are competing to sell products to a relatively smaller market. As Easterlin, Schaeffer, and Macunovich put it, the

"baby boom" generation, on reaching working age, caused a sharp upswing in the supply of young workers, with marked adverse effects on their relative wages, rates of employment, and prospects for upward job mobility. In contrast, the baby boom generation's parents had been the beneficiaries of an unusually favorable labor market situation, due in part to their relatively scarce numbers. (1993: 497)

These and other analysts show that income per family member for at least the early boomers did not fall as much as labor-market logic should suggest, largely because more households have dual earners than before, and families are having fewer children than the boomers' parents did (Easterlin, Macdonald, and Macunovich 1990; Sabelhaus and Manchester 1995; Crystal and Johnson 1998; Radner 1998). To some extent, having fewer children may even be seen as a more pleasant life. But a given income with two people working does not go as far as if only one person earns it, since the second job "creates increased work-related expenses such as child care, transportation, and clothing" (Crystal and Johnson 1998: v). The extra costs of two jobs and the strains of child-rearing in those circumstances suggest that the increase in "adjusted family incomes" hides a loss in well-being due to unfavorable labor-market conditions.

Moreover, the increase in the number of dual earners on average will lower boomers' future Social Security pensions, relative to their families' lifetime contributions. The earnings of males grew much more slowly (if at all) among the boomers than for their parents' generations. Yet, on average, the wife's total earnings remained well below the husband's, both because of lower wage rates for women and because women are likely to spend some time out of the labor force, bearing and raising children. In a study of those baby boomers born before 1954, Crystal and Johnson (1998) therefore found that Social Security benefits for most women are likely to be based on their husband's income. Put differently, those families will have lower actual replacement rates than if the whole income had been earned by the primary earner. In this instance, Social Security is not favoring the boomers at all.

Asset Markets

The effects of generation size on experience in asset markets is less straightforward than the effect on experience in the housing and labor markets.

The stock market boomed from 1982 into 1999. That boom would seem to indicate that larger generations are good for the market. We should expect that, as the baby boomers are in the prime of their working lives, they are trying to save and invest for retirement. As a large generation, they are presumably competing to buy stocks and thus driving up prices. Higher stock prices, of course, are rarely considered a problem, since higher prices raise the putative value of those portfolios.[5]

Eventually, the demographics may be expected to change. Then the baby boomers, instead of being net purchasers of financial assets held either individually (through personal savings plans) or collectively (through employer pension plans), will be net sellers—in a big way. Hence prices are likely to fall. The situation for personal assets in equities is analogous to the pressures on Social Security. As Sylvester Schieber writes, "The boomers' retirement will make claims through upward pressures on the payroll tax as they draw Social Security benefits and downward pressures on financial markets as they sell their accumulated assets by cashing in their pension promises and selling other assets accumulated during their working lives" (1997: 269). Effects of demographic trends in the United States should not be mitigated by the possibility of selling assets overseas, because most of the developed world will be undergoing similar demographic trends at the same time (Schieber and Shoven 1997b: 239; Heller 1998: 10–11).

Unlike the labor and housing-market effects, the financial market effects of demography are not evidently a disadvantage to a larger generation. But the demographic effects on asset prices suggest that those price movements themselves can be deceptive. Unusually high increases during the period when the baby boomers are likely to be saving most are likely to turn into less favorable price trends when they need to sell off their assets. Smaller cohorts should have less effect on market prices, in either direction.

Implications of the Broader View of Life Chances

The "unfairness" of Social Security and Medicare to post-baby-boom cohorts therefore must be significantly offset by other demographic effects that relatively favor those cohorts. It would be much easier to argue that the boomers are being exploited by previous cohorts than that the boomers will be exploiting their children. Looking backward, housing and labor-market effects go in the same direction as the burdens of paying for Social Security and Medicare. The boomers are paying much higher taxes for those programs than previous cohorts paid and will be receiving lower Social Security replacement rates.

But that just provides more reason to be wary of claims about intergenerational inequity. The boomers' parents did have to pay extra to raise the boomers. They also were more likely to have experienced the struggles of the Depression while growing up; their income growth began from the low Depression base; and a lot more Americans fought in World War II than in Vietnam (where only persons born before 1956 could have fought at all). Those who sacrificed most in World War II did not live to collect Social Security or Medicare or to benefit from the economic boom of the 1950s and 1960s. Others who fought and came home had experiences that most people in my age group can only guess at from reading and a few movies (since the parents did not talk much about their horrifying experiences). If we hesitate to suggest cutting benefits to pensioners right now in pursuit of "generational equity," that may indicate that, deep down, we realize that the standard comparisons in financial terms are inadequate.

There is a lot more to "intergenerational equity" than the pattern of Social Security and Medicare contributions and benefits. The ways in which those programs favor the baby boomers over later cohorts will be significantly offset by the disadvantages experienced by boomers in the family and market economies.

The Fairness of Benefits

Imagine that Social Security and Medicare were abolished. Clearly, the future burdens on taxpayers would be reduced. Would that be "fairer"? Fair should not mean just nice for workers (never mind the fact that workers would face new burdens and risks for their own parents, burdens that would be distributed in unfair ways). Making the lives of the elderly much more miserable in order to reduce burdens on workers is not evidently "fair" in principle.

A balanced assessment of the equity of Social Security and Medicare must therefore consider the benefits of those programs. Can they be cut in a way that maintains fairness between workers and seniors in the future?

We can exclude Disability Insurance from the discussion because its benefits go to people of working age. Looking at OASI and Medicare alone, the right question then would be, Does the fact that paying currently promised benefits requires taking a larger share of future workers' income justify reducing the promised benefits for elderly people? We have already seen that workers are projected to have substantially higher net incomes, even after Social Security and Medicare taxes, on average. What would be the effect of benefit cuts on recipients?

Medicare

It would be hard to justify any reduction in Medicare benefits. As I showed in chapter 4, Medicare provides less financial protection against medical care costs than is offered by the vast majority of employer-sponsored insurance plans (Thorpe 1998: 11; Aaron and Reischauer 1995: 11). Its enrollees have substantially greater health-care costs than the national norm. Insurance protection that is well below the norm, for people with greater-than-normal need, cannot be unfairly large. American workers do extensively subsidize the health benefits of American retirees. That is, however, entirely normal. There is no major industrial country in which much of the health costs of the elderly is not financed by younger citizens, because elderly persons have much higher costs but do not have higher incomes (on average). What makes American workers' subsidization of insurance for the elderly unique is that some of those workers do not themselves have coverage. The real inequity is between workers who have insurance and those who do not.

Social Security

Social Security is a much more complicated case, because its benefits are intentionally different for different individuals, according to their previous incomes and family situations. We also need to distinguish monthly or annual pension income from the total benefits received over a lifetime. From the standpoint of adequacy, the monthly payment is more important; in terms of return on contributions, total payout matters more. There is a further difficulty: how to assess future benefits without knowing what future notions of a "decent" standard of living will be. Standards do change over time. What seems like abject poverty to many Americans today includes luxuries unimaginable to Americans a century ago—such as refrigeration to store food.[6]

One simple approach would be to compare Social Security with the guaranteed pensions in other countries. If Social Security were more generous, that might seem an argument for cuts. Although comparisons are complicated in many ways, R. Kent Weaver summarizes that Social Security appears to be relatively ungenerous, especially in its level of minimum guarantee to older retirees (1999).[7]

Social Security is not out of line by this measure, but maybe most countries are going to be unfair to future workers. That brings us back to the analytical difficulties involved in assessing future fairness. Fortunately, we can cut through a few of these analytical Gordian knots by looking at projected changes in the relationship between Social Security benefits and workers' incomes. If, as we will see, monthly payments relative to workers' incomes are going to fall, then it seems reasonable to conclude that benefits will be no less "fair" to workers in the future than they are today. That will allow us to focus on current benefits for the rest of our analysis.

The Decline in Future Relative Benefits

Benefits are compared to beneficiaries' own earnings in terms of the replacement rate, the portion of previous earnings that benefits replace at the

下

TABLE 7.1

Estimated Social Security Replacement Rates under Current Law, by Earnings History, for Workers Retiring at Age 65

Year of Retirement	Steady Low Earnings/[a] (%)	Steady Average Earnings/[b] (%)	Steady High Earnings/[c] (%)
1995	58.2	43.2	34.5
2000	57.2	42.5	34.4
2005	54.7	40.7	33.4
2010	52.4	39.0	32.2
2015	52.4	39.0	32.2
2020	51.8	38.5	31.8
2025	48.7	36.2	29.9

SOURCE: Advisory Council on Social Security 1997a: 223–25, tables RR.1–RR.3.

NOTES: These calculations were made on September 13, 1996, and included an expected change by the Bureau of Labor Statistics in how it would calculate the Consumer Price Index that is used for benefit COLAs but no other changes in existing Social Security law. The "replacement rate" as defined here is the percent of earnings in the last year of work that is replaced by benefits in the first year of retirement. The projections showed no further decline in replacement rates after 2025, as the various legislative changes that produce the decline (such as raising the normal retirement age to 67) will have been implemented by then. The economic assumptions are from the trustees' intermediate cost scenario.

[a] Equivalent to earnings of $15,000 in 1995.
[b] Equivalent to earnings of $25,000 in 1995.
[c] Equivalent to earnings of $40,000 in 1995.

time that an individual retires. If wages grow more quickly than prices (as they are projected to do), then, during retirement, a given individual's pension will decline relative to average workers' incomes. As people live longer, they will, on average, see their relative pensions decline more. So replacement rates at the time of retirement can only overstate the generosity of benefits compared to workers' future earnings.

As table 7.1 shows, under current law replacement rates are expected to decline slowly until about 2025. The absolute real value of pension income will rise more slowly than workers' incomes because of the scheduled increase in the Normal Retirement Age. From 2000 to 2025, while average wages are projected to grow by just over 25 percent, the benefit for workers at average or lower wage levels will grow by barely half of that.[8] These figures do not include the further effects of provisions that will automatically increase the taxation of benefits, which could be viewed as a further benefit cut.

We may conclude that, unless you believe benefits are unfairly high now, they cannot be unfairly high in the future. Are Social Security benefits unfairly high now?

Different Benefits for Different People

That might depend on whose benefits we are considering. People who earn more contribute more and are supposed to get more back. Compared to people with lower incomes, those with higher incomes are also more likely to have private pensions, should have higher private pensions than those held by lower earners, and should have greater separate retirement savings. For all these reasons, those retired Americans who receive higher Social Security benefits probably also have higher non-Social-Security incomes and could seem to have less "need" for Social Security benefits at all.

Yet *that is not a failure of the system; it is part of the point of the system.* The same people who get the larger checks each year and seemingly "need" them less also contributed more each year, relative to their eventual pensions, than did other beneficiaries. Although the effect of lower replacement rates in lowering the return to higher-earners' contributions is countered by the fact that higher earners tend to live longer, higher earners still, overall, collect a smaller proportion of their contributions (Panis and Lilliard 1996: 13, 26; Advisory Council on Social Security 1997a: 199–205). Put differently, the people who get the highest Social Security benefits contributed proportionally more, in the past, to pay other people's benefits.

So we might have different standards for different people's benefits. First, what kind of standard of living could be bought with the average benefit? We might agree it was too high if it seemed that many people would be happy to live on that alone, because then the average American would find no reason to save. Second, is the low end of benefits adequate at all? If it can only finance a very meager existence, perhaps it is too low. Third, at the high end, how does the lifestyle that can be financed by Social Security alone compare to its beneficiaries' lives before retirement? It ought to buy a much reduced standard of living, but the payments ought not to be so small as to make Social Security seem like a total rip-off to its more fortunate beneficiaries.

Social Security benefits depend on many factors besides earnings, especially whether one is married or single and the age at which the primary earner retired. Because their needs are different, we must look at couples and single persons separately.

Benefit levels and poverty. One standard way to look at benefit adequacy for low-income individuals and couples is to compare benefits to the federal government's definition of poverty. Yet the poverty threshold is a very meager standard of living.[9] A wide range of studies of the threshold for nonelderly families has shown that what most people would call an adequate level of consumption requires significantly higher incomes.[10] In 1981 the Bureau of Labor Statistics calculation of the "lower family budget" for a family of four was 165 percent of the official poverty threshold. Asked what the minimum income needed for a family of four might be, Americans in surveys in the 1980s continually provided a median answer of at least 140 percent of the official figure. Most respondents with family incomes up through 150 percent of the poverty threshold, when asked by Gallup Polls in 1984 and 1987, reported that there had been times during the year when they were unable to afford food, clothing, or medical care (Schwarz and Volgy 1992: 33–40; see also Renwick and Bergman 1993).

This information should provide some perspective on the fact that a single worker who retired at age 65 in 1996, after working full time at the minimum wage for at least thirty-five years of earnings, would have received $584.40 per month. The poverty threshold was $627.08 per month (*Social Security Bulletin* [1997], annual statistical supplement). So, though not officially poor while working, such a worker would be poor when he retired (unless he had somehow saved significantly from his low working income). Social Security pays 50 percent more for couples than the worker's entitlement alone, whereas the official poverty formula says two can live less than 1.5 times as expensively as one. Therefore the minimum-wage couple after retirement would not be officially poor, but the couple's benefits would be only 12 percent higher than the threshold—well below more reasonable measures of adequacy.

That is the formula; what about actual benefits? Table 7.2 is based on the Social Security Administration's records of benefits earned by each contributor. Such records, unfortunately, do not tell us the benefits for couples, because both members of the couple may be listed as "retired workers." Nonetheless, they show that in 1996, 34.7 percent of retired workers had benefits below $600 per month, clearly below the poverty threshold. The low end of Social Security benefits could not possibly be considered excessive.

Nor are average benefits excessive. In 1996 the average monthly benefit among all OASI (not disabled) beneficiaries was $690.70 per month; retired workers averaged $744.90 per month. This average was significantly reduced by individuals taking early retirement, and to the extent that that is a choice,

TABLE 7.2
Social Security Benefit Levels, 1996

Average Monthly Benefit:	$672.80
OASI	690.70
DI	561.80
Average Benefit for	
Retired Workers	744.90
Men	838.00
Women	643.60
With Reduction for Early Retirement	678.30
Retired at Age 65	779.30
With Delayed Retirement Credit	1,030.20
Surviving Widows and Widowers	707.20
Spousal Benefit Only	369.00
(Wives)	385.50
Percentage with Benefits	
Below $600 per Month:	
All Retired Workers	34.7
Early Retirees	40.5
Age 65 or Later Retirees	20.2

SOURCE: *Social Security Bulletin* (1997), annual statistical suppl., tables 5.A1, 5.A3, 5.B1, 5.B2, 5.B6.
    NOTE: The data in this table is based on a 10% sample of all beneficiary records. No more thorough count exists, and given this sample size (over 4 million cases), the margin of error is likely to be miniscule.

the data may make Social Security seem less generous than it is. The average retiree's benefit was, however, only 19 percent higher than the poverty threshold for individuals age 65 or over, and even the average benefit among those who retired at age 65 was only 25 percent more than the threshold.

The spousal benefit makes the program more generous to couples than to individuals. That does change the picture a bit (though we should remember that after one member of the couple dies, the other is back at the individual benefit level).

Table 7.3 reports data about families, statistics that the Social Security Administration created by matching its data files to records from the Bureau of the Census Current Population Survey for March of 1996. The different poverty threshold reduces the share of couples in poverty. Also, the higher earner in a couple generally has higher earnings than do single people (whether marriage increases income, or income stress breaks up marriages, I hazard not a guess). Even so, table 7.3 shows that 33.9 percent of couples over age 65 had benefits below a figure ($12,000) that is only 26 percent higher than the poverty standard. Even the median benefit for couples in 1996, $14,352 per year, was only 51 percent above the poverty threshold—a figure that the other data cited above suggests is barely adequate. So the low end of Social Security benefits is clearly inadequate, and even the average benefit for couples would not make any normal person think there was no need to save for retirement.

If there is any case for significantly reducing Social Security benefits, then, it must be made among the minority of beneficiaries with the highest benefits, at some figure significantly above the median.

Benefits for higher earners.   Maximum benefits in 1996 would have been $1,286.10 per month for a single worker who had earned at or above the income threshold for thirty-five years and $1,929.15 for a couple with a primary earner at that level. That sounds a lot better (though, as we shall see, it is hardly lush living). A third of the couples receiving Social Security benefits in 1996 collected between $15,000 and $19,999 per year; 12 percent received more, with 3.3 percent receiving more than $25,000 (SSA/ORES 1998a: 64).

In order to assess these benefits, we must remember, first, that they finance

TABLE 7.3
Income from Social Security Benefits, by Family Unit Type, 1996

	Married Couples		Nonmarried Persons	
	Age 62–64	Age 65+	Age 62–64	Age 65+
Number (in thousands)	1,086	8,872	994	13,378
Median Income	$9,754	$14,352	$6,926	$8,298
Percentage under $7,000[a]	31.4	9.3	50.3	34.3
Percentage under $9,000[b]	42.6	16.1	71.7	59.6
Percentage under $12,000[c]	74.3	33.9	93.0	87.4

SOURCE: SSA/ORES 1998a: 64, table V.A.2. Some figures are author's calculations from summing percentages reported for smaller categories, so there may be small random rounding errors.

NOTES: The data in this table, unlike those in tables 7.1 and 7.2, are based on a smaller survey (the March 1996 Current Population Survey). The figures for ages 62–64 include some disability beneficiaries, rather than only retirees and persons receiving survivor benefits.

[a]The poverty-level income for a single person age 65 or over in 1996 was $7,525 per year. It was higher for younger persons. So individuals with benefits below this level receive Social Security benefits distinctly below the poverty level.

[b]The poverty-level income for a couple age 65 or over in 1996 was $9,491 per year. The poverty level for younger couples was higher. So couples with benefits below this level receive Social Security benefits distinctly below the poverty level. It also represents an income 20% above the poverty level for individuals age 65 and over.

[c]This figure represents 126% of the poverty level for a couple age 65 or over.

a much lower standard of living than these retirees had while working (as is shown by the low replacement rates recorded in table 7.1). Second, at the very top level of benefits, couples are quite likely to have had two incomes or a primary earner who worked past age 65.[11] In either instance, the higher benefits would be caused by particularly high contributions, compared to either single-earner families or people who worked only until age 65. The highest level of benefits for couples, then, may be especially justified as preventing the system from being unfair to dual-earner families or individuals who work past age 65.

Even if there are special reasons for the highest level of benefits, it might seem, to some, too high. But is it? Not in Montgomery County, Maryland (where I lived while writing much of this book). In 1993 the county government reported that the pretax income needed for a couple to meet a "minimum standard of need" was just over $19,000 per year (Community Action Board 1993: 11). The comparable figure in 1996 could only be higher. Even the high end of Social Security benefits for couples in 1996, therefore, could buy only slightly more than a "minimal" standard of living in that part of the country.

Costs are lower in many other places, but not so much lower as to make Social Security benefits, on the whole, seem excessive. Table 7.4 illustrates estimated costs for what we might call a "very minimally middle-class" lifestyle for an elderly couple, in different parts of the country. I have estimated the costs for 1996 so that we can compare them to benefit levels in that year. Some readers may consider this budget to be excessive, but I doubt that most would agree.[12]

This budget assumes that our couple lives in a one-bedroom apartment. It spends the amount for food that would be allowed under the U.S. Department of Agriculture's "low-cost food plan" for a family of two, both age 51 years or over. Poverty-level budgets often assume that the family does not own a car. That, however, is clearly inappropriate for a budget that is supposed to reflect what most middle-class people would consider even a barely adequate living standard. So I assumed that this couple buys a small car only once every ten years, drives it less than the average household, and must pay for automobile insurance.

The average senior couple, as we have seen in chapter 4, pays quite a lot for medical care, in spite of Medicare. Table 7.4 assumes spending of $2,000 per

TABLE 7.4

Illustrative Costs, by Community, of a Very Minimally Middle-Class
Lifestyle for an Elderly Couple, 1996

County (Town or City)	Monthly Expenses	Annual Expenses
Knox County, Ill. (Galesburg)	$1,348	$16,181
Kanawha County, W.V. (Charleston)	1,390	16,685
Rice, Minn. (Northfield)	1,427	17,125
Orleans, La. (New Orleans)	1,452	17,419
Montgomery, Ala. (Montgomery)	1,452	17,421
Pierce, Wash. (Tacoma)	1,458	17,491
Pima, Ariz. (Tucson)	1,467	17,601
Johnson, Iowa (Iowa City)	1,470	17,641
Duval, Fla. (Jacksonville)	1,485	17,823
Sonoma, Calif. (Santa Rosa)	1,611	19,335
Cook, Ill. (Evanston)	1,664	19,973
Norfolk, Mass. (Brookline)	1,725	20,699
Orange, Calif. (La Mirada)	1,726	20,715
Montgomery, Md. (Rockville)	1,734	20,813

NOTE: See the text for discussion of and references for the assumptions made in constructing this table. The figures given here are not perfect but should be close to the truth, and I have tried to estimate costs on the low side. Further research, whether supportive or critical, would be much appreciated.

person in 1996. The table includes $30.00 per month for local phone service and occasional long-distance conversations with children or other relatives. Energy costs were projected based on the Department of Energy's figures for the smallest residences for which it provides data, those with heated floor space less than one thousand square feet. Any budget also should include some amounts for other necessities, such as clothing. Montgomery County's 1993 estimate of $1,500 per year for clothing and miscellaneous personal-care goods and services is unlikely to be excessive in 1996. It includes a very minimal amount of reading, recreation, and entertainment expense. Two dollars per day per person for all these expenses does not seem like living large.

Some of these costs, such as housing and energy, will vary greatly across communities. Others, such as medical care and food and the cost of buying an automobile, may vary less. In the table I accounted for variation where I could get data (housing and energy) but not where I could not (such as for auto insurance). I then calculated estimates for fourteen communities across the country, in order to establish the range that I illustrate here.

This budget is not only pretty skimpy, but also I have attempted to estimate costs conservatively.[13] As the table shows, where housing is extremely cheap (such as in Galesburg, Illinois), our very minimally middle-class lifestyle

might cost as little as $16,000 per year. But not many of the elderly popula-
tion live in places like Galesburg. Many live in places like Orange County,
California; Montgomery County, Maryland, or Norfolk County, Massachu-
setts, where the same lifestyle would cost over $20,000 per year. And many
others live in places like Jacksonville and Tucson, where this lifestyle would
cost between $17,000 and $18,000.

In short, for most elderly couples, benefits totaling $18,000 per year in 1996
would have barely paid for a minimally middle-class lifestyle: one small car
purchased every ten years, with little bad luck in maintenance or insurance
costs; a one-bedroom apartment; low energy consumption; few long-distance
phone calls; a skimpy food budget; average medical care costs; and about four
dollars per day (two dollars per person) for anything else. No airplane trips or
Winnebagos; few gifts for grandchildren; and not even any state or local taxes
(people living on just Social Security would not be paying income tax). Many
seniors could barely afford that lifestyle even with maximal Social Security
benefits of, in 1996, more than $20,000 per year.

The figures here do not represent a scientific survey of living standards. But
they should show that the higher range of benefits for couples is not enough
to convince any middle- to upper-middle-class person to forgo saving for retirement. It does not remotely approach providing a standard of living that
would replace what they had before retirement.

It is possible to argue that Social Security expenses could be marginally reduced for persons at the upper level of benefits. But it makes little sense, given
the figures here and the projections that benefits will decline relative to workers' wages over the next three decades, to call major benefit reductions a matter of "equity."

Prospects for the Future and Intragenerational Equity

Any serious examination of the effects of generation size on life opportunities
must be confounded by the fact that, independent of demographics, different
times offer different opportunities. All other things being equal, a smaller generation may have advantages in the labor market. Yet all other things may not
be equal: there may be more productive inventions at some times than at others, or more competition from foreign low-wage labor, or higher or lower real

interest rates, or many other factors that make the economic experience of persons born a decade or two or three apart quite different.

When we look at some of those other effects, they reveal that the supposed inequities caused by the effects of cohort size on the burdens of paying for entitlements for seniors are far less significant than other factors.

Real Interest Rates and the "Moneysworth" of Social Security

Real interest rates determine the difference between what an individual could have earned by investing her payroll contributions in financial markets and the "return" that is implicit in the Social Security benefit formulas.

The Social Security Administration actuaries have calculated the "moneysworth" of individuals' payroll tax contributions for people with different family and income profiles, born at different times. These moneysworth figures understate the value of OASDI benefits: for example, they do not express the insurance value of protection against disability or longer-than-average life span, or the value of creating annuities without the overhead costs of private annuity markets. However, since those caveats are true of benefits for all recipients, comparison of moneysworth for people born at different times provides a good indicator of the change in the effect of Social Security across cohorts.[14]

The SSA analysis shows that moneysworth ratios can be divided into three periods. The first period, which includes persons born around 1950–55 or before, began with very high ratios that then declined as "the OASDI program was maturing and increasing payroll tax rates resulted in reductions from initially extraordinarily high ratios of benefits to contributions." But the decline was intensified by the fact that "interest rates from the late 1970s through the late 1990s exceeded the growth rate in wages to an historically unusual extent—as a result, cohorts with earnings during this period and benefits after this period have extraordinarily high present value of contributions as compared with the present value of benefits" (Advisory Council on Social Security 1997a: 177).

The trend was expected to reverse and the moneysworth of contributions to grow for individuals born between around 1955 and 1970. "This increase occurs because payroll tax rates are essentially stable among these cohorts, life expectancies are increasing," and interest rates are expected to fall to more historically normal levels. In short, both demographics and economic factors would improve. Then, for individuals born after about 1970, moneysworth figures would decline "due to the increasing payroll taxes starting 2030" (Advisory Council on Social Security 1997a: 197).

The first thing one should notice about this description is that it does not break out on simple "baby boomers versus others" lines. The trend changes toward the middle of the baby boom, not before or after. Moreover, the moneysworth of Social Security for individuals born in 1973 (nonboomers) is higher in *all* categories of earnings and marital status than for the boomers born in 1949. Almost all categories of workers born in 1997 also do better in moneysworth terms than the 1949 group, though not by so wide a margin. For almost all marital status and earnings level combinations, the moneysworth of Social Security for the baby boomers who do best (those born in 1964) is exceeded for everyone born afterward until around 1991, and it is not until sometime after 2000 that individuals are born for whom Social Security was expected to offer a worse return than for the baby boomers who did worst, those born around 1950 through 1955.[15]

In short, trends in real interest rates mean that, viewed purely as an investment (as it is in many criticisms), Social Security has been less fair to baby boomers than to many succeeding cohorts. Notions that "Generation X" cohorts will be exploited through Social Security by the baby boomers are dead wrong.

Stagnation and Inequality of Wages

The moneysworth calculations reflect not only high real interest rates for most of the past three decades but also low wage growth during the same period, which lowers the benefits created by the Social Security formulas (Radner 1998; Mishel, Bernstein, and Schmitt 1997).

Income Stagnation

If we look more closely at wage trends, we can see that the early baby-boom cohorts have higher incomes than preceding groups not because income grew quickly for the boomers but because the boomers started at a much higher level than their predecessors did, as a result of economic growth that occurred before most of the boomers entered the workforce (i.e., until the oil-price shock of 1973). After entering the workforce, however, baby-boomer cohorts in general saw lower wage growth than did the cohorts twenty-five years before. Another way of looking at the same effects is this: after the first baby-boom cohort, later groups did not have higher incomes (in real dollars) at comparable ages. Income at ages 20–24 for the cohort born in 1961–65 was barely higher than the income at the same ages for the 1946–50 group; and income for the cohort born in 1971–75 was lower (Radner 1998: 12, 13).

To put this another way, there was hardly any real growth in starting incomes for twenty-five years, from 1970 to 1995. If we were to worry about "generational inequity," we might better look not at the boomers versus younger cohorts but at the steady, secular decline in income prospects from the beginning of the baby boom on (Schrammel 1998).

Income Inequality

Not only did wage levels stagnate, but earnings in general also became substantially less equal over the past quarter-century. For instance, the median wage (in inflation-adjusted dollars) declined even when the average (mean) wage rose. That means that even when the total wage bill rose, most people did not end up with more money. The benefits of any growth accrued only to the higher-income population (Mishel, Bernstein, and Schmitt 1997; Galbraith 1998).

There is a lot of dispute about the reasons for the growing inequality but none about the fact. Some claim that education has become more important to productivity, causing the less-educated to do much worse financially; changes in government aid may have made education less accessible as it became more important; others think computers must have something to do with it; others believe increases in international trade drive down wages for Americans who compete with foreigners (such as manufacturing workers) but do not affect Americans who do not (such as doctors and lawyers and economists).[16] Fortunately, we do not have to explain either the stagnation of real wages or the growing inequality. All we need to know, for a discussion of the ostensible entitlement crisis, is that these trends in pretax earnings surely were not caused by the future costs of Social Security and Medicare. If the trend of inequality continues, it will have far more significant effects than the projected future rise in tax burdens to pay for Social Security and Medicare.

Dean Baker (1998) estimated income distributions if average wages fol-

TABLE 7.5
Potential Effects on Workers' Incomes If Income Inequality Increased after 1995 in the Same Way as before 1995

	Estimated After-Tax Hourly Wages (Constant 1995 Dollars)				
	1995	2010	2030	2050	2070
Without Increasing Inequality					
First Decile	$4.67	$5.40	$6.34	$7.54	$9.14
Third Decile	6.82	7.89	9.26	11.02	13.35
Median	9.36	10.81	12.69	15.10	18.30
Seventh Decile	13.20	15.25	17.90	21.31	25.82
Ninth Decile	20.64	23.85	27.99	33.33	40.38
With Increasing Inequality					
First Decile	$4.67	$4.62	$4.53	$4.45	$4.40
Third Decile	6.82	6.75	6.62	6.50	6.42
Median	9.36	9.53	9.73	9.94	10.23
Seventh Decile	11.06	11.44	11.91	12.42	13.03
Ninth Decile	20.64	23.33	27.38	32.14	38.00

SOURCE: Baker 1998: tables 1, 4.

lowed the intermediate path in the Social Security trustees' projections but the distribution of income followed the trends observed from 1973 through 1995. Table 7.5 summarizes some of his work.[17] It lists after-tax hourly wages at five points of the wage distribution: the tops of the first, third, fifth, seventh, and ninth deciles. (The top of the first decile is the income at which 10 percent of wage earners earn less and 90 percent earn more; the top of the fifth decile is the median, and the top of the ninth decile is the income at which 90 percent earn less and only 10 percent earn more.) All his figures are adjusted for inflation and are therefore reported in 1995 dollars.

The first half of table 7.5 presumes that income inequality does not continue to increase as it did from 1973 through 1995. In that case workers at all income levels see after-tax real wage increases of, for example, 36 percent from 1995 to 2030. The second half of the table provides estimates at the same deciles if, instead, the trend of inequality continues. Workers at the first and third deciles have lower real incomes in the future than they had in 1995. Even those at the top of the seventh decile (with earnings higher than two-thirds of the rest of the population) would have only a 12 percent increase in the thirty-five years from 1995 to 2030.

By any reasonable standard, therefore, the recent trend in wage inequality has been and would be something far more like a crisis, for most Americans, than the supposed future crisis caused by the costs of Medicare and Social Security. Stagnation and inequality in wage growth did great damage to families' economic prospects beginning in 1973; and if those inequality trends were to continue, they would do much more damage to the economic prospects of most Americans in the future.

This chapter has shown why the third major accusation against Social Security and Medicare, that they create insupportable generational inequities, is false. Longer life expectancy does not in itself make pay-as-you-go social insurance unfair. The peculiar effects of the baby-boom bulge in the population do raise legitimate issues. But because of many factors, the legitimate concerns caused by unequal cohort sizes do not justify radical reform.

First, Social Security and Medicare benefits and burdens are only a portion of life chances. In other ways, smaller cohorts can be expected to do better than larger ones.

Second, fairness should not mean only whether workers at one time will be contributing more to social insurance for the elderly population than workers at other times (they will). It should also involve comparing living standards of workers and seniors at each point in time. Slashing benefits so that seniors would be much worse off, relative to workers, than they are today might seem fair from the first perspective but not the second. Our analysis of benefit levels showed good reason to believe they will not be excessive. Thus, one cannot expect that cutting benefits would make ours a more equitable society.

Finally, other economic factors are far more important than Social Security's and Medicare's terms. The high real interest rates of the 1970s and 1980s mean that, if viewed purely as an investment, Social Security has actually been a worse deal for baby boomers than for a number of the subsequent cohorts. Wage stagnation and growing inequality have had far more negative effects on most Americans, and inequality if continued would have much worse effects, than the supposed inequities created by pay-as-you-go financing of Social Security and Medicare.

There is a modest case for making the baby boomers contribute a bit more to the costs of their future pensions and Medicare than they would under a pure pay-as-you-go system. The best way to do that would be to pay a bit more and consume a bit less through government now, which would reduce the federal debt so that future workers will pay less for interest costs. That is exactly what the current accumulation of Social Security surpluses is supposed to accomplish: *the right policy is already in place.*

More radical steps that have been promoted as ways to make society more "fair" would, however, do nothing of the sort. Significant cuts to, or "restructuring" of, Social Security and Medicare would put the low-income families who benefit most from Social Security and Medicare at greater risk. The cure for the supposed equity problem could easily be worse than the disease.

PART III

Reforms That Would Not Be Improvements

EIGHT

Privatizing Security?

The most prominent proposals to "reform" Social Security involve replacing some portion of the current program with a system of mandatory contributions into individually owned pension accounts. Mandatory private accounts adopt one of the rationales of social insurance: that people have to be forced to protect themselves.[1] But they are not well fitted to two other purposes of social insurance: (a) to soften the trade-off that lower earners face between saving enough for retirement and having a decent standard of living while working and (b) to guarantee a specific amount of retirement income, regardless of individuals' luck with investments.

Privatization advocates nevertheless argue that replacing all or part of the program with private accounts would improve on traditional social insurance for the following reasons:

1. Private accounts inherently are funded instead of pay-as-you-go. Thus, they would be less of a burden on future taxpayers. In most versions of this analysis, funding pensions would increase national savings and thereby eventually improve economic growth.

2. The rate of return on personal investments is likely to be so high that they would be a much better deal on average for contributors. Even many people who do worse than the average could get a higher return than from pay-as-you-go social insurance.

3. Equity or adequacy problems that remain could be addressed with separate, means-tested government transfer programs, such as a tax-financed base pension.[2]

Critics of privatization challenge each of these arguments.

Types of Privatization Proposals

Estimated effects of any given plan must depend on its details. There have been many plans, and their sponsors keep changing them. I will refer to individual plans, therefore, only to illustrate key issues. But it seems useful to distinguish two basic characteristics of plans.

The first is whether a plan explicitly cuts the amount of pension that is absolutely guaranteed. Most of the plans being discussed in early 1999 did so; although their sponsors argued that supplementary private accounts would more than replace the lost guarantee for most recipients, they did create an evident risk of getting less.[3] Some plans, however, created private accounts and then used them to offset Social Security benefits. In this approach, guaranteed benefits would be reduced only to the extent that private earnings were available to replace them.[4]

The second major difference involves how the new accounts would be financed. Of the major privatization proposals, only the plan proposed by Advisory Council chair Edward M. Gramlich did not worsen the federal government's immediate budget position, because Gramlich would have financed private accounts from new contributions. Most other plans diverted some of the payroll taxes that were already going to Social Security into the private accounts.[5] And some, such as economist Martin Feldstein's 1998 plan, would have financed the accounts through reducing general revenues. Feldstein offered workers a tax credit to cover their contributions (CBO 1998c; Samwick 1998).

All plans are subject to questions about the likely rate of return on investments. Plan designs make different trade-offs between risks to beneficiaries and to the federal budget. In all cases we need to consider how well an idea, however theoretically attractive it might be, could be implemented.

Rate of Return on Investments

Arguments about rate of return should involve evidence and inference based on the U.S. economy. Some privatization advocates have claimed that Chile's privatization of pensions after 1981 shows that such an approach would work in the United States (Tanner 1996; "Social Security's Savings" 1997). But Chilean experience is much more mixed than they claim; moreover, the "successes" cited by privatizers had little to do with the kinds of market forces that would be relevant to predicting experience in the United States (White 2001; also Kritzer 1996; Vittas 1995; Utthoff 1993; Diamond, Lindeman, and Young 1996). Therefore, we will focus on U.S. evidence, which poses enough difficulties.

Overhead Costs and Return on Investments

It is necessary, first, to distinguish average returns in the markets from what an individual would realize in his or her account. The costs of administration for a system in which employees chose among a wide range of privately managed funds, as in the Feldstein proposal, would include activities such as record-keeping, marketing, collection and management of the money, and education of investors about their choices. The consensus among studies by reputable sources such as the Social Security Administration actuaries, the Employee Benefit Research Institute, and the National Academy of Social Insurance is that such costs could easily amount to 1 percent of assets per year. Because that 1 percent would be charged against a given year's contribution every year from when it was made until the worker retired, the net effect of charges over a forty-plus-year career would be to reduce accumulations by about 20 percent. Even the most efficient (and bare-bones) imaginable administrative structure, which would give employees less choice than in most proposals, would be equivalent to a front-load charge of between 5 and 11 percent for the average earner.[6]

There are also costs at the point of retirement. In order for benefits to be analogous to Social Security, especially in providing protection against the risk of outliving one's earnings, they would have to be converted into an inflation-adjusted annuity. At present, private annuity purchase is subject to significant adverse selection: the people who purchase annuities are those who most expect to live longer than the average person. Since they will be paying for a longer period of time than average, insurers offer lower monthly payouts than could be afforded for the average retiree. We might expect, then, that annuities in a mandatory system would be a better deal than in the current private market.[7] Yet there would still be administrative and overhead costs. One careful study showed that, excluding adverse selection and compared to a port-

folio fairly similar to Martin Feldstein's assumptions, annuitization in 1998 reduced the portfolio value for 65-year-olds by about 13 to 15 percent (Poterba
and Warshawsky 1998: table 2).[8]

The implication of these administrative-cost and annuity-purchase figures
is that even with minimal estimates of these overhead costs (say, 15 percent
combined), the return to investors will be significantly lower than the average
earnings on assets. If costs resembled those for current investments and annuities, even without adverse selection, benefits for plans with substantial
choice could be reduced by at least 30 percent.

Return on Equities

The second major issue related to rates of return involves what the earnings
on investments would be before subtracting overhead costs. Most analyses by
advocates of privatization, and even estimates by the Social Security Administration actuaries, have presumed that stocks will return the historic average
"equity premium," about 4.3 percentage points above the interest rate on Treasury securities, or 7 percent real growth per year. Yet there are very good reasons to believe that that is too optimistic.

Timing and Demographics

The simplest reason is timing. Stock market values in 1999 reached record
highs, as did the ratio of stock prices to corporate earnings, the "price/earn-
ings ratio" (P/E ratio) (Samuelson 1998). When P/E ratios are especially high,
the market has tended to be a poor investment over the following decade
(Wessel 1997a). Such a decline might be delayed if the large baby-boom population, while in the saving phase of their lives, were to continue to pour funds
into the markets, which would lead to higher prices. But eventually that would
have to end, and then both unfavorable demographics and high P/E ratios
could lead to a long period of stagnation.

The Baker Critique

More fundamentally, economist Dean Baker has argued, the "claim that
stock market returns will match past performance is inconsistent with the decline in economic growth predicted by Social Security's Trustees." If economic
growth in fact will be "more than 2 percentage points slower over the next sev-

enty-five years than it has been during the past seventy-five years," how could investment earnings be the same (1997a: 3)? As he points out, if the growth forecast were revised upward, there would be no inconsistency. But there would be no or hardly any shortfall in the existing program, either, as faster wage growth paid for the benefits.

The return on equities consists of dividends and price appreciation. The former depend directly on corporate earnings, and the latter has tended to be related to earnings (the P/E ratio). Total corporate earnings, in turn, ought to be related to the growth of the economy. If economic growth slows, then one would expect corporate earnings to slow, and therefore return on investment would be expected to slow.

Large fluctuations are possible over time. In the long run, however, the mismatch between the trustees' growth-and-return assumptions, Baker argues, means that either the P/E ratio would have to rise to absurd levels or the corporate-profit share of the economy would have to do so. For example, all other things being equal, the P/E ratio would be 34:1 in 2015 (not impossible compared to 28:1 in 1999), 79:1 in 2035 (hmm . . .) and 216:1 in 2055 (oops). Instead, he wrote, if P/E ratios were kept constant at their late-1996 levels, so that the assumed investment returns were financed by an increase in the capital share of national income, "by 2055, real wages would have to fall to just 18 percent of the levels projected in the Trustees' report, and by 2070 they would actually turn negative" (1997a: 19).

Dean Baker's arguments set off a furious debate among economists ("Taking Stock" 1999). The return on capital cannot depend solely on the level of economic growth. It should also depend on the supplies of capital and labor and thus rise if the ratio of capital to labor declines.[9] The trouble with this objection to Baker's analysis is that, although it may indeed help explain the run-up in P/E ratios from 1973 to 1999, neither part is supposed to be true to a significant extent in the future. Labor-force growth is supposed to decline—that is the demographic problem. And privatization advocates claim that savings will increase.

Economists who disagreed with Baker also argued that, though his scenario may make sense for a closed economy, much of the current earnings by major corporations are earned overseas and should not depend on domestic economic growth. Moreover, there is a whole lot of labor overseas relative to the amount of capital that could be invested there. Yet the assumed levels of investment earnings overseas, extrapolated far enough in the future, also become, in the words of economist Burt Malkiel at Princeton University, "a far-fetched prospect" (Passell 1997a).

More Modest Estimates

By 1999, therefore, the balance of analytical opinion strongly favored lower assumptions about future earnings on equities. The Employee Benefit Research Institute adopted much of the Baker logic, substituting a lower projected rate of return on investments, in its modeling of the effects of privatization plans (Olsen et al. 1998). The Committee on Investment of Employee Benefit Assets (1999), using work by four major investment firms, projected that future returns are likely to be about 1 percent to 3 percent higher than the return on Treasury securities, instead of 4.3 percent higher. The General Accounting Office (GAO 1998a) used both the SSA assumption and an alternative, with returns a percentage point lower, for its work.[10]

In September of 1999, Peter Diamond, an MIT professor who is one of the nation's most eminent experts on public finance and social insurance, issued the most thorough analysis of the rate-of-return issue. Considering a wide range of factors, including many not mentioned here, he concluded that the historic average might be achieved—*if real stock market prices were to first drop substantially over the next decade.* For instance, if dividends remained a constant share of GDP, and the real value of stocks fell by about a third over the next decade, then a 7 percent real return in subsequent years would be plausible.

To the average worker, Diamond's scenario might not be any more attractive than Baker's. It seems rather unlikely that privatization would be attractive to voters if they were told, "By the way, your investments will lose value for the next ten years." They might say, "OK, let's wait, and if that happens, we'll privatize ten years from now." And after a decade they might want to see market values climb for a while before privatizing.

The bottom line of Diamond's analysis, then, is that the standard projection of returns *beginning today,* which has been used in all advocacy for privatization and even some neutral analysis, is too high. Long-run projections should probably use an equity premium of 3 percent or slightly less—which would still be higher than in some current estimates. If, according to investors' usual practice, private portfolios were diversified into a mix of equities and safer investments (such as corporate bonds and Treasury bills), the return would be lower.

Privatization, Risk, and Inequality

Privatization changes a portion of Social Security from a defined-benefit (DB) plan to a defined-contribution (DC) plan. That has two fundamental effects: the DC contributions guarantee no specific level of benefits, and individuals who make the same contributions could receive different benefits. The former is a security issue, the latter an equity issue.[11]

Approaches that promise to maintain current benefits as a minimum provide less of a risk to adequacy. But they rely on subsidies from the federal budget that, at a minimum, do not represent the logic of a private account; and they still pose the equity problem.

Risk and Security

Economist Alicia Munnell, a former member of President Clinton's Council of Economic Advisers, argues that "uncertain outcomes may be perfectly appropriate for supplementary retirement benefits, but not for the basic guarantee." She quotes the late Herbert Stein, who chaired the council for President Nixon and who made this point most clearly:

> If there is no social interest in the income people have at retirement, there is no justification for the Social Security tax. If there is such an interest, there is a need for policies that will assure that the intended amount of income is always forthcoming. . . . Retirement income that depends on one's skills and luck as an investor is not consistent with the goals of a mandatory Social Security program. (Munnell 1998: 8)

The issue is not just what degree of individual risk is acceptable but what amount and form of variation in return is acceptable in a government program in which participation is required by law. The current Social Security system includes some differences in return that are quite intentional, in line with the concern for adequacy in social insurance. What of the differences that would follow from different investment results?

Risk and Equity

It seems fair to say that the performance of investments depends on both the skill and the luck of the investor. Some readers may feel that skill is so paramount that people whose investments did poorly would deserve their fates. Those who feel that luck is more important will be less comfortable with making pensions depend on it.

The most serious concern involves the time trend of market values. Two people might follow the same investment strategies but have different results because they invested at different times. As Gary Burtless writes, in the two years leading up

> to January 1975 the Standard and Poor's composite stock market index fell 50% after adjusting for changes in the U.S. price level. The value of stock certificates purchased in 1972 and earlier years lost half their value in 24 months. The average real rate of return on a worker's lifetime investments in the stock market plunged more than 3 percentage points (from 8.6% to 5.3%) in a very short period of time. For a worker who planned on retiring in 1975, the drop in stock market prices between 1973 and 1975 would have required a very drastic reduction in consumption plans if the worker's sole source of retirement income depended on stock market investments. (1998a: 5–6)

Burtless calculated replacement rates for workers retiring after forty-year careers if they had invested in stocks and then purchased annuities. Replacement rates vary not only because of differences in return on the investments while a person is working but also because the conversion of a balance into an annuity amount depends greatly on the interest rate at the time of conversion.[12] People who retire when interest rates are low will receive lower pensions for the same amount of savings as people who retire when rates are higher. Adjusting for both factors, Burtless found that replacement rates may be relatively stable for more than a decade (e.g., from the late 1950s through the late 1960s or during the 1980s) and then either plummet or rocket upward. He concluded that "Social Security pensions have been far more predictable and have varied within a much narrower range" and that "traditional Social Security provides a much more solid basis for retirement planning and a much more reliable foundation for a *publicly mandated* basic pension (7; his emphasis).

The problem here is not just the variation but also the lack of any principle to justify it. Why should people who were born in 1910 (people who would have been on the wrong side of the 1973–75 stock-market slump) have systematically lower pensions than people born in 1908?[13]

Effects on Redistribution

Privatization also is highly likely to reduce the redistribution that Social Security presently provides. Private accounts should give higher returns to people who invest more, for two reasons. Flat management fees, which are common, take a larger proportion of smaller savings. People with less to invest tend, because of concern about maintaining a minimum income, to choose less risky portfolios, which have lower returns, than do people with more to invest.[14]

Redistribution by Family Type

Private accounts also would not give higher returns on the same contribution to individuals with larger households to support, as Social Security now does. Nor would they favor one-earner households. Favoring such households makes child-rearing easier and is one reason why "family-values" advocates are leery of privatization. As Gary L. Bauer writes, "no matter what the market does, why do we think the nation will be better off by forcing workers to put their money into stock rather than, say, spending it on rearing children?" (1997). The ways that Social Security favors single-earner families may seem unfair to some dual earners, who might get a higher return from the investment of one spouse's earnings.[15] Nevertheless, people who favor the effects of the current rules should be skeptical of privatization.

Privatization and Disability Benefits

Private-account proposals also have lowered disability benefits. The current formula for disability insurance is based on the defined retirement benefits. If the latter are cut, the defined disability benefit will fall; but the disabled, who will be younger and will have accumulated savings for much less time, are much less likely to have accrued large enough private accounts to make up for the cut in the standard benefit.[16] Disability benefit cuts could be prevented by using a portion of private-account contributions to purchase supplementary disability insurance. But that would reduce the "rate of return" at retirement, which may be why it has not been proposed.

Racial Inequalities

Privatization advocates from the Heritage Foundation have argued that private accounts would actually be better than the current system for minorities (Beach and Davis 1998a,b,c). They do make some important points. No estimation method is perfect, and the distributional calculations used by the Social Security actuaries do have weaknesses.[17] In addition, because whites on average live longer than blacks, they collect benefits, on average, for a longer time. Hence, "for an African-American worker, [the retirement portion of] Social Security offers a worse deal than it does for a white worker with an identical income and family structure" (Beach and Davis 1998c: 13). But, sad to say, African American and white workers do not on average have the same incomes and family structures.

The methods used in the Heritage Foundation analysis misrepresent the effect of different life expectancies on both retirement contributions and benefits.[18] They exclude survivors' benefits in a way that excludes much of the advantage of Social Security to black families "who need it before retirement age precisely because blacks do not live as long" (Fierst 1998).[19] African Americans are disproportionately likely to be Disability Insurance beneficiaries, being 19 percent of the total, and the study excluded DI.[20]

On balance, the available evidence suggests that rates of return in the old-age portion of OASDI alone might have been slightly better for whites than for blacks but that the program as a whole has favored the latter (Kijazaki 1998; Panis and Lilliard 1996).

Political Risks to Redistribution and Guaranteed Benefits

In one way or another, most privatization plans attempt to address distributional concerns by making the remaining defined-benefit program more redistributive, in order to compensate for the effects of the defined-contribution plan.

For example, the Personal Security Account (PSA) plan proposed by five members of the 1994–96 Advisory Council would have turned traditional Social Security into a system that paid "a flat retirement benefit for full-career workers which is scaled to years of work and financed on a pay-as-you-go basis. This benefit would be financed (together with disability and survivor benefits) by 7.4 percent of the current 12.4 percent social security payroll tax" (Weaver 1998: 12). In other words, there would be no relation between taxes paid and benefits received; if one worker contributed four or five times as much as another, he would get no higher benefit.

One has to be skeptical of the survival prospects of such an arrangement. As Jonathan Chait writes,

> If you add on individual accounts, then each American would have two things: first, a regular Social Security account, parts of which are being siphoned off for current retirees, the disabled, and low earners; and second, an individual account, the benefits of which accrue solely to you. Can there be any doubt as to what would happen next? People would look at their two accounts—one of which was being sucked away to help complete strangers, the other of which was nicely compounding into a nest egg—and demand that Congress reduce the public account and increase the private one. (1999a)

The remaining traditional Social Security would look like a terrible deal for higher-income persons (Aaron and Reischauer 1998a: 158). For example, under the PSA plan, maximum earners would receive 80 percent of their retirement benefits from their 5.0 percent of payroll contributions to their personal accounts and only 20 percent of their retirement benefits from the 7.4 percent they paid for traditional OASDI (Advisory Council on Social Security 1997a: 47).

Privatizers claim that their reform is necessary because people are not getting a good enough return on their money when they give it to the government for Social Security. So they would be more satisfied, and Social Security would be protected from "political risk," if voters "owned" their own accounts. But if that is the reason to privatize partially, why on earth would voters maintain a remaining Social Security program that was a much, much worse deal?

Very similar political concerns would apply to the plans that explicitly guarantee to maintain existing benefits. They say, essentially, that individuals would own personal accounts. These accounts would accrue earnings, at a rate of return higher than that on contributions to the remaining traditional Social Security (if they did not, privatization would have failed totally). But then

much of the income from the private accounts would be denied to their owners, taken back in order to offset Social Security benefits.

How would this look to beneficiaries? Robert Greenstein worries that they
are likely to perceive that they would be receiving "only a modest Social Security benefit, which would equal the difference between the annuity payment
from their individual account and the Social Security benefit level to which
they are entitled" (1999: 2). This benefit, relative to contributions, would look
like a very bad deal, causing the same political troubles as in the PSA plan.
Moreover, the basic system of reducing earnings from the private accounts in
order to offset Social Security benefits would be very hard to sustain. In the
Feldstein plan this would look like a 75 percent tax on earnings, and in the
Archer-Shaw plan, for most retirees, it would be a 100 percent tax. "After being told the individual accounts are their property," Greenstein notes, "American workers would see their accounts entirely taxed away when they retired"
(3). This, too, does not look like a politically sustainable policy.

Effects on the Federal Budget and the Economy

That brings us to the next issue, the effect of privatization on the federal budget and the economy. Except for the Gramlich plan, all of the privatization
proposals involve reducing federal revenues in the short run. The Feldstein
and Moynihan-Kerrey plans, for instance, would have reduced revenues by 2
percent of payroll, roughly 0.8 percent of GDP (though in different ways).

Normal logic suggests that such plans should reduce national savings. Thus,
in estimating the effect of the Feldstein plan for Personal Retirement Accounts
(PRAs), the CBO reported that

> government saving would decline because the tax credit would reduce the sur-
> plus and, in later years, increase the deficit. Although private saving would rise,
> it would not rise enough to completely offset the loss in revenue. The proposed
> tax credit would have to be deposited in a retirement account, but even so, it
> is unlikely that private saving would go up by the full amount of the credit.
> Other saving most likely would fall because PRAs would increase workers' re-
> sources and would reduce their need to save in other forms for their retirement.
> (1998c)

Feldstein and Samwick asserted, instead, that all the investments in the PRAs would represent extra national savings. Better yet, the extra growth caused by the extra savings would increase corporate earnings so much that, by 2030, higher corporate tax collections would finance the tax credits (Samwick 1998).

Arguments That Privatization Would Increase Savings
"It Would Just Get Spent Anyway"

How could they make this assertion? By claiming that if their plan did not pass, politicians would find some other way to eliminate the portion of projected budget surpluses that was represented by the contributions to PRAs. If the money was not going to be there anyway, the PRA plan could not worsen the budget situation (Samwick 1998: 3). This is the right-wing version of the argument the Clinton administration made for its proposal to double-count Social Security surpluses—and no more defensible. As chapter 3 explained, there is reason to seek procedures to prevent future Social Security surpluses from distorting other budget decisions. But it is at best perverse for advocates of privatization to turn the fear that that might happen into a self-fulfilling prophecy.

"It Will Be Paid For, Somehow"

Feldstein made the further assumption that after the surpluses ended but before economic growth burgeoned enough to pay for the tax credits, those credits would be financed by other tax increases or spending cuts. As CBO commented, "there is no basis for making that assumption" (1998c).[21] Sponsors of the Archer-Shaw plan also had a period of several decades during which subsidies for individual accounts would exceed the amount of the Social Security surplus, with no evident way to pay the costs (Greenstein 1999: 1–2).

Contradict Yourself or Ignore the Obvious

At their worst, advocates of privatization have stretched logic to a breaking point. Professor Feldstein assumed that private accounts that promised higher retirement benefits would not reduce other personal savings. This is an especially interesting position for him to take, since he has argued strenuously for decades that one of the negative effects of Social Security is that people reduce their personal saving in response to their expectation of Social Security payments. As Robert Greenstein and his colleagues comment, "if Feldstein is correct on this score, then the plan he has proposed would discourage other saving to a greater degree than the current Social Security system since his plan promises workers they will receive more retirement income than the current system provides" (1998: note 16).[22] Feldstein even counted the administrative costs of private accounts as extra saving (CBO 1998c).

Borrow Now, Save Later

To their credit, the sponsors of the PSA plan did not make such unreasonable arguments. They explained that some Social Security shortfall was already built into the estimates; we could borrow now or borrow later; and that they were suggesting borrowing earlier in order to create a system that would require much less borrowing later.

Yet there is also something a bit too easy about financing the transition to private accounts with extra federal borrowing (or, under the new budget environment, less federal saving). "In essence," Gary Burtless and Barry Bosworth explain, in the PSA sponsors' projections,

> workers' well-being has improved because they can borrow (through the U.S. government) at a 2.3 percent interest rate and earn returns that exceed 5 percent. If this magic works when 5 percentage points of the payroll tax is diverted into individual accounts, it is natural to ask why the diversion should be limited to 5 percent. Why not divert the entire 12.4 percent tax into individual accounts? (1997: 11–12)

The question is rhetorical, but the point is not: profits from using federal borrowing to finance private accounts depend on the attractiveness of federal debt as a risk-free investment, which is a strange basis for privatization.

The Likely Balance of Effects

The PSA advocates do have a point. Because they would eventually reduce government obligations, most privatization plans would eventually improve the government's savings position and thus (presumably) the nation's. In addition to the eventual effects of lower government spending, analysts have argued that, since all profits on savings would be within accounts that (supposedly) could not be touched until retirement, the *earnings* on the investments would be entirely saved (unlike other earnings) and would raise net national savings.[23]

But "eventually" in this case is a very, very long time away. In plausible estimates, savings become positive at least thirty and sometimes many more years in the future.[24] Any positive economic effects, then, would be a few decades later. In the meantime the government would have less money to pay for other expenses, such as Medicare. So this kind of financing approach does not fit any serious concern with entitlements as a whole.

The bottom line is that there are small possible economic and budgetary advantages from privatization, but unless privatization is financed with extra money (as in the Gramlich plan), these are uncertain, could be expected to occur only quite far in the future, and are likely to include more negative budgetary effects for the first three decades.

Implementation Issues

Privatization also poses major administrative challenges. A report by the Employee Benefit Research Institute put the task in perspective: "Adding individual accounts to Social Security could be the largest undertaking in the history of the U.S. financial market, and no system to date has the capacity to administer such a program" (Olsen and Salisbury 1998: 1–2).

The basic difficulty is how to keep track of both contributions and who has a claim to the proceeds of the accounts. Currently, most employers send both payroll taxes and income tax withholding as *lump-sum payments* on a semiweekly or monthly schedule to Federal Reserve Banks or other authorized institutions. They do not provide a breakdown of these sums into credits for individual employees until the end of the calendar year. So, as the same study notes, "it can take a year or more for some payroll taxes paid on behalf of an individual employee to be identifiable as such" and "up to 16–22 months before the aggregate taxes they have sent over the year can be separated into payroll taxes and federal income taxes" (Olsen and Salisbury 1998: 13–14). Since figures do not need to be correct until a person retires, the design works for the current system. But deposits into private accounts would need to be credited much more quickly and precisely, in order to invest the right amounts of money and earn for as long as possible.

Perhaps individuals could be credited with estimated payments. But then what would be done about the differences between the estimations and reality? How would money be taken back or added into accounts, on what assumptions about returns? If an employer paid too little, that would deprive workers of the earnings on the missing payments. Who should pay for the difference? The employer? The government?

Alternatively, individual payments could be recorded much as they are in current 401(k) plans. Unfortunately, "millions of employers . . . do not offer [401(k)] plans and therefore do not have the administrative infrastructure in place" to do the same for Social Security individual accounts. Moreover, this service would be especially burdensome for small employers (Olsen and Salisbury 1998: 16). Dallas Salisbury, the president of the Employee Benefit Research Institute (EBRI), therefore "does not think that an individual account system for over 140 million workers, with less than an 18 to 24 month lag in account recording, is feasible at acceptable administrative cost in the absence of new technological developments, including moving 5.5 million small employers from paper filing to automated filing" (NASI 1998: question 3 n. 1).

Individual accounts also raise difficult consumer-protection issues. Arthur Levitt, chairman of the Securities and Exchange Commission, argued that "if we are to have self-directed individual accounts, we must be ready to undertake an unprecedented level of broad-scale policing of the equity markets. Without such policies, fraud and sales practice abuses may be perpetrated against an army of novice investors. And many of those novice investors are our society's most vulnerable citizens" (1998; see also Stevenson 1998). These risks, he explained, have been demonstrated clearly by the "mis-selling" controversy in the United Kingdom's version of pension privatization, in which "abusive sales practices, coupled with inadequate regulation, led to billions of dollars in losses for investors" (Levitt 1998).[25]

Some of these risks could be greatly reduced if the government limited investments to a few broadly indexed options. Yet that is not what most privatization advocates have proposed. In short, privatization poses huge challenges in the matters of collecting and accounting for the money and protecting investors. At best this will be expensive; at worst it might be impossible; most likely, it would involve some painful mistakes before the problems were solved.

Projections of Outcomes from Privatization

Given the variety of plans and their provisions and the many uncertainties about issues such as rate of return to equities and costs of administration, it would be impossible to predict the effects of privatization per se with any credibility. Different plans have different trade-offs: for example, privatization will seem to yield better returns to individuals to the extent that it imposes greater costs on the budget. Nevertheless, there have been some careful efforts to analyze effects, and they do reveal some patterns that can be generalized to the basic choice.

In order to evaluate privatization plans, we need some assumption about what would otherwise be done about the projected shortfalls. The standard approach is to assume that taxes would be raised as needed. I follow that approach here because that is how other people have done the calculations, because it would be the purest form of continuing current policy, and because it is basically how shortfalls have been addressed in the past.

Analyses tend to focus on two different figures, the level of benefits and the rate of return. These can have different profiles, mainly because raising taxes would not reduce benefits but would lower rates of return; most privatization plans emphasize stabilizing contributions and thereby at best improve benefits much less than they improve rates of return. So privatization, to the extent that it offers any advantage, would offer less of one in terms of adequacy than in terms of rates of return.

We need to remember that stated rates of return constitute an incomplete standard for a social insurance program. From a social standpoint, because of the insurance and redistributive aspects of Social Security, the "moneysworth" ratios understate its value; even for an individual, the insurance aspects make it worth more than the figures project. We focus on rates of return here because they are the main subject of advocacy for private accounts.

The analysis here is based largely on work by the 1994–96 Advisory Council on Social Security, which compared both the Gramlich and the PSA plans to a range of alternatives,[26] and by the Employee Benefit Research Institute, comparing both some generic approaches and some of the actual plans to more traditional reforms (Olsen et al. 1998; Copeland, VanDerHei, and Salisbury 1999). These analyses themselves, however, include some very different assumptions.[27]

Patterns
Privatization Should Raise Returns—Eventually

In both analyses the versions of privatization that are designed to have the highest returns do, indeed, provide significantly higher returns, for some cohorts, than those cohorts would receive if Social Security were financed by pay-as-you-go tax increases. In the EBRI best case, a generic privatization plan would raise the "payback ratio" for single individuals born in 2026 by 50 percent for men and 30 percent for women, compared to raising taxes only (Olsen et al. 1998: 13). In the Advisory Council analysis, the "moneysworth ratio" for the PSA plan would be 18 percent higher for "composite workers" born in 1973 and 35 percent higher for composite workers born in 1997 (1997a: 199).

In both cases, however, privatization is not so beneficial for older workers. As a worst case, in EBRI's generic scenario, workers born in 1976 would do significantly worse under privatization than with a "raise taxes only" approach. In the generic privatization scenario, those workers pay the entire cost of the transition, and that overwhelms the higher returns on private investment.[28]

Borrowing to Finance the Transition Makes Privatization Look Better

The SSA's estimate of the PSA plan and EBRI's estimate of Moynihan-Kerrey also showed that financing the transition with extra borrowing does, indeed, make the rate of returns look better. Yet both plans would still be worse than raising taxes only for individuals born before sometime around 1960 (Advisory Council on Social Security 1997a: 210; Copeland, VanDerHei, and Salisbury 1999: 9).[29]

More Privatization Yields Higher Returns on Average

A third point is most obvious from the Advisory Council figures for returns on the PSA plan as opposed to the more modest privatization in the Gramlich plan. As Gramlich himself (1996: 65) points out, to the extent that the point of privatization is to gain a higher return on private securities than on government bonds, one gains more from doing more. This is just a matter of mathematics.

So why do not all proposals include at least 5 percent of payroll for private accounts—or even more? There are two basic problems: privatization on a larger scale means both higher transition costs and subjecting a bigger portion of retirement income to the various risks associated with the market.

Extrapolating to Policy Choices

The available data do not tell us what the results would be if a privatization plan did not rely on as large subsidies from reducing projected budget surpluses as in the PSA and similar approaches but also was not financed in as draconian a manner as EBRI's generic scenario. Assuming that the outcome would be somewhere between these two sets of estimates, however, it seems likely that privatization would be inferior to pay-as-you-go finance for all but the youngest current workers; it would provide higher returns, on average, for those workers and people born later. In other words, the break-even point would be somewhere around the individuals born in 1976. If we believe that greater risk would lower the value of returns, the break-even point would be a bit later.

Which is more important? Although the conventional wisdom is that "our grandchildren are more important," we should remember that under the current estimates, the rates of return for many of the baby boomers are worse than for younger workers, and the further one projects into the future, the higher individual and family real incomes are expected to be. So there is reason to doubt that reforms should favor future cohorts over nearly all current workers.

The Diversification Alternative

There is one more reason for skepticism about privatization: much of its merits might be achieved by an alternative. That alternative would be to invest some portion of the Social Security trust funds in equities on behalf of the Social Security program itself. Then the government would have more money with which to pay for benefits. The money invested in equities, having been spent, would not be available for tax cuts or increases in other spending and so could not be "wasted." Government investment, or "trust-fund diversification" is therefore favored by many, though not all, critics of privatization.[30]

The Advantages of Government Investment in Equities

Advocates of trust-fund diversification agree with privatizers that there should be a higher return on stocks than the growth of wages and that measures that would raise the rate of return are more attractive than benefit cuts or tax increases that would lower it (Ball 1998: 15).

Yet diversification advocates see major advantages over privatization. Having the government invest in the markets in order to increase accumulations in the OASDI trust funds would not expose individuals to market risks. Benefits would still be defined in advance, but they would be financed by a mix of taxing, borrowing, and earnings, rather than just taxing and borrowing. Government revenues eventually would be higher, because higher debt would be more than offset by the earnings on the private investments. The return on investments should be higher than for privatization because the vast majority of the costs of administration of accounts and annuitization of benefits would be eliminated. Moreover, the privately invested portion of the trust funds could be invested entirely in equities and thereby earn a higher return before administrative charges than most people could risk individually. The reason is that within any plausible government investment design, the earnings from investments would ultimately represent only a small part of the total financing of benefits. The rest of the "portfolio" on which benefits would be based would be the government's taxing power—the safest portfolio imaginable.

If the return on investment by the government would be higher and safer than the returns on private accounts and would also give the government extra revenues compared to the current policy of using Social Security surpluses to reduce national debt, why would anyone object?

Objections to Government Investment

The basic objection is that government ownership of shares in corporations sounds too much like socialism. Aside from worrying that this would make the government too powerful, critics also claim that the government would invest inefficiently, lowering the return on investments (Mitchell 1998; Tanner 1998).

Lower Return?

Federal Reserve Board chairman Alan Greenspan, for example, has expressed his fear "that we would use those assets in a way that would create a lower rate of return for Social Security recipients . . . it would create suboptimal use of capital and a lower standard of living" (Walsh 1999: A1, A12). That view is echoed by a chorus of critics who cite examples of "distorted" investing by other public funds. For example, public pension funds have been pressured not to invest in tobacco companies or not to invest in companies that did not follow the "Sullivan Principles" for doing business in South Africa. In some cases, state or local pension funds have been invested in local businesses, such as a Colt firearms factory in Connecticut or a savings-and-loan in Kansas (Baldauf 1999).

But there are big flaws in this criticism. Proposals for private investment of Social Security moneys assume a much different structure and investment pattern than has been used for state and local funds. All proposals presume that the funds will be invested in broad stock market indices. That leaves no funds for targeted investments in local companies. It is certainly possible that Congress could require some deviations from an index: as political scientist R. Douglas Arnold puts it, the Wilshire 7000 index minus three tobacco companies ("Taking Stock" 1999: 8). But however desirable or undesirable such policies might be for other reasons, excluding a small portion (here, less than 1%) of a large index could have no more than minuscule effects on rates of return. Any plausible reduction in return from "social investment" decisions under the proposed frameworks could not compare to the overhead savings of government compared to individual investment.

Moreover, it is possible to design a limited investment scheme (as I suggest in chapters 11 and 12) in which the amount of new investment in the trust funds each year is small compared to the total economy. In 2008, for example, I suggest investment of $50 billion out of a total projected GDP, according to the Congressional Budget Office in 1999, of $13 trillion. Even "suboptimal use" of this capital is unlikely to make a significant difference to the economy, especially because most of it would be invested in index funds.

In fact, state and local pension plans' investments in equities already are sub-stantial, and they are more subject to concerns about distortion than any SSA investment plan based on index funds could be. Yet, as Alicia Munnell and Pier-lugi Baldizzi write, "although one can criticize some aspects of state and local government investment activity, they have hardly caused major disruptions of the equity market or distorted corporate decision-making" (1998: 6).

The purely economic arguments about the "inefficiency" of the govern-ment investing in the stock markets therefore are not a substantial objection. That brings us back to the political stakes.

Excessive Government Power

Worries about the political effects of the government investing funds in the stock market (or other private property) influenced the early decisions about whether Social Security should be pay-as-you-go or funded. Indeed, a decade ago Aaron Wildavsky and I wrote that Social Security could not be entirely funded in advance because it would have to own too large a part of the U.S. economy. "Who would control the fund?" we asked, "Or, whom would the fund control?" (1991: 316; see also Myers 1998).

But there is a huge difference in scale between what we were discussing then and current proposals. Funding a small fraction of total benefits is a lot differ-ent from funding the whole program. Moreover, we wrote at a time when much less thought had been put into how to design government investment, and there was less experience on which to base arguments that safeguards against political distortion of decisions should be adequate.

Henry J. Aaron and Robert D. Reischauer (1998a: 110–14) have proposed a design based on the current Thrift Savings Plan for federal employees. Other discussions make similar suggestions (NASI 1998; GAO 1998a; American Academy of Actuaries 1998b). They begin by placing management of the So-cial Security reserves in a "Social Security Reserve Board" (SSRB) appointed in the same manner as the Federal Reserve. That is, members would have stag-gered fourteen-year terms, so any given Congress and president would have little direct influence on the board majority. As Aaron and Reischauer note, the Federal Reserve "has sustained its political independence for eight de-cades" (1998a: 111) even though managing the nation's money supply is at least as politically charged as investing some Social Security funds.

The SSRB would be required to select fund managers on the basis of competitive bids, and fund managers would be required to invest only in broad market indices. These indices would have to match services that the managers were offering to individual investors, so the trust fund investments would be "merged with funds managed on behalf of private account holders." As the funds grew, the number of managers with which the SSRB contracted could also be expanded, so that voting rights for shares would be spread among multiple managers.

Thus, there would be three levels of insulation of fund management from control by elected officials. The method of appointment of SSRB members would insulate most members from particular politicians. The limitation of investments to passively managed funds would insulate fund managers from the SSRB. Diffusing voting rights among multiple managers and pooling the trust-fund assets with other assets (assets that are subject to the restraints of normal fiduciary rules) would further inhibit the use of voting rights to influence corporate policy in directions desired by some factions within the government.[31]

Could Congress still interfere, for example by changing the rules? Of course it could. The real question, though, is whether the safeguards would be strong enough to prevent more than marginal violations. With rules for investment set in law, any deviations would require passing new laws. In that process, however, as Aaron points out,

> Congress already holds the cards. It enacts tax policy, regulatory policy. It can put in place prohibition mandates. It can raise or lower tariffs. It has the ability to grant or withhold credit guarantees, or credit itself, for export. If Congress wants to interfere or influence private decision-making by American businesses, it has instruments that are part of its normal portfolio and that would arouse no unusual sense that rules were being flouted." ("Taking Stock" 1999: 4)

Why should members of Congress who want to attack, say, tobacco companies do it through trust-fund investment policy, which would be seen as messing around with Social Security benefits as part of another agenda, rather than through some other method? Manipulating the trust funds looks like a way of buying extra enemies, namely the people who do not care about tobacco but do worry about paying Social Security benefits.

In addition, as Reischauer argues, critics of trust-fund diversification discuss the issue "as if we had only one branch of government, and that was the legislative branch, and it was peopled by totally undisciplined folks who are listening to their polls and saying, somebody in my neighborhood doesn't want us to invest in this company because they degrade the environment, so let's write that one out, and so on" ("Taking Stock" 1999: 222). This would be a cartoon version of government. What you learned in high school is more accurate: there is a whole system of checks and balances, with a president and courts and a Congress that is itself divided and does not pass legislation very easily. Under these conditions, the odds that direct interference in trust-fund investment decisions could occur without strong public support seem quite low. If such strong public support did exist, Congress and the president could attack whatever industry they did not like in other ways.

The only thing Social Security investment accounts might add to government's ability to interfere with businesses is the force of guilt. Perhaps voters could feel especially bad about benefiting from the profits of a highly unpopular industry and would want to salve their consciences by disinvesting, even if they did not want to attack the industry in other ways. In order for this to make a real difference to the economy or returns on trust-fund investment, however, we would need a very large industry, with high returns compared to the average (so that divesting would lower returns), that would be affected because nobody else would invest when the government sold its shares (in spite of the high returns) and that the public hated enough to divest but not enough to punish in other ways. This cannot happen enough to justify forgoing the advantages of trust-fund diversification.

Other Objections

Coming from a different perspective, some observers fear that trust-fund diversification would make the government more dependent on "the markets" (NASI 1998). If Social Security benefits depended substantially on the returns on equity investment, the government might be especially loath to take steps that would spook investors; therefore, it might favor investor interests over labor.

So what else is new? For at least the past twenty years, political discourse and action have favored "the markets" over labor. The era of panic over budget deficits began, in 1980, with a Democratic president worried about the bond market; and President Clinton's own attack on the deficit was motivated by the same concerns (White and Wildavsky 1991; Woodward 1994). At least, with trust-fund investment, the object of that policy would be to limit payroll taxes and preserve benefits and thus would be in the interest of working people. To put this another way, if the economy is expected to develop in a way that favors capital over labor, then it makes sense to give labor a small piece of the capital pie. Privatization is promoted as a way to do that, but trust-fund diversification would do so more surely and more safely.

A related concern involves how government's stake in the markets could affect other policies. "What a spectacle it would be," one reporter commented, "if the Social Security trust fund had a large position in the Microsoft Corporation as the Justice department was pursuing a vigorous antitrust case against it" (Morgensen 1999: A19). Not really. After all, if invested in index funds, the Social Security trust funds will have positions in Microsoft's competitors as well as in Microsoft, so the funds' financial interests would not be so clear.

A final concern has to do with how the government would respond to any dramatic drop in stock market values. As the General Accounting Office reported, "the more the trust fund is counting on stock sales to pay promised benefits, the greater its vulnerability in the event of a general market downturn" (1998a: 35). Given a financial stake, "would the government have an ever greater incentive to control market fluctuations, if not the market itself?" (Levitt 1998).

Well, yes. This, and the other concerns, are reasons to limit the size of the trust fund's investments, so that earnings on those investments represent only a relatively minor portion of Social Security's financing. But they could represent as much as 1 percent of GDP, thus about a sixth of the program's costs in the year 2030, and leave the government in a position where the extra borrowing that might be required by a decline in those earnings would have only minimal effects on the economy.[32]

On balance, a modest amount of trust-fund diversification could offer some of the advantages of privatization with none of the disadvantages; and the political risks of diversification could be managed with sensible governance structures and limits on the size of the investments.

Risks, Opportunities, and the Purpose of Social Security

The best available evidence and analysis suggest that, compared to simply raising taxes to pay eventual benefits, privatization plans should provide a better return on some individuals' contributions to Social Security. It appears that this would be most true for workers born after around 1976 and mostly false for workers born earlier. But the precise date depends on specific plans and estimating assumptions.

It is not clear that policy should favor the younger workers over the older ones. Baby boomers, in the standard estimates, already are getting lower "returns" from Social Security than will workers born in the last two decades of this century. We have also seen that under privatization benefits would be much less certain, in ways that are unlikely to seem fair. Partial privatization would add a new form of inequality to pensions: inequality between people who happen to retire at only slightly different times but on different sides of market swings.

Advocates of privatization claim that their plans would maintain Social Security's protections for the individuals whom it currently is designed to especially help: those with low working incomes, women who do not have full careers in the labor market, dependent survivors, and disabled persons. Their methods to do so, however, put the remaining defined-benefits portion of the program at great political risk by making it seem like a really bad deal to many voters.

Finally, partial privatization poses significant new administrative challenges, which may both be difficult to solve and raise doubts about the integrity of the system.

This does not mean private saving is a bad idea. Of course it is a good idea. All but the poorest citizens should be making some private provision for their retirement, through private pension plans or individual savings. But privatization would make such accounts a much larger portion of people's pensions, and security, than they are today. That does not seem wise.

As Lawrence H. Thompson argues, the ideal pension system would "provide a stable, predictable, and adequate source of retirement income to each participant" (1998b: 1). We might add that stability is especially important for a guaranteed minimum.

The choice between public and privatized pensions cannot be separated from another issue, the difference between defined-benefit plans (like Social Security) and defined-contribution plans (in which return depends solely on earnings on the contributions). As Thompson argues, both government-sponsored defined-benefit pensions and either privately or publicly sponsored defined-contribution pensions have risks. Voters can choose to cut the benefits in a plan like Social Security, and returns in the market can vary. Legislative stalemate might block necessary adjustments (such as, for example, tax increases to pay reasonable benefit levels) in a defined-benefit plan. Yet a government-sponsored defined-contribution pension might be reduced even by measures that are sought by the beneficiaries, such as exceptions that allow withdrawals to pay for buying a house, education, or other popular goals—as has, in fact, occurred with American voluntary defined-contribution plans, such as IRAs.

The logical response to such a situation is to have a mix of DB and DC pensions. In nations such as Germany and France that have relied almost exclusively on the DB approach, Thompson argues, that could justify a shift toward defined contributions. But "the United States already has a mixed public/private and defined-benefit/defined-contribution system" (1998b: 5). In fact, as we saw in chapter 7, our defined benefits through Social Security are already pretty low.

Privatization, by moving America's total pension package toward a nearly exclusively defined-contribution approach, would increase uncertainty by unbalancing the risks. The choice remains one of individual values. But we have seen in earlier chapters that no "crisis" requires radical reform. In this chapter we have seen that partial privatization is likely to be a worse deal, even in investment terms, for a large majority of people in the workforce today. It clearly will provide less protection against a wide variety of risks. My personal opinion is that the point of a mandatory pension is to guarantee a social minimum. Both the economic and the political threats to that guarantee, from partial privatization of what is already a relatively small defined-benefit program, are too great.

NINE

Medicare Vouchers: Not Ready for Prime Time

The most prominent current proposals for Medicare reform would transform Medicare from a system in which separate HI and SMI coverages guarantee a package of benefits for which enrollees pay only the SMI premium to a system in which enrollees would choose from a selection of combination plans and pay the difference between those plans' premiums and some government premium support. Such proposals were supported by the majority of the now defunct National Bipartisan Commission on the Future of Medicare and by a wide range of academics, including some of the most respected students of health care and social insurance (Aaron and Reischauer 1995; Wilensky and Newhouse 1999; Pear 1999; Goldstein 1999a; Vladeck 1999; Altman and Tyson 1999).

If vouchers to choose among combination plans were a good idea, one would expect experience with combination plans so far to make that clear. Yet chapter 4 established that experience with the Medicare Risk program was quite mixed. In this chapter I will show that the practical and theoretical evidence for assuming that vouchers would provide the basic Medicare benefit package more efficiently than traditional Medicare can do so is extremely weak.

The current Medicare program has holes, particularly in the benefits package, that combination plans might help fill. But it is not so inadequate, and voucher approaches have too many potential problems, to justify switching to a voucher system before most of those problems are solved.

Why Switch to Vouchers?

Some scholars argue that Medicare must move to vouchers so that seniors will enroll in managed-care plans like most workers have, on the grounds that it is politically unacceptable for seniors to have less restrictive insurance than their children (Aaron and Reischauer 1998b: 69). Yet, regardless of the merits, there is a powerful "backlash" against managed care already.[1] Perhaps the average voter's reaction to having Mom or Dad pushed into managed care more slowly than everyone else someday will be, "Hey, that's unfair, do it to them, too." But it might just as well be, "At least someone's system is still O.K." As I wrote this book there was nary a shred of evidence that workers thought that if something was wrong with their own health care, that should be inflicted on seniors as well.

If they did, they should never have supported Medicare in the first place. After all, Medicare, unlike workers' own insurance, is mandatory and guaranteed to all. People who earn less contribute less for the coverage. Sicker people do not pay more. Workers contribute yet do not immediately and directly benefit. All these provisions might seem just as "unfair" to workers as the fact that seniors are not forced into managed care, but nonetheless, Medicare has been extremely popular.

So the political argument in favor of vouchers is peculiarly unconvincing. The case for vouchers must be made on policy merits: the proposition that they would give better value for the government's, and the citizens', insurance dollar.

Cost-Control Performance and Methods

What, then, has been the cost-control experience of Medicare, compared to the rest of the American health-care system? And what is the prospect that vouchers would reduce costs?

Cost Control Experience and Projections

Medicare must be more expensive per person than other insurance, simply because elderly and disabled people have more medical problems than other citizens. So we need to compare the rate of increase in costs, not absolute levels. Differences in the benefits covered by the two systems might then bias the comparison of trends. For instance, hospice and home health benefits are a more significant factor in Medicare than in private insurance, so fast growth in those costs helped make Medicare look worse in the early 1990s (Levit et al. 1996). But when pharmaceutical benefit costs increase more quickly than others (as appears to be happening at present), that will make private insurance look worse. As of the end of 1998, therefore, the standard comparisons simply looked at the growth of costs per enrollee over time.

In 1998 the National Health Statistics Group of the Health Care Financing Administration's Office of the Actuary reported that

> Medicare and private health insurance benefits (personal health care expenditures) per enrollee actually have grown at comparable annual rates from 1969 through 1997 (10.4% and 11.4%, respectively). . . . However, two periods marked significant growth differences in spending between the two funding sources. The first period was 1985–1991, when average annual growth in private health insurance spending per enrollee exceeded the Medicare rate by 4.5 percentage points. The second was 1993–1996, when average annual growth in Medicare spending per enrollee exceeded that of private health insurance spending by 5.2 percentage points. However, in the past two years Medicare per enrollee growth has been trending down, while private health insurance per enrollee growth has trended up, narrowing the gap to two percentage points by 1997. (Levit et al. 1998b: 107)

Medicare's superior long-run performance does not fit a story about inherent private-sector superiority. So advocates of the efficiency of private insurance have to argue that something that occurred in the 1990s permanently altered the cost-control comparison in favor of private institutions.

That private-sector advantage in the mid-1990s developed in part because of much better cost-control performance in the private sector and in part because of peculiar political barriers to Medicare cost-control legislation. The major deficit-reducing package in this period, in 1993, included few Medicare savings because President Clinton was saving such reductions to help finance his initiative to guarantee health insurance for all Americans. The next round of attempted budget-deficit reductions, by congressional Republicans in 1995, was vetoed by President Clinton in part on the grounds that it would have cut and restructured Medicare too much. The deadlock was not broken until 1997 (Longrest 1998: 229–30).

Just as traditional Medicare controlled costs relatively poorly in the mid-1990s because of unusual circumstances, some of the private-sector successes were due to causes that should be regarded as temporary.

First, employers switched employees in large numbers from relatively "unmanaged" indemnity plans to versions of managed-care organizations that either regulated utilization more, paid less per service, or both. But switching to the less-expensive form of private insurance is a one-time saving that cannot be repeated.

Second, providers of all sorts, in virtually all circumstances, began accepting lower prices from purchasers. Data from Congress's independent commissions that analyze both Medicare hospital and physician payments shows the decline in prices paid by private insurers, compared to Medicare (PPRC 1996: 216; ProPAC 1997b: 22–25). Caregivers appear to have become extremely worried that in the future they could lose access to large numbers of (paying) patients and hence might be unable to stay in business. Publicity about "managed competition" and the Clinton health plan was one likely factor; publicity about Republican plans for Medicare was probably another. For years, providers were told that they would have to join managed-care networks to survive. So they did, at discounted fees.

But it is widely agreed by analysts of the current health-care market that employers since the mid-1990s have been responding to employees' demands for wider networks. Indeed, insurers have become very defensive, insisting that their goal is to provide wide networks.[2] In 1997 health-market analyst Jeff Goldsmith suggested that "when providers realize that the threat to exclude them from networks is less credible with each passing year, it may be difficult for health insurers to continue getting that level of panic-driven discounts" (CSHSC 1997: 4). And many observers of the health-care market argue that the discounting pressure has weakened (Weinstein 1999b; Zelman and Berenson 1998).

The most clearly temporary cause of slow premium growth was that insurance companies lost money on their medical lines. This tends to happen as part of the "underwriting cycle," in which premiums are higher than costs for a while, insurers then compete more and premiums fall below costs, insurers insist on higher prices (even at the expense of market share), and premiums rise above costs again. But 1998 was the fourth year of a down cycle, and that had to end.

As the unusual circumstances that spawned it have disappeared, so has the private-sector advantage in cost control. Total Medicare spending did not grow at all between 1997 and 1999, which means that costs per enrollee declined (Board of Trustees 2000c: 40, 42). Both CBO and HCFA projections in 1999 included quite slow growth through 2002, and the HCFA figures extend that trend for the next thirty years. The reasons for this change remain unclear. Perhaps the cost-saving measures in the Balanced Budget Act of 1997, described below, worked even better than was anticipated in the early estimates. It is likely that highly publicized investigations or prosecutions of health-care providers for questionable Medicare billings, particularly the federal government's onslaught against the giant Columbia/HCA hospital chain, had a "sentinel effect." That is, hospitals especially were scared into billing more conservatively (CBO 1999: 72; Board of Trustees 2000c: 10–11; Kleinke 1998; "Feds Triple Health Fraud Cases" 1999).

Meanwhile, costs for private-sector insurance began to rise again. Such increases had been projected, a bit too pessimistically, before (CSHSC 1997; Ginsburg and Pickreign 1997; Ginsburg and Gabel 1998). Nevertheless, the balance of evidence and analysis suggested somewhat faster premium growth in the future. At the beginning of 1999, a series of surveys and commentary indicated that the premium growth in 1999 could be about 3 percentage points faster than in 1998.[3] Premiums in the California Public Employees Retirement System (CalPERS) rose by 7.3 percent in 1999; premiums in the Federal Employee Health Benefit Program (FEHBP) rose by 10.2 percent (Merlis 1999: 5, 11). CalPERS and FEHBP are two of the systems most frequently cited by advocates of the superior cost control possible from having competing plans.

Clearly Medicare's cost-control performance was better than that of private insurers in 1998 and 1999, and it is very likely to be better in 2000. What about later years? In 1998 the Health Expenditures Projection Team of HCFA estimated that Medicare would maintain an advantage into the next decade (Smith et al. 1998). They may have been too pessimistic about private-sector trends. But even Paul Ginsburg (1999), one of the most cogent critics of the HCFA study, argued that the most plausible scenario for the private sector was the one the Congressional Budget Office projected in January 1998. That

CBO analysis projected premium growth of about 1 percent over GDP growth, still slightly higher than the 1999 Medicare forecasts of trends from 1997 to 2002. Actual private-sector experience at this writing was not so good. We have already seen in chapter 6 that Medicare should be able to do that well without switching to a voucher system.

The data, therefore, do not fit the common claim that a system of competing private plans could be expected to control costs better than Medicare's other methods. Would a "reformed" market do better than the ones experienced so far? There can be no empirical refutation of an argument that some nonexistent private arrangement would do better, but there also can be no empirical support for the argument. "Belief in the private sector's ability to hold down costs of care," as Marilyn Moon notes, is "a strongly held philosophical viewpoint," even if "not backed up with facts" (1999: 10).

Different Systems, Different Methods

Specific individuals or interest groups might still prefer the cost-control methods that are likely to be used by managed-care plans, compared to cost controls in traditional Medicare, even if the resulting totals were the same. Analysts associated with right-wing think tanks argue that the methods used in traditional Medicare are "price controls" and therefore inherently inefficient (Butler 1998).[4] Even some nonconservatives assert that managed care would make medical care more efficient than Medicare's traditional methods (Aaron and Reischauer 1998b).

The assumed association between "regulation" and irrationality and of "managed care" with efficiency is based on a myth. The myth is that managed care is simply a way to deliver the right care to the right people in the right amounts at the right time and that it therefore derives its savings entirely from avoiding wasteful care (Ignagni 1998: 28). Yet much of the savings has been based on extracting discounts (lower prices) from providers in return for including them in a network, which involves no management-of-treatment decisions. The defining characteristic of one entire class of managed-care organizations, the Preferred Provider Organization (PPO), is that providers are "preferred" if they accept lower fees.

At the same time, some cost-control methods within traditional Medicare

are designed to improve efficiency. Under the Prospective Payment System (PPS) for hospital care, hospitals are paid a fixed fee (with adjustments for factors believed to be out of the hospital's control) for services according to the patient's primary diagnosis (Diagnosis Related Group [DRG]). Hospitals that provide care more efficiently will make more money, and that is why many Republicans were able to rationalize the creation of PPS as a "market-related" reform in the 1980s (Smith 1992; U.S. House, Committee on Ways and Means 1998: 1039–1110).

This book would be much longer if we discussed all the possible methods of health-care cost control, how well they might fit into traditional Medicare or managed-care plans, and their merits and demerits. Besides, I have done that elsewhere (White 1997, 1999d). But a few points seem clear enough.

First, however spending is reduced, that results in less income for medical providers. Academic Medical Centers, for instance, might be paid lower fees by Medicare or by private insurers and might lose patronage by private insurers. Whatever the cause, providers object to lower incomes. Second, the methods used will affect which providers lose how much. But no analysis shows that the distributional effects of spending reductions from competing plans are superior to the effects from Medicare's traditional methods of cost control.[5] Third, any system of multiple insurers must have higher administrative costs than traditional Medicare. Medicare's costs are so low because it does not have to market, or make profits, or borrow in the capital markets. Private insurers do all that and more. And in any voucher scheme, the government would have to pay out additional funds to prevent abuses of the competition, such as by regulating marketing to limit cherry-picking. In order for a voucher system to be more efficient in terms of medical care for the money, therefore, it has to do more with fewer dollars, not just the same dollars.

There is no systematic evidence, and little evidence of any sort, that the methods that private plans would use to control costs in a voucher system would be more effective or have fewer negative side effects than the methods available to traditional Medicare. As chapter 4 describes, Medicare's own experience with "Risk Plans" through 1997 was unfavorable. The Balanced Budget Act of 1997 expanded private plans within Medicare, while adding provisions intended to correct some of the problems experienced in the past. We turn, therefore, to the BBA and its implementation.

Learning from the Balanced Budget Act of 1997

Medicare provisions in the 1997 Balanced Budget Act (hereinafter, BBA-97) evolved out of two years of political battle between President Clinton and Congress over the terms of any budget-balancing bill, during which Medicare was one of the centers of controversy (Maraniss and Weiskopf 1996; see also the *Congressional Quarterly Almanac* for 1995, 1996, and 1997). One key issue was whether Medicare could and should be made more like the private sector through encouragement of competing plans. The alternative was to save money through some mix of tightening Medicare's previous cost-control systems and extending them to services such as SNFs to which they had not been applied, and perhaps higher charges to beneficiaries. The political answer was "Both!" BBA-97 saved money in the traditional way, while including measures to move Medicare toward a voucher system.

Savings

The BBA's savings included dozens of provisions, and we will look only at the most significant.[6]

Reductions in HI and SMI System Costs

Most simply, the law reduced the update factors for PPS payment rates. The Prospective Payment Assessment Commission had reported that hospitals had managed to increase their profit margins on Medicare patients to a level at which they could afford a substantial cut (ProPAC 1997a: 15–25; also Guterman 1998). BBA-97 also ordered HCFA to implement new prospective payment systems for other HI services, including inpatient rehabilitation services, most skilled nursing facility benefits, and, perhaps most significantly, outpatient services from hospitals. The creation of new PPS systems is, however, technically quite difficult; so the law provided backup cost controls in case HCFA was not able to implement all the mandated reforms on time (as has been the case).[7]

The law also reduced payments for noninsurance functions of Medicare, such as capital payments and the Indirect Medical Education (IME) and disproportionate share hospital (DSH) adjustments. Combined with restraint of the updates for the existing PPS payments and the new systems for outpatient care and SNFs (which sometimes are owned by hospitals), BBA-97 could have significant effects on hospital incomes.

Within SMI, the law reduced scheduled updates for physician fees and altered some of the workings of the physician fee schedule. BBA-97 got more of its savings from nonphysician services. It slowed increases in fees for durable medical equipment and froze fees for laboratory services through 2002.

In a provision that would affect both HI and SMI costs, BBA-97 required that the secretary of HHS establish a prospective payment system for home health services and implement it by October 1, 1999. The law also required limits on total payments per visit and per beneficiary.

These and other changes to HI and SMI payments were accompanied by some expansions in benefits for preventive care such as mammograms, pap smears, and prostate cancer screening. The net effect of all these measures was estimated as $72.1 billion in savings over five years and $186.6 billion over ten years (O'Sullivan et al. 1997: 66–68). In essence, the standard price regulation measures were tightened where they already applied, and they were applied to areas where they had yet to be implemented. In the view of Marilyn Moon and her colleagues, "Medicare has been a leader in hospital and physician payment restructuring, and this legislation finally allows it to establish sound payment policies for the other parts of the program where it had been reimbursing the old-fashioned way—on the basis of costs and charges" (Moon, Gage, and Evans 1997: 6).

Increased Charges to Beneficiaries

BBA-97 increased the Part B premium in two ways. The premium was set permanently at 25 percent of costs, rather than being allowed (in theory), as under existing law, to grow only at the (normally slower) rate of increase of Social Security COLAs. In addition, the shift of home health services to Part B, by increasing Part B costs, automatically increases premiums. These two measures were projected to raise the premium to $67.00 instead of $51.50 in 2002 and to $105.00 per month in 2007.[8]

This premium increase raised concerns about affordability for lower-income beneficiaries. Although BBA-97 includes a program for assistance in addition to the preexisting Qualified Medicare Beneficiary (QMB) and Specified Low-Income Beneficiary (SLMB) programs, it is very limited.[9] However, since Congress had continually acted to maintain the 25 percent standard, and since most of the estimated premium increase resulted from its doing so, it is unreasonable to view most of the increase as a new choice to target the poor.

Savings from Combination Plans

The third major category of savings involved reduced payments to combination plans. The basic problem, remember, was that plans were paid 95 percent of the Adjusted Average Per Capita Cost (AAPCC)–based rate, but the available data suggested that the people who joined the plans would have cost about 90 percent of that rate if they had stayed in traditional Medicare.

Under BBA, payments to plans were to be restrained automatically, and indirectly, by the savings in traditional Medicare, for the latter would lower the costs in the AAPCC calculation. If enrollees in the combination plans were likely to incur only 90 percent of the average level of costs had they stayed in traditional Medicare, it also seemed reasonable to move the payment from 95 percent toward 90 (though not all the way); BBA-97 did that.[10] Because the plans were not passing graduate medical education (GME) funds on to hospitals, it also seemed sensible to take those funds out of their premiums and pass them directly to the hospitals.

Other provisions of BBA-97 altered the rules for paying plans in ways that were supposed to be budget-neutral. A few more, meant to expand the use of new forms of combination plans, were expected to lose about $4 billion over five years (O'Sullivan et al. 1997: 53).

Overall Pattern of Savings

Exactly none of the savings measures in BBA-97 were based on expanding the use of combination plans. In fact, the measures to increase the use of combination plans were estimated, in and of themselves, to raise Medicare costs. This does not exactly suggest that vouchers would "save" Medicare by controlling costs. Yet BBA-97 was designed to help the case for vouchers, because some other provisions might show that the weaknesses in the Medicare Risk program could be overcome.

Medicare + Choice

The most basic difficulties are

risk selection and adverse selection,

the fact that the geographic bias of combination plans toward high-AAPCC areas has meant low availability in much of the country,

distrust of HMOs, which means that vouchers would be more popular if they gave access to other kinds of plans, and

concerns that the elderly population, which includes a large number of persons with cognitive and other disabilities, would be bewildered and bamboozled by a requirement to choose among plans.

The Medicare + Choice program created by BBA-97 has provisions to address each of these problems.

Biased Selection into Plans

One way to limit selection effects is to regulate enrollment and disenrollment. Plans were required to accept any eligible enrollees, though with some escape hatches, and were forbidden to terminate enrollees except for nonpayment of premiums, "disruptive behavior," or in the event that a plan left the Medicare + Choice business for an entire area.[11] A more significant change restricted when individuals could choose combination plans. As of November 1, 2001, Medicare beneficiaries will be allowed to choose Medicare + Choice plans once a year (in November, for the following calendar year). They will then have three months to change their minds. As Marilyn Moon and her colleagues summarize, "locking beneficiaries into their choices for the year will reduce the current problem of paying monthly premiums for beneficiaries while they are healthy but traditional claims when they become ill and disenroll" (Moon, Gage, and Evans 1997: 12). This measure is clearly appropriate, but elimination of the disenrollment safety valve does mean that consumer protections for enrollees will become more important.

BBA-97 also ordered the secretary of HHS "to implement a risk adjustment methodology that accounts for variations in per capita costs based on health status by no later than January 1, 2000" (U.S. Senate Committee on Finance 1997: sec. 9). It would be difficult not to improve on Medicare's previous risk-adjustment methods, and if plans in fact were cherry-picking, better risk adjustment will save money.

Unfortunately, the most promising technical approach is to adjust payments based on data about individuals' health status. The requisite data, however, is not so easy to find. Hospitalization data is much more prevalent than other sources, but it only distinguishes some conditions. Also, if plans get paid more for people who are diagnosed as being sick, they will lose much of the incentive to keep people healthy that is supposedly one of the points of HMOs. Expenses in a given year also may not predict costs in the next year so well (MedPAC 1998a).

Given these obstacles, but a congressional mandate, HCFA's Robert A. Berenson, M.D., explained that "risk adjustment is so fundamental to giving the correct incentives to plans that we need to move forward, even if it's imperfect" (Iglehart 1999: 148). HCFA would start with hospitalization experience and phase in ambulatory data as it became available. The real problem from the plans' perspective was that even though risk adjustment was by some accounts supposed to be budget-neutral, it is hard to imagine how any effective approach could be so if the plans had members who were healthier than average. HCFA announced on January 15, 1999, that it would phase in the risk-adjustment plan over five years. As a result it would reduce average payments to plans in the year 2000 by only 0.76 percent. Nevertheless, the American Association of Health Plans and the Health Insurance Association of America both condemned HCFA's announcement, on the grounds that reducing payments to managed-care plans would reduce supplemental benefits to their members.[12]

Geographic Distribution of Plans

Under the BBA, federal payments to each plan would still be based on the AAPCC figures but with complicated modifications intended to lower payments in areas that have high fee-for-service costs and raise them in areas where those costs are low.

The removal of graduate medical education payments from the rates has that effect because teaching hospitals tend to be in higher-cost areas. But there are other, more direct, measures. One is a slow and partial shift of the basis of payment from local costs to national averages, which will raise payments in areas with costs below the average. This new blended payment is constructed in a way that is intended to reduce the extent to which areas with higher utilization are rewarded with higher premium contributions (MedPAC 1998a: 14).

The BBA then guaranteed low-cost areas a minimum monthly payment (the "floor"), which was set at $367 for 1998. This raised the payment in a third of all counties, which accounted for 14 percent of the Medicare enrollees. In 8 percent of counties, the local AAPCC figure was $300, so the payment increase was quite significant; however, those counties were home to only 2 percent of enrollees (Moon, Gage, and Evans 1997: 12). The adjustment upward to pay minimum premiums in low-cost areas was supposed to be budget-neutral, so increases in those areas would require lower premiums in the higher-cost areas.

Although these measures were supposed to encourage combination plans in low-cost areas, they could fail for two reasons. First, the other requirements for managed care, such as having enough physicians to allow selective contracting or a large enough patient base to justify a separate insurance pool in that area, may not be met. Second, when costs are already low because of low utilization and prices, managed-care organizations may not be able to improve on that performance. Meanwhile, CBO (1997c) estimated that Medicare would lose as much as $750 per person by paying more than the cost of traditional Medicare to some plans. The best one can say for BBA-97's higher payments in these areas is that it makes more sense to subsidize supplemental benefits in areas that consume low levels of the basic Medicare package than in areas that consume high levels of the basic package.

The good news, from a budgetary perspective, is that the risk of higher payments seems to have been blunted by the remaining obstacles to setting up combination plans in low-cost areas. Little if any of the intended expansion occurred in the first three years.

New Types of Plan

Instead of being basically limited to HMOs, the new set of choices can include HMOs with or without a point-of-service option, Preferred Provider Organizations (PPOs), Provider Sponsored Organizations (PSOs), private fee-for-service plans, and Medical Savings Account (MSA) plans. The first three types are referred to as "coordinated care plans" and are subject to different regulatory oversight than the MSAs and private fee-for-service. This can be justified on the grounds that plan managers interfere more with the physician-patient relationship in the former plans.

There is a pretty strong case, on its face, for including PPOs among Medicare options. They are a major form of managed care, so offering them can be justified as based on experience with managed care in the private sector. And they have lots of members.

The theory of Provider Sponsored Organizations, on the part of doctors at least, is that PSOs would avoid the high overhead of other restrictive systems and would be provider friendly. But PSOs have not arisen in the private market because physicians have not had the capital to meet state regulatory requirements for insurance companies. The BBA-97 allowed the secretary of HHS to waive such state laws, applying less rigorous standards (MedPAC 1998b: 23–25, 38–39). If any are created, the PSO design might encourage risk selection, as physicians who are stakeholders in the PSO would have strong incentives to steer healthier (thus cheaper) beneficiaries to the PSO and less healthy patients back into HI and SMI. The CBO (1997c) therefore estimated that the PSO option would increase Medicare's costs by $1 billion over five years, or between $300 and $400 per expected enrollee.

The two forms of uncoordinated care plan, Medical Savings Accounts (MSAs) and private fee-for-service, are more controversial. MSAs have been promoted by conservatives and the American Medical Association for years, with a widely skeptical response from mainstream health-policy analysts.[13] The concept is that, instead of HI and SMI, enrollees would choose "catastrophic" coverage that applied to all costs over a high deductible (no more than $6,000 in 1999 and indexed to inflation). The expenses being counted must include all HI and SMI benefits but may include many other benefits at the plan's option. In order to help pay the deductible, individuals could set up "medical savings accounts." All contributions to and earnings from these accounts would be tax-free, and withdrawals would be tax-free so long as they were applied to any service considered medical care under the Internal Revenue Code. Medicare would contribute to enrollees' accounts each year the difference between its local contribution rate for risk plans and the premium for the catastrophic insurance associated with the MSA.

MSAs may or may not save money *for their enrollees* compared to other cost-control methods; they may seem more attractive in other ways to some potential enrollees and health-care providers. But there is little doubt that they threaten severe risk-selection and equity problems. Healthier people would have clear incentives to choose MSAs and collect cash from Medicare. So would richer people, who could cover shortfalls (up to the deductible) if they guessed wrong about their health. Most people with chronic illness, expecting to spend the deductible each year, would know that they would pay more out of pocket in the MSA system and so, with their high costs, would stay in traditional Medicare.[14] Given fervent Democratic objection and equally fervent Republican support for MSAs, BBA-97 limited this option to a "demonstration" that could include no more than 390,000 enrollees. Nevertheless, CBO (1997c: table 4B) estimated that demonstration would raise Medicare's costs by $1.5 billion over five years, or about $950 per enrollee.

The question about private fee-for-service is why it should exist at all, since HI and SMI already offered fee-for-service coverage in a way that must have lower overhead costs than any plan that has marketing expenses. One possibility is that a private plan would offer a broader benefit package, serving essentially as a comprehensive Medicare-plus-Medigap plan. But that could encourage packages designed to risk-select, for example by offering some form of health club benefit. Private fee-for-service (FFS) might also allow high-prestige physicians to escape the Medicare fee schedule. They would make it clear that they would be more open to serving patients in the private FFS plan, for which their pay rates would be higher. And in markets with costs currently below the payment threshold, perhaps providers could organize fee-for-service plans that had no restrictions but took the extra money available to plans and split it among providers, as extra fees, and enrollees, as supplemental benefits. This possibility explains why even some proponents of a voucher approach to Medicare were skeptical of the private fee-for-service option (Wilensky and Newhouse 1999: 99–100).

In theory, therefore, the extra options provided in Medicare + Choice seemed to offer as many difficulties as improvements. In practice, they have had virtually no effect. In the first two years no private fee-for-service plans were approved for participation, even in low-cost areas. Nor were any MSA plans, and only two PSO plans were accepted. Even PPOs had not burgeoned, perhaps because PPOs "may not be able to conform to the requirements for information on quality and outcomes" (Wilensky and Newhouse 1999: 98; see also Neuman and Langwell 1999).

Under the circumstances, it would be hard to show that BBA-97 demonstrated the merits of offering Medicare enrollees choices other than HMOs.

Consumer Protection

BBA-97 requires that HCFA distribute extensive public education materials about plans' offerings. Plans are also required to market to more risky populations (e.g., disabled people); give members direct access (without gatekeepers) to some specialists, such as gynecologists; pay for emergency and poststabilization care out-of-network; have extensive internal quality assurance plans; and provide appeals processes that members could use if denied a service. Some of these provisions were put directly into the legislation (for example, that plans pay for emergency care so long as a "prudent layperson" would have gone to the emergency room with the symptoms in question); others were to be developed by HCFA as regulations.

Many of these measures resemble some adopted for the commercial managed-care market in some states. Whether and in what sense they will be sufficient remains to be seen. Consumer advocates identify significant weaknesses, whereas advocates for health plans argue that they are too onerous (Dallek 1998; MedPAC 1998b). As with other reforms, therefore, it is too early to say that the consumer protections in Medicare + Choice will be satisfactory.

Implications of BBA-97 and Its Implementation

The Balanced Budget Act of 1997 was produced by a clash between two visions. The status quo, traditional Medicare, was a system with one main insurance pool, whose members all paid the same premiums (save for special help for the poor) and had access to virtually all medical providers. In that system, which remains the norm, costs are controlled (somewhat) by a mix of cost-sharing for beneficiaries and fee schedules and prospective payment systems that apply to all providers of a given type of service. In the alternative vision, individuals would receive a voucher that they would use to pay (most of) the costs of insurance. They might have to pay much more than the Part B premium to purchase the Medicare package. Through their plans, Medicare beneficiaries would most likely face restrictions in the providers to which they would have access.

In a voucher plan, the main form of cost control for the government arises from setting the voucher amount. In other words, voucher plans explicitly or implicitly raise the question of whether Medicare is to be converted from a defined-benefit plan to a defined-contribution plan.[15] Because the current Medicare package does have holes, which means that access to and costs of supplemental benefits are quite unequal, moving to a voucher approach would not increase insecurity and inequality as much as the stark contrast suggests. But it still involves a very different vision of Medicare from what has prevailed to date. Since beneficiaries would have to pay the difference between the contribution and the premiums for whichever plans they bought, the defined-contribution approach would shift the risks of higher health-care costs from the government to beneficiaries.

BBA-97 did not include a defined contribution—and therefore did not get its savings from encouraging enrollees to switch to combination plans. It did seek to encourage that model by offering fixes to some of the problems previously observed in combination-plan performance. We have seen that none of those measures have been in place long enough to show that they work. Some, such as encouragement of plans other than HMOs, had clearly not worked in the first two years.

In fact, BBA-97 may not have encouraged combination plans at all. In principle, if Medicare has been subsidizing HMOs, measures that reduced the subsidies should discourage enrollment. Similarly, making fee-for-service Medicare less costly should reduce HMOs' ability to gain savings with which to finance extra benefits and recruit members. Targeting payment reductions on high-cost areas, if compensating increases in low-cost areas cannot attract plans because of other obstacles, should further dampen the move to combination plans.

BBA-97's combination of measures threatened to cause very low premium increases in high-cost areas. The act therefore guaranteed an increase of 2 percent in each county. Although this was at least an increase, whereas average payments per person in the fee-for-service sector declined in 1998–99, it was much less than HMO managers in general believed necessary to finance their previous levels of extra benefits (MedPAC 1998a: 14–18).

Because of the implementation of new risk adjusters in 2000, combined with further blending of the rates, many plans expected to receive less than they desired in 2000, even though basic increases would be higher. The financial prospects of combination plans therefore looked a lot less rosy after

BBA-97 than before. The result, at the end of 1998, was a spate of publicity about insurers dropping out of the program. Enrollment in combination plans continued to grow, though much more slowly, through late 1999. But then it stopped.[16] Plans began paring back the supplemental benefits that they offered.[17]

Ironically, the BBA, as I wrote, had not reduced payments to combination plans as a share of local spending on traditional Medicare. Payments to plans in calendar year 2000 were "about 95.5 percent of the average amount paid in the Medicare [fee-for-service] sector" (HHS Inspector General 2000: iii). Relative payments did not fall because the minimum increase for combination plans was higher than the average increase in fee-for-service costs. That means any negative effect on payments to HMOs was caused by the successful cost control in traditional Medicare. HMOs were having trouble providing extra benefits at traditional Medicare's costs because the traditional program was, for the moment, outdoing them at cost control.

In spite of what should be viewed as a dismal record from the perspective of voucher advocates, BBA-97 did have one more provision that in theory could provide important evidence about whether vouchers can improve on the current system. Yet its fate to date also is not encouraging.

Analysts of all stripes agree that basing payments on the AAPCC is a bad idea. Ideally, plans would compete, offering their packages at market prices, and competition would drive premiums below the AAPCC-based figures. Interestingly, both friends and foes of the voucher idea would like to see that idea tested. If it worked, voucher skeptics might rethink their positions. If it failed, we would at least know that the market, not "government price-setting," explained why vouchers did not save money.

BBA-97 therefore instructed HCFA to implement, by January of 1999, four demonstrations of methods under which plans' prices within a given market would be set by competitive pricing. But plans' managers tend to like competition rather less in practice than in theory. Congress had previously been induced to block demonstrations in Denver and Baltimore. As of mid-1999, the best HCFA had managed was to plan demonstrations beginning in 2000 in two cities, Kansas City and Phoenix. In the face of political objections, those were postponed until at least 2001 (Jones 1999; Dowd, Coulam, and Feldman 2000; Nichols and Reischauer 2000).

The practical difficulties of a competitive pricing system for combination plans can seem daunting even in advocates' accounts (Feldman and Dowd 1997). That makes the experiments even more important. They could yield important information about how a sort-of market for plans might be structured, with what results. Yet, if the experiments ever do occur, it will surely take more than a year or two of experience, in more than two markets, to develop meaningful information. For example, plans might bid low in a first year, discover they lost money, and seek large increases in the next. In that scenario the first year's bids would be very misleading. Or all the plans in a market might bid fairly high, making the market look like a failure from a cost-control perspective. Yet if the plans were doing well, eventually some might lower prices in search of a larger market share. Even if they occurred, we could not expect the demonstrations to help solve the "how to pay the plans" conundrum for at least a few years. The fact that the experiments have been blocked should create some doubt among the advocates who claim that vouchers would work given proper regulation and use of market incentives. What if those conditions cannot be created?

Not Yet, and Maybe Never?

The evidence in this chapter shows why there is great doubt that a voucher approach is ready for implementation in Medicare or ever will be advisable.

Yet combination plans still offer a distinctly better deal for supplemental benefits, for many enrollees, than they could hope to obtain any other way. Though they might offer less value in the future, so might other supplemental policies, which also would be affected by factors such as soaring costs for pharmaceuticals. The stagnation of enrollment in Medicare + Choice plans as of 1999 could reverse if other sources of supplemental benefits unravel. We do not know how the implicit competition between combination plans and other Medicare supplements will develop.

We also do not really know what effects the more traditional cost controls in BBA-97 are having. Providers claim to be hurt, but that is to be expected. Even if some, especially academic medical centers (AMCs), are losing dangerous amounts of income, that does not mean that a voucher system would be better for them. After all, one of the reasons AMCs may be dependent on federal funding is that private payers are paying them less. One of the main cost-control measures of "managed care" is to reduce hospitalizations, especially, if possible, in high-cost hospitals.

We do know that HCFA faced a huge task in implementing the act. In June of 1998 the Medicare Payment Advisory Commission issued a report that indicated "the enormous scope and complexity of the tasks that must be completed to implement the provisions of the BBA." At the beginning of 1999, a bipartisan group of policy analysts issued an open letter calling on Congress and the administration to provide more resources to HCFA, lest it fall behind "in its implementation of many of the significant reforms mandated by the Balanced Budget Act" (Butler et al. 1999).

In short, both implementation and adaptation of BBA-97 could and probably should take years. In the course of that activity, we may learn more about both how a voucher system might work and how best to make it work. In the meantime, as this book was written and edited, the evidence that Medicare should be expected to control costs less successfully than private insurers could do so was extremely weak. Medicare's costs were on a pretty favorable path. The overall budget situation was even better. Given those conditions, what to do about Medicare would, by normal logic, seem obvious: do as little as possible while the system deals with the 1997 reforms.

There is simply no basis for more radical action. Adopting vouchers with so little evidence either that they could work or about how to make them work defies common sense.

TEN

Too Young or Too Rich for Social Insurance?

Privatization arguments have been most prominent among Social Security and Medicare reform proposals because they offer, according to proponents, some gain to go with policy pain. Yet many other ways to reduce the expected gaps between Social Security and Medicare revenues and obligations have been included in privatization plans. These other measures have been proposed both because the "savings" from privatization were not in themselves large enough to meet the goals of those plans' proponents and, in the case of Social Security, to finance the transition to private accounts.

One important question is whether particular measures would fundamentally change the nature of the programs. Privatization would alter part of the pension created by Social Security from a defined-benefit plan to a defined-contribution approach. We have discussed how the remaining defined benefits under a privatization plan might, if concentrated on low-income enrollees, fundamentally change the program's politics. But there are also ways in which other commonly prescribed savings would radically alter the entitlements to Social Security and Medicare.

In this chapter we discuss three common reform proposals. Two alter the entitlement in obvious ways: (a) by changing the age of eligibility and (b) by creating versions of a means test. Most proposals of these types would be bad news, but there is room for the development of less dangerous reforms, and I will suggest how that might be done. The third proposal, reducing the automatic cost-of-living adjustments for Social Security, looks more like a straightforward benefit cut. But it would change the basic way in which Social Security offers protection against the risk of a longer-than-average life span and is simply a bad idea.

Raising the Age(s) of Eligibility

"Raising the retirement age for Social Security and Medicare," the *Wall Street Journal* reported, "is one of the most popular ideas among experts looking for long-term savings" (Calmes 1997b). Life expectancies have increased since Social Security was created and can be expected to increase further. As a result, retirees are collecting for a larger portion of their lives. On average, people are healthier at any given age, and fewer jobs involve hard physical labor, so it may seem "only reasonable . . . that more years of life should translate into more years of work" (Wildavsky 1998: 1561). As Edith U. Fierst, a member of the 1994–96 Advisory Council, put it, "raising the normal retirement age is the intuitive way of curbing the costs of longer life" (Advisory Council on Social Security 1997a: 138).

Compared to some other proposals, raising the age of eligibility also is distinctly less threatening to one of the major purposes of entitlements for seniors, which is to provide insurance against outliving one's savings. Social Security or Medicare would protect people who are age 85 whether benefits begin at 65, 67, or 70.[1]

The case for some adjustment of age of eligibility is strong. Yet it is stronger for Social Security than for Medicare and requires modification even for Social Security.

Social Security

Before going further, we need to remember what the normal retirement age (NRA) really means. It is the age of retirement *with full benefits.* Workers can choose to retire as early as age 62 with actuarially reduced benefits. At present the reduction is about 20 percent per month; when the NRA rises to 67, individuals who retire at age 62 will receive benefits that are reduced by 30 percent per month. Since most people retire before age 65, the major effect of raising the NRA itself would be to lower their benefit checks, though some

TABLE 10.1
Life Expectancy Increases

Calendar Year	At Birth		At age 65	
	Male	Female	Male	Female
Historical Data				
1940	61.4	65.7	11.9	13.4
1960	66.7	73.2	12.9	15.9
1980	69.9	77.5	14.0	18.4
1995	72.4	79.0	15.3	19.0
Projected Data				
2010	74.9	80.4	16.3	19.5
2030	76.5	81.7	17.1	20.4
2050	77.8	82.9	17.9	21.2
2075	79.3	84.2	18.8	22.2

SOURCE: Adapted from Board of Trustees 1998a: 60, table II.D2. Projections follow the trustees' "intermediate" forecast of economic and demographic trends.

persons may delay retirement because the reduced monthly check seems inadequate.

Some proposals include raising the early eligibility age (EEA) as well. One reason is precisely to ensure that early retirement does not, when the NRA is raised, make monthly benefits too likely to be inadequate (Burtless 1998b: 5). The other is that the available evidence suggests that the age at which retirement can be taken, not the NRA, has the strongest effect on actual retirement behavior, and delaying retirement is seen as a good thing (Quadagno and Quinn 1997).

The average voter is distinctly uninterested in delaying retirement (Wildavsky 1998). Yet, the likely future shortage of workers relative to the elderly population leads many scholars to promote policies that would give people incentives to work longer. Jill Quadagno and Joseph Quinn thus write that "encouraging workers to stay active in the labor market longer than they currently do . . . may be just what we need" (1997: 146). As Richard Burkhauser puts it, "in a world of difficult choices about the use of tax dollars, it is no longer sensible policy to encourage the vast majority of healthy, employed workers to leave their job via the Social Security system at age 62" (Wildavsky 1998: 1564).

Supporters of raising the retirement age can also claim, using data such as in table 10.1, that they would not be changing the promise made in 1935. For example, the National Commission on Retirement Policy (NCRP) plan would have raised the NRA to 70 by 2029 (1998: 6). But life expectancy at age

65 increases by more than five years between 1940 and 2030 in the table; thus, ostensibly, the higher age would still provide the same length of retirement. That is not quite true, because when Social Security was adopted, its sponsors knew full well that life expectancies decades later would be higher than in 1940, and they still chose 65. Yet the trend does support raising the retirement age somewhat, eventually.

Unfortunately, in spite of the analytic justification for raising retirement ages, there is an obvious objection that, as the *Wall Street Journal* (Calmes 1997b) reported, is identifiable by economists, politicians, and plain old citizens:

> That's easy for white-collar workers like us to suggest. But talk to laborers. (Economist Barry Bosworth)

> It might be fine for somebody like me, who's always had a desk job. But what about the people who have laboring jobs? What about people who really work with their hands and their backs? (President Clinton)

> Might be okay for somebody who sits on their butt all the time. (Kate Wilke of Bayonne, N.J., wife of a printing press operator)

Right. Raising the retirement age clearly would favor what we once called the middle class or upper middle class over the working class. That is not what Social Security is supposed to do.

The class bias is partly a matter of attitudes. "I've always thought this is a favorite proposal of workaholics and not a favorite proposal of anyone else," commented Marilyn Moon, one of the two public trustees of the OASDI funds (Wildavsky 1998: 1563). Marilyn and I may love our jobs, but our jobs may be relatively easy to love. Does the guy who drives a Federal Express truck want to work to age 70? Do you want him to?

Blue-collar workers may have especially good reasons not to want to work into their late sixties. For example, according to Bureau of Labor Statistics data, workers age 65 and older "are five times as likely to have a fatal transportation accident, 3.8 times as likely to get killed by objects and equipment, and 3.4 times as likely to die in an assault" (Moss 1997). Blue-collar work actually is more dangerous for older workers.

The class bias is also a matter of opportunity: does Federal Express want to employ 69-year-old drivers? How long one works is not just the worker's choice. Even white-collar workers may have difficulty staying employed so long. In economic theory, as younger workers become scarcer, employers will recruit older workers more heavily, but the current trend is the opposite. Senior executives who were asked the age of peak productivity for workers lowered their estimate from age 56 in 1994 to age 48 in 1997. In the recession of the early 1990s, older workers were more likely than younger ones to be laid off. In 1997 Julie Kosterlitz of the *National Journal* reported that

> when top officials in 20 companies were interviewed for a recent study conducted for the AARP, the virtues employers most commonly ascribed to older workers—such as loyalty and lower absenteeism—were considered to be of *substantially* less value than traits they thought older workers lacked, such as flexibility and the ability to learn new skills. . . . The result is likely to be a sorry mismatch of supply and demand. Those with the most skills and education will be the most needed, but also the most able to retire; those with the least education will have a greater need for, but slimmer prospects of, continued work. (1997: 1884–85) (emphasis in original)

Proposed responses to this dilemma leave much to be desired. One option is to ease the definition of disability, and therefore access to DI benefits, for persons between ages 62 and 64 if the early eligibility age is raised to 64. Another would be to lower the age of eligibility for Supplemental Security Income (SSI) (Burtless 1998b; Wildavsky 1998). Any compensating measure, however, would pose two problems: how to administer it (who, exactly, would be "disabled" because of being blue collar?) and what its implications for Social Security would be. If the point of Social Security is to be a basic retirement system, it should be basic for everybody.

There is some basis for encouraging later retirement. Any such change does need to be legislated long in advance. But the possible inequities caused by raising the ages of eligibility are severe. What can be done?

It is time to consider changing the basis of eligibility from age alone to a mix of age and years in the workforce. Such a combination is common in private pensions, including those of many government workers. It would take advantage of the fact that people with desk jobs, on average, spend more time in school, and blue-collar workers, in general, spend less. Therefore, the former begin full-time work later, and hence (other things like unemployment experience being equal), at any given age have been in the workforce for fewer years.

A system that allowed retirement based on either years in the workforce or calendar age therefore could allow earlier retirement for blue-collar workers.

For instance, if the law entitled people to full benefits in 2030 at age 68 or with 46 years in the workforce, that would make no difference to a person who graduated from college at age 22 and worked steadily. But a lawyer (presumably with a higher-than-average income but not entering the workforce until around age 25) would have to work until age 68 for full benefits, and a blue-collar worker (having begun work at age 18) could, if continually employed, get full benefits at age 64.

This basic approach leaves many questions to be answered. For instance, what should be done about women who leave the workforce to raise children? What should be the age and years-in-workforce standards, both for normal and early eligibility? Whatever the difficulties, however, it makes more sense to address the demographics by changing the entitlement to benefits in a way that considers both age and time in the workforce than to simply raise the age thresholds.

In order to give proper consideration to the relevant issues, either the Social Security Advisory Board (SSAB) or a specially convened group could be given a target range of savings and asked to report options. The proper response to rising life expectancies is the most significant issue on which there is reason for structural change, but it makes sense to take the time to find the best response rather than to legislate hastily.

Medicare

Raising Medicare's eligibility age is at least as high on the political agenda as raising Social Security's NRA. The Senate voted to raise Medicare's eligibility age to 67 as part of its version of the Balanced Budget Act, although the provision was dropped from the final legislation. Yet raising Medicare's eligibility age is less defensible than raising Social Security's.

First of all, it would be a very severe and concentrated benefit cut, especially for low-income seniors. Remember that the real effect of raising the NRA is to lower monthly pension payments for beneficiaries who retire early. So the cut is spread over the entire period of retirement. In contrast, 65- or 66-year-old persons who had to purchase a replacement for Medicare in 1997 would have lost between about $3,500 and $4,500 per year for an individual and $7,000 to $9,000 for a couple.[2] Many low-income elderly people would not have the cash to pay those premiums. Employers are unlikely to pick up the slack. Most advocates of a later retirement age say not that individuals will continue with their old careers but that there will be "bridge," often part-time, jobs (Quadagno and Quinn 1997; Burtless 1998b). Part-time jobs are particularly unlikely to include medical insurance. Indeed, high medical insurance costs for the elderly may already be one reason that companies are not eager to hire them.

Labor unions fear that employers not only would not cover the newly uncovered workers but would reduce some of their present coverage for retirees. In 1997 Richard Lesher, then president of the U.S. Chamber of Commerce, agreed, commenting that "lots of companies, you know, take it right up to the Medicare threshold, and that means adding two more years into their plan, and lots of companies are not going to like that at all. Small companies don't do that to begin with, so you're really talking about medium- and larger-sized companies who won't be too excited about that at all" ("It's Your Business" 1997).[3] The most thorough analysis of raising the eligibility age for Medicare to 67 concludes that that measure "would affect a substantial fraction of beneficiaries without having a commensurate effect on expenditures, even in the long run . . . upwards of 500,000 persons ages sixty-five and sixty-six would be left without any insurance, and even more would not be able to afford coverage with benefits similar to those of Medicare" (Waidmann 1998: 156).

In order to raise the Medicare eligibility age without having extremely dangerous implications for low-income seniors, the government would have to plug at least some of the gaps itself. A common proposal is to expand Disability Insurance (and thus access to Medicare through DI).[4] But that would create a new set of issues. The current law that allows DI beneficiaries to go on Medicare after two years would have to be altered—raising the question of why, if 65-year-old DI beneficiaries could get immediate Medicare coverage, 45-year-olds should not. How would inability to hold a job be distinguished from inability to get one with insurance? Why should able-bodied people who cannot get a job go without insurance or pay a high financial penalty to get it? There would be a flood of new DI applications, creating serious administrative burdens. And of course, the extra DI costs would require some sort of adjustment in OASDI financing.

The more likely way to plug the gap would be to create some new program to help those who were no longer eligible for Medicare purchase insurance. The most obvious approach is to allow them to "buy in" to Medicare, with subsidies according to income for premium costs. That, however, would start to look a lot like a means-tested Medicare program. One might wonder, quite reasonably, why Medicare was means-tested for some people but not others.

There is reason to look at measures that would alter the age of eligibility for Social Security. But the same approach to Medicare is just a bad idea.

Means-Testing

Not so long ago, it was generally agreed that means-testing a social insurance program changes it so fundamentally that it could not be called "saved." As late as 1982 the Greenspan Commission unanimously rejected "proposals to make the Social Security program a voluntary one or to transform it into . . . a program under which benefits are conditioned on the showing of financial need" (Kingson and Schulz 1997b: 45). Yet means-testing is now on the policy agenda.

The Old Means-Testing Was as Bad as Critics Feared

Eric Kingson and James Schulz summarize the experience with means-testing:

> Major problems that have been documented repeatedly are the high administrative costs, the imprecise targeting (i.e. including or excluding the wrong people because of the typical complexities of rules and procedures), the stigma related to receiving benefits, the abuse of power by those determining eligibility, and the consequent low participation rates of those who are eligible. (1997b: 46–47)

A major means-tested national cash program for the poor, Aid to Families with Dependent Children, was created as part of the Social Security Act. Unlike Social Security, however, the value of AFDC's benefits dropped by 40 percent between 1970 and 1993, and the entitlement itself was abolished as part of "welfare reform" in 1996 (46).[5] Supplemental Security Income (SSI) for very poor individuals who are old, blind, or disabled has been uncontroversial. But if SSI has not had the political weaknesses of means-testing, it has exemplified the administrative ones. The income and especially the asset tests for eligibility are extremely complex (U.S. House, Committee on Ways and Means 1996: 263–68). They have led to "major administrative problems," and about 40 percent of those who are eligible for SSI benefits are not enrolled in the program (Kingson and Schulz 1997b: 47; Derthick 1990). Medicaid is another means-tested program that seems to have survived political attack. Yet that entitlement also was almost eliminated in the budget battles of 1995. Moreover, it has some of the same administrative problems as SSI. In 1996 less than half of the children eligible for Medicaid were actually covered by the program.[6]

The New Means-Testing

In spite of this history, what Kingson and Schulz call the "New Means-Testing Approach" is being promoted now. The new means-testing innovates by saying not that only people with particularly low means should receive benefits but that people with higher-than-average means should be denied or have reduced benefits. Peter G. Peterson (1996) has labeled his version of this approach as not a "means test" but an "affluence test."[7] As Peterson explained his proposal, the

> test would progressively reduce benefits to all households with incomes over $40,000. . . . Households with incomes under $40,000 would retain their full government benefits. Higher-income households would lose 10 percent of all benefits that raise their total income above $40,000, plus 10 percent for each additional $10,000 in income. Thus a household with $50,000 in total income and $10,000 in federal benefits would lose 10 percent, or $1,000, of its benefits; a household with the same $10,000 in benefits and $100,000 in income would lose 60 percent, or $6,000. (1996: 167–68)

Advantages of the New Means-Testing

The Peterson proposal has some merits and demerits that we need not examine in detail here.[8] It also exemplifies two advantages of the new means-testing. First, most voters would still receive benefits. Hence the political disadvantage associated with traditional means-tested programs would not be as strong. Second, Peterson's approach would have to be administered through the income-tax system. Taxing back a universal entitlement at least presumes that people get entitled in the first place, so it would not exclude eligible people. Since the costs of the IRS already exist, the system would also not have extra administrative costs as large as in traditional means-testing. There would be no special process of applying for benefits and therefore much less (if any) stigma for receiving them.

Effects on Saving

Although the new means-testing clearly would be less threatening than the old kind, it still poses versions of the same problems. The old means-testing, for example, was frequently condemned on the grounds that it provided the poor with incentives not to work. The new means-testing could give higher-income people incentives not to work or save.

Eugene Steuerle, who has argued extensively for entitlement reform, nonetheless reports that many aspects of the current benefit structure and tax law already combine to create the equivalent of high marginal tax rates on work by, or extra investments by, seniors. The new means-test approach would add "yet another form of benefit reduction or taxation" (1996: 170) on top of what in some cases is already, by his calculations, a more than 50 percent marginal tax rate. Gary Burtless adds that the new means-testing sends "comparatively affluent workers a clear message: If you increase your private saving for retirement, the state will sharply reduce your Social Security pension" (1996a: 179).

New Inequities

Steuerle also points out that "means tests that operate only after ages sixty-two or sixty-five create some unusual inequities in the law: they force older workers to face much higher tax rates than are faced by younger workers with the same levels of income" (1996: 171). Peterson and the Concord Coalition may rationalize that on the grounds that elderly people are unproductive and undeserving, but the rest of us might not agree. Besides, Peterson's proposal would penalize any elderly person who was productive (who earned above his or her threshold). In addition, people who did not save, or who hid their assets by transferring them to their children, would receive benefits paid for in part by people with equal lifetime incomes who were more provident (saved

more) or honest (hid less). "Finally," Steuerle points out, "there is the fundamental philosophical issue of what individuals might reasonably expect when
mandated to participate in a partial insurance system. . . . If it is mandated
that individuals put money aside for retirement, then it is questionable
whether some of them should simultaneously be told that they are going to
get nothing back out of that money later" (1996: 171–72).

Political Effects

Most generally, the new means-testing threatens to destroy the existing balance between the goals of equity (defined as some sort of personal return on
contributions) and adequacy (of income or benefits for those who do not do
so well in the marketplace). Kingson and Schulz fear that there would be
"good reason to believe that the introduction of such a means test would, in
the long run, undermine the political support, the legitimacy, and ultimately
the financial viability of Social Security" (1997b: 54–55).

The validity of these fears would depend on the specific proposal. Yet they
are surely significant, and the same distributional ends could be achieved with
less risk. For instance, if wealthier people were believed not to be paying their
fair share in society, the income tax could be made more progressive. Or, since
the elderly are more likely to be consuming and less likely to be saving, the tax
system could target consumption more and income less. Any of these approaches would have a distributional justification similar to that of the new
means-testing, without making Social Security and Medicare themselves seem
like bad deals and thus threatening their support.

In short, even the new means-testing would fundamentally change the rationale of Social Security away from the idea that contribution entitles people to benefits, thus endangering the program.

Means-Testing and Medicare

Medicare is not so clear a case because of the form and origins of Part B. The
new debate raises old issues about the basic nature of the program.

Support for Means-Testing

In 1997 the Senate Finance Committee adopted, by an 18–2 vote, a re-
markably bad idea, a means-tested *deductible*. After much self- congratulation,

senators awoke to the perversities of that approach (helpfully explained in a scathing op-ed by Robert Reischauer) and replaced it with a means-tested Part B premium (Havemann 1997a,b; Pear 1997a; Reischauer 1997d).⁹ This provision, adopted by a vote of 70–30 on the Senate floor, would have increased the percentage of Part B costs paid by wealthier beneficiaries beginning with incomes of $50,000 for single people and $75,000 for couples. The premium would have been raised on a sliding scale from 25 percent of program costs (about $540) to 100 percent (about $2,160) for individuals with $100,000 and couples with $125,000 income (Georges 1997; Pear 1997b).

Not only did the Senate support the idea strongly, but also President Clinton endorsed the concept in principle and said he would be "happy to defend the vote of any member of Congress, Democrat or Republican, who votes for this" (Mitchell 1997). Reischauer wrote that "There is little reason to provide large Medicare subsidies to the most affluent 5 percent of senior citizens. It should be enough to provide these fortunate seniors with access to a non-cancelable insurance plan with very low administrative costs at an actuarially fair price." He argued that wealthy elderly people should "bear a bit more of Medicare's burden through the fair, feasible and effective mechanism of relating Medicare's premiums to participants' incomes" (1997d).

Put that way, few advocates of social insurance would disagree. Yet the Senate proposal was hotly opposed on the grounds, in Ted Marmor and Jacob Hacker's words, that it transformed, "a reasonable sentiment—that social programs should be progressively financed—into a truly bad idea" (1997).

Part B and Social Insurance

The key to the Medicare means-testing debate can be seen by asking whether Reischauer's argument for charging beneficiaries would sound as plausible if applied to Part A. If ability to pay was all that mattered, there would be no more excuse for helping people with HI than with SMI. Indeed, means-testing Part A would seem to make more sense, since it would actually help the HI trust fund. Yet it is not even on the policy radar screen, because affluent elderly people are seen to have "contributed," through their payroll taxes, to Part A in particular.

Proposals to means-test Part B contributions are thus the logical result of the 1965 compromise. Part B is designed as a voluntary program with individuals subsidized from general revenues. Steuerle's point about the unfairness of denying benefits to people who have made mandatory contributions applies to Part A but not, at least directly, to Part B.

Nevertheless, the presumption that wealthier seniors have no real claim to Part B benefits may be considered unrealistic for two basic reasons. First, a dedicated contribution may not really be necessary in order to create the kind of moral entitlement associated with social insurance. Canada's national health insurance arrangement, for example, is mandatory but financed by the general revenue of the federal government and the provinces and, in a few provinces, a partial premium paid by beneficiaries. So its financing is much the same as Part B's, yet universality is one of the basic provisions of the Canada Health Act, and hardly anyone in Canada would see a new-fangled means-test as a modest policy change. Similarly, SMI has been viewed as a program for all the elderly for a generation, clearly different from means-tested Medicaid because everyone is covered regardless of income, and as something people deserve after a lifetime of work.

Second, technicalities and origins aside, how many people really think of Parts A and B as separate programs, rather than as aspects of a single program called Medicare? Certainly not the supporters of significant cuts! When Republican politicians from 1995 to 1997 claimed that reform was necessary because of "Medicare's" impending bankruptcy, they did not point out that only Part A, HI, could go bankrupt—and indeed, they proposed cuts in Part B as part of the "rescue." At the beginning of 1999, the chair of the National Bipartisan Commission on the Future of Medicare was emphasizing that Medicare needed to be reformed sooner than Social Security, because "Medicare"—not HI—was going to go broke by 2008.[10] The two programs are treated separately for the technical purpose of making the HI trust fund more solvent. But when that includes, as it did in 1997, transferring an expense from HI to SMI, critics attack such provisions as shams because they do not reduce total Medicare spending.

Practical Effects

In 1998, under the Senate's 1997 proposal, about 3 million Medicare enrollees would have paid some extra premium, and about 1.3 million of those would have paid the full actuarial value of Part B coverage.[11] Considering extensive administrative costs, net savings would have been small, and the affected population seems too small to have impacted Medicare's political viability (Pear 1997c). So what was the brouhaha about?

The catch was what would happen over time. The thresholds in the Senate proposal were not indexed. As the years passed, more and more couples, for example, would have incomes above $75,000 and would pay some extra premiums, or above $125,000 and would have to pay the full cost of Part B. By 2008 the share of Medicare beneficiaries paying any extra premium would have doubled, and the share paying the full cost would have more than doubled.[12] Moreover, those couples that paid the full cost would have been paying more than $10,000 per year.[13] By 2030, more than a third of enrollees would have been paying some extra premium, and just less than 20 percent would have been paying the full cost of Part B. Under the estimates at the time, this cost would have been nearly a quarter of income for a couple at the $125,000 level (which would mean a lot less than it does today).[14]

In short, once the savings became big enough to be significant (i.e., help "save" Medicare in 2030), so would the other consequences (i.e., reduced political support for Medicare in 2030). Higher-income seniors might believe that Part B offered them little; and higher-income workers would expect to get nothing from the program. These two groups would be likely to begin to resent paying general taxes to support only other people's medical insurance. Faced with having to pay an actuarially fair premium, the healthier well-off elderly person might choose instead to buy the same coverage for less money from risk-selecting private plans. Then Part B not only would not collect the extra premiums for those people but would be left with a sicker group of enrollees.

Why, then, did President Clinton express support for the idea and offer political "cover" to legislators? Because he endorsed a version of the idea, not the exact proposal. In negotiations with congressional Republicans over what would be included in the final version of the BBA-97, the administration's suggestions differed from the Senate plan in significant ways. First, the White House wanted higher income thresholds, so that the proposal would affect fewer people. Second, it wanted the thresholds indexed to inflation. The population that would be required to pay more than the 25 percent premium would still have grown, because wages grow more quickly than inflation, but it would have grown much more slowly. Third, and most significant, President Clinton opposed charging any more than 75 percent of the full value of Part B coverage. By preserving a "subsidy" of 25 percent of Part B costs, this provision would have ensured that even high-income enrollees got something for their tax dollars and would have significantly reduced the incentives for anyone to opt out and seek private coverage at a lower price (Georges and Calmes 1997).[15]

President Clinton's proposals would have been safer, but the most important implication of the difference between his version and the Senate's plan is that there are many ways to relate contributions to income.

True Income-Related Premiums

If their goal was to increase equity by more directly relating contributions for Medicare to ability to pay, means-test proponents would not alter the Part B premium but abolish it. Then Part B would be financed entirely by the moderately progressive general revenue system. A surcharge on the income tax could provide any desired amount of extra funding.

If the goal of policy instead was to relate contributions to income but also maintain a dedicated premium for Medicare coverage, the logical approach would be to merge Part A and Part B, make participation in the consolidated program compulsory, and require that enrollees contribute a percentage-of-income premium for the consolidated coverage. A premium for Medicare as a whole would reverse the current strange policy of having beneficiaries pay for Part A coverage only when they are not receiving it (while in the workforce) and pay nothing when they are receiving it. As a matter of principle, it would suggest that individuals who live longer, and therefore receive more protection from Part A, also should contribute more.[16]

Medicare would then be financed by three streams of revenue: a dedicated payroll tax from workers, a percentage-of-income premium from beneficiaries, and a subsidy to the system as a whole from general revenues. The Medicare contribution could be charged either against all income or Social Security benefits. The French and the Germans, among others, collect a small percentage of pension income from retirees as their specific contributions for their benefits, on the principle that solidarity means that everybody should contribute (Fielding and Lancry 1993: 749; Glaser 1991: 121–24).[17]

The great advantage of a percentage-of-income premium, as opposed to a means-tested one, is that the former can be lower than the present flat rate, not just higher. A premium of 3 percent of income in 1998, for example, would have been only $300 per year for a single person with an income of $10,000, as opposed to $525.60 under current law. A couple with the same income would have paid $300 instead of $1,051.20. So percentage-of-income premiums can collect more from those who can afford more and less from those who can afford less. They follow the basic logic of social insurance, in which people contribute according to their ability to pay.

Both percentage-of-income and means-tested premiums would pose administrative challenges. Yet the challenges are much the same for both approaches: how to measure income and collect the contributions.[18] The major administrative difference is that the percentage-of-income approach might reduce costs by limiting or eliminating the need for separate, Medicaid-related premium subsidies for the elderly poor.

On balance, charging one income-related premium for Medicare as a whole, rather than a means-tested premium for Part B, has clear advantages. Most evidently, because wealthier enrollees do benefit substantially from Part A, there would be less reason for them to believe they were getting no benefits for their money. Converting enrollee charges from a flat rate to a percentage of income would also visibly put enrollees on the same basis as workers.

Reducing COLAs

Reducing cost-of-living adjustments sounds like a relatively politically attractive way to cut Social Security benefits, because nobody's check would be reduced from one time period to the next. Instead, people would receive smaller increases—a change that would be much less visible. Policymakers took advantage of that fact when they delayed COLA adjustments by six months as part of the 1983 Social Security rescue package. This was, in essence, a small but permanent benefit cut.

Implications of a Permanent Change in the COLA Formula

A one-time COLA cut or delay, however, is much different from the proposals being made in current debate. The latter involve permanent alterations of the formula to update benefits. In the most common version, each year benefits would be increased not by the increase in the cost of living as calculated by the Bureau of Labor Statistics (BLS) but by that figure minus one percentage point. So a 3 percent rise in the Consumer Price Index (CPI) would yield a 2 percent increase in benefits.[19]

If you believe that the CPI in fact reflects the cost of living, then adjusting by less than the CPI is a hidden way to cut the real value of benefits.[20] Any COLA cut would have its most significant effect on older retirees. For example, if the inflation rate were 3 percent, and each year benefits were raised by only 2 percent, then after ten years real benefits would have fallen by 9 percent. After twenty years, they would have declined by 18 percent. Older beneficiaries are disproportionately in poverty and rely more than younger beneficiaries on Social Security (SSA/ORES 1998a: 104, 131). Erosion of their other assets over time is one reason they are more likely to be poor. Therefore, *COLA reductions target benefit cuts on those people who can least afford them.* If we believe that one of the major purposes of Social Security is to serve as insurance against the risk of outliving one's savings, then a policy of adjusting benefits by less than the rate of inflation must be a basic change in the program's purposes.

The only way to justify systematically reducing COLAs as "saving" Social Security is to believe, like Senator Daniel Patrick Moynihan (D-N.Y.), that the Consumer Price Index systematically overstates inflation. If it does, then COLAs equal to the CPI increase each year would be real benefit increases, and smaller adjustments would still hold beneficiaries harmless.[21]

The Cost-of-Living Debate

There is indeed reason to believe that the Bureau of Labor Statistics has, in the past, calculated the Consumer Price Indices in ways that slightly overstated inflation. The BLS therefore has been implementing a series of changes that are expected to reduce measured rates of inflation in the future. These changes alone, without any policy changes, will improve Social Security's expected finances by reducing projected future benefit increases relative to wages.[22]

Implications of the Boskin Commission Report

Why, then, should adjustments be made by fiat, rather than by the BLS altering its methods as it has in the past? Moynihan and other advocates of

COLA reduction responded that we know that the CPI overstates inflation and that 1 percentage point is a good ballpark estimate of the error. So, rather than waste money now, the government should make the fix and let the measurements catch up.[23] They cited the report of a commission that the Senate Finance Committee appointed in +1995 to review the issue. This commission, chaired by Michael Boskin, who had been chair of the Council of Economic Advisers for President Bush, estimated that the CPI overstated inflation by about 1.1 percentage points per year.[24] Yet if the Boskin Commission's figures were true, there would be no problem needing solution.

If inflation projections for the future are high by 1.1 percentage points per year, then real-wage growth would be that much higher each year. If that was true, Dean Baker estimates, then before-tax average real wages, instead of growing by 40 percent from 1995 to 2030, would more than double. "Even after factoring in the necessary increases in payroll taxes they still will have risen by 98%" (1998: 22). Then paying higher taxes for Social Security and Medicare would not be a serious burden on future workers, because they would be so much better off than average workers today.

Indeed, if the CPI adjustments have been so excessive, then the past quarter-century has been a much more pleasant time, economically, than virtually anyone has realized. Both wages and productivity have grown much more quickly. There has been no productivity crisis caused by lower national savings (or anything else).[25] But maybe times have not been so good. There are lots of reasons to doubt the Boskin Commission figures.

Critiques of the Boskin Estimates

To begin with, they are high compared to other estimates. If we add the Boskin Commission estimates to the corrections made by the BLS in 1995–96 and scheduled for 1997, the previous error would be as much as 1.79 percentage points.[26] By way of comparison, a Federal Reserve Board study before the BLS actions expressed the possible range as 0.4 to 1.5 percentage points; the Dallas Federal Reserve Bank suggested that the figure would be less than 1 percent; and the Congressional Budget Office reported that available empirical studies might support an overestimate of between 0.2 and 0.8 percent (Abraham 1995: 61–62; see also CBO 1994).[27]

Boskin and his colleagues also took some logical concerns to illogical extremes. One instance involved "substitution effects." If the price of one product goes up, so that you buy another, what you as a consumer lose is not the difference between the new and old prices of the first product but something more like the difference between how you valued the original product at its old price and the substituted product at its old price. This has to be less than the difference between the old product's old and new prices (or you would have just paid the new price for the old product, instead of substituting). As Boskin puts it, "by substituting chicken, you partially insulate your family from the rise in beef prices" (1996).

Yet there must be some limit on "substitution" logic. One critic of the Boskin report commented, "A chicken/beef example makes it too easy. . . . If the price of gasoline should soar again, and consumers switch to public transit, bicycles, and walking, should such substitution 'fix' the CPI weights to make gasoline inflation disappear?" Indeed, research in 1972 showed that some elderly persons were substituting canned dog food for meat, "a cheaper substitute that they considered sanitary because it was canned" (Freedman 1996: 61). Was price no problem for those seniors?

The report also emphasized that some prices rise because of quality improvements. Automobiles are more reliable, and televisions have clearer pictures, than they did in the past. Yet the BLS does make quality adjustments. In 1995 these were so extensive that "the reported rate of inflation was reduced by 1.9 percentage points—to 2.5 percent from 4.4 percent—according to BLS calculations" (Berry 1996: E10). On what basis, then, could the five economists on the commission show that their judgment was more accurate than that of the bureau?[28]

Not much. Experts can differ on, say, the "quality improvement" from the invention of Honey Cinnamon Cheerios (Deaton 1998: 38; yes, they actually argue about such things). But critics identified clear errors in the commission's work. For instance, it assumed that the CPI procedures did not consider improvements in automobile durability, when in fact they did (Abraham, Greenlees, and Moulton 1998: 32). The commission also assumed that residential rents should rise proportionally with square footage as a "quality improvement," whereas real estate professionals assert that "price per square foot goes down as square footage increases." Boskin replied that "for every one of these things someone can quibble about on the downside, we left out as many on the upside" (Berry 1996: E10). But why would they do that? In fact, how would he even know that? If he could count mistakes, why were they made? One outsider commented that the BLS, under attack for its own estimates, would have had much more trouble defending itself "had the Commissioner had to defend in public testimony the sort of fragmentary research estimates on which the Boskin Commission based its conclusions" (Deaton 1998: 38).

Quality in some areas may have increased but in others may have declined. As one critic asked, "Has no member of the commission taken an airplane trip recently? Had any difficulty making a reservation, getting a seat, fitting into it, trying to schedule trips in the most time-efficient way? Has no member of the commission been hungry on an airplane . . . ?" (Freedman 1996: 6). Critics also point out that most of the goods for which quality may have improved greatly are more relevant to higher-income persons. Computers have improved, and there are more prepared foods in the gourmet section, but "meat and potatoes are still meat and potatoes" (Berry 1996: E10).

Therefore, although some economists believed the Boskin report's estimates were reasonable,[29] they in no way represent a consensus analysis of trends for the population at large. Moreover, costs of living for seniors appear to rise slightly more quickly than for the population at large, because what the elderly actually consume is different.[30]

COLA Changes Should Be Left to the Experts

The 1994–96 Advisory Council reported that "maintaining full cost-of-living adjustments (COLAs) throughout the period of benefit receipt is one of Social Security's most important contributions to individual security." Social Security is one of the very few pension sources with inflation-proof benefits; thus, it is a safety net even for people with relatively good private pensions. The Advisory Council added that

The Council . . . supports current efforts to remove bias from the CPI and believes that the Social Security cost-of-living adjustment (COLA) should follow the changes in the CPI made by the Bureau of Labor Statistics (BLS) wherever they may lead. The Council, however, does not support changes in the COLA motivated by political considerations. No matter how well-intentioned or even how accurate such changes might later prove to be, the Council believes it would be a bad precedent. Changes should be made only as a result of careful expert consideration by the government agency charged with that task. (Advisory Council on Social Security 1997a: 17–18)

Rather than correcting a technical flaw in benefit calculation, automatic reductions of COLAs below the measured increase in the cost of living would threaten Social Security's most basic functions: insuring all retirees against economic risk (inflation) and demographic risk (outliving one's other savings). It is the worst possible way to cut benefits.

Of the three proposals discussed in this chapter, only legislation of smaller cost-of-living adjustments should be dismissed out of hand.

The "new means-testing" approach to Social Security and Medicare is far more dangerous than its proponents will admit. Yet the net benefits of Medicare should be related more closely to income. This could best be achieved by combining Parts A and B and charging an income-related premium for the combination. This new premium could be set at a level that would increase Medicare's revenues.

Raising the age of eligibility for Medicare would endanger the many persons who could obtain no comparable insurance. Yet, nothing in the case for social insurance determines at what age individuals should be eligible for pensions, so raising the age of eligibility for Social Security is a less radical reform than, say, than means-testing. Nevertheless, raising the normal retirement age or the early eligibility age for Social Security would pose significant problems for those workers who do not "sit on their butts all day."

The best response to this dilemma, on the benefit side, would be to change the basis of eligibility from age alone to a mix of age and years in the workforce. That is common in other pension plans and would eliminate much of the class-based inequity that is inherent in basing eligibility on age alone. Because that would be a significant change in the rules of eligibility for Social Security, however, it would require more study and development before any proposal could be debated and adopted.

This chapter has identified two areas, income-relation of Medicare premiums and the basis of eligibility for Social Security benefits, where early action should be considered but immediate action would be unwise. Time is needed to work out the best approaches.

PART IV

Responsible Reform

ELEVEN

Moderate, Though Hardly Modest, Reforms

After all the dramatic ideas such as privatization and changing the entitlements to Social Security and Medicare have been considered, there remain the traditional ways of controlling or avoiding deficits in those programs: spending less on benefits or collecting larger contributions.

I have argued that Medicare benefits are too limited to justify cuts. There are many dangerous ways to cut Social Security benefits as well, such as reducing COLAs. Yet there are other, more moderate measures, that are less dangerous and more justifiable.

Privatization of Social Security is too dangerous, but a modest amount of diversification of the trust funds could be helpful. I have argued that privatization of Medicare, whether by a defined contribution or by "premium support," is an idea whose time has not come. Yet Medicare has some attributes that might best be reformed even if we were not worried about costs. If these reforms also help solve some of the problems of a premium-support type approach, all the better. There are reasons not to rely on payroll taxes to cover all future cost increases for social insurance. Yet we can justify scheduling small increases in revenues that would at least reduce future shortfalls in each program.

This chapter therefore suggests a moderate reform agenda for Social Security and Medicare. Taken as a whole, it is not so modest at all. It provides plenty of potential work for American politicians and policy commentators. The possible roads to and consequences of this reform package are considered in chapter 12.

Incremental Reforms to Social Security

Although the 1994–96 Advisory Council on Social Security produced three different comprehensive reform plans, all three included some common elements. Each of these elements has its critics, but they nevertheless should be adopted.

In chapter 3 I explain why it makes more sense to estimate overall reform packages on a pay-as-you-go basis than in the common terms, which describe how reforms would improve long-term actuarial balance by some fraction of taxable payroll. As I note there, however, individual provisions are best explained in the standard terms, because that allows us to compare provisions most easily.

Cover All State and Local Workers

All three factions of the Advisory Council recommended that participation in Social Security be made mandatory for employees of state and local governments. Inclusion has not previously been made compulsory because of "an earlier belief that Federal compulsion of the States to participate might not be Constitutional" (Advisory Council on Social Security 1997a: 19). Recent court decisions, however, have led most observers to believe the courts would uphold mandatory inclusion of state and local employees (GAO 1998b: 19–20).

At present, about 70 percent of state and local workers are already covered anyway, but the rest, about 5 million workers, are not.[1] The Advisory Council argued that

> To the extent feasible, everyone who works for pay should be covered by the Social Security program. Every occupational group contains substantial numbers of people who at one time or another will need the protection of the program. Over the course of a lifetime, it is impossible to foresee who will and who will not need this coverage. Moreover, all Americans have an obligation to participate, since an effective Social Security program helps to reduce public costs for relief and assistance, which, in turn, means lower general taxes. (1997a: 19, 20)

Advocates of including state and local employees can also point out that if you see the program as an intergenerational compact, workers who are not part of the system are not contributing as they should for their own parents.

The most immediate practical reason to include all state and local employees, however, is that almost all of them end up being included, either as workers or as dependents, anyway. But, as the General Accounting Office reports, if their government job is their main career, their second job will likely have relatively low earnings even if their career did not, so they would be favored by the benefits formula even though their earnings were in fact higher than average. If they qualify as spouses, they will often get spousal benefits even though, if they had contributed to Social Security instead, the pensions based on their own earnings would have exceeded the spousal benefit. Congress's efforts to reduce such "windfalls" to state and local government workers have proved very difficult to administer. Mandatory coverage would have some administrative costs of its own, but in the long run it would reduce the inequities of the present situation (GAO 1998b: 10, 12).

Mandatory coverage of state and local government employees would improve Social Security's finances both because of the elimination of windfalls and because the newly covered employees would contribute for many years, raising surpluses and thus interest earnings, before collecting benefits. The Social Security Advisory Board estimated in 1998 that it would save about 0.21 percent of taxable payroll.

This proposal would have negative impacts on either state and local governments or pensioners, because the former in essence have been financing pensions for their employees without contributing to the costs of current Social Security benefits. GAO guesstimates that additional costs for state and local governments (or employees, in higher contributions or lower eventual benefits) would be between 2 and 7 percent of the affected payroll, probably closer to the latter. There would also be some difficulties in integrating Social Security benefits with those pensions that are currently available to some workers, especially police officers and firefighters, well before the Normal Retirement Age; and transition issues for some advance-funded state and local plans (1998b: 13–19). Yet the fairness arguments for including all state and local employees seem strong, as is shown by the fact that all members of the Advisory Council endorsed the proposal.

Lengthen the Period for Benefits Computation

Another option calls for increasing the averaging period for calculating average indexed earnings (AIME) from 35 years to 38. Under current law, people
count their highest 35 years of earnings; the effect of adding three more years
can only be to lower the average and, as a result, reduce benefits. On average,
the SSA actuaries project that lengthening the period for the AIME calculation to 38 years would reduce benefits by 3 percent.

This reduction would be larger for people with intermittent earnings. For
example, a Congressional Research Service (CRS) report noted,

> A worker retiring at age 65 in 1998 with a 35-year career of average earnings
> would receive a monthly benefit of $938. If the averaging period were 38 years
> in length, this worker would have 3 years of zeros in his or her earnings record,
> and . . . the worker would receive $885 in monthly benefits, representing a
> 6 percent reduction from the current law level. (Koitz 1998: 11)

Edith Fierst dissented in the Advisory Council report, on the grounds that
women are especially likely to have interrupted work records, and "the option
of child care provided by the mother, especially in early childhood years, is a
choice families should be able to make" (1997: 137). That objection, however,
should be put into the perspective of the entire Social Security program, which
already leans toward favoring women, including those who work in the home.
The average benefit reduction for men would be 3 percent and for women 3.9
percent.

As benefit reductions go, this one may seem relatively justified. People who
work more are affected less. That can be contrasted to privatization schemes
in which, on average, people with higher salaries get more. Moreover, there is
no obvious class-based effect: it is possible, for example, that high-income people who take time off would be at least as affected as low-income people. The
only very clear bias is that people like myself who spend too long in graduate
school would lose. But, to the extent that such people have desk jobs, they are
the people who should be able to work past age 65 more easily. Because people with hard physical jobs are likely to have started work earlier, the 38-year
rule seems unlikely to discriminate against them. So, on balance, this is a fair
benefit cut, and it was estimated in 1998 to reduce the long-term actuarial im-

balance by 0.25 percent of taxable payroll (Social Security Advisory Board 1998).[2]

Increase the Taxation of Social Security Benefits

There is also particularly good reason to alter the taxation of Social Security benefits so that the tax is modestly increased. At present, benefits are taxed only if they raise the adjusted gross incomes of individuals above $25,000 and of couples above $32,000. And only 85 percent of those benefits are subject to tax even so. As the Advisory Council explained,

> the goal was to tax Social Security recipients in a way similar to the recipients of other contributory defined pension benefit plans—that is, including as taxable income recipients' benefits to the extent that they exceed what workers had paid in. However, Congress chose a proxy of 85 percent of benefits as representing amounts not attributable to employee contributions, rather than having taxes on benefits computed individually. (1997a: 20–21)

All members of the Advisory Council proposed phasing out the income thresholds. The Advisory Council estimated that 30 percent of beneficiaries still would pay no taxes on their benefits because their incomes would be below the thresholds for income taxation anyway. Eight of the thirteen Advisory Council members also proposed replacing the 85 percent rule with a more exact calculation. This measure should slightly favor higher-income beneficiaries, but accuracy still seems desirable when achievable.[3] The Social Security Advisory Board estimated in 1998 that combining these measures would save 0.35 percent of payroll.

It is hard to imagine a more easily defensible benefit cut or tax increase (take your pick). It does not violate the original promises of the program; it will mostly affect people who can afford it; it is hardly discrimination to treat Social Security benefits like other pension income; and it may be the "fairest way to ask present retirees to share in the cost" of improving Social Security's financial condition (Advisory Council on Social Security 1997a: 20).

Benefits of These Broadly Acceptable Reforms to Social Security

Some other reforms may be worth enacting, even if they do not yield estimates of significant savings. For instance, seniors might be allowed to take the extra benefits from working past the Normal Retirement Age as a lump-sum payment rather than an increase in each month's benefit spread over many years. The prospect of cash on hand may be more attractive than increased monthly payments, even if their actuarial values are equal. The extra work effort then would (very modestly) increase national income (Etheredge 1999: 85–86).

It was estimated in 1998 that the Social Security provisions discussed in this section would reduce the long-term actuarial imbalance by 0.81 percent of taxable payroll. Chapter 12 provides a rough estimate of their usefulness on a pay-as-you-go basis. But if we compare the standard figure to the estimated shortfall at that point of 2.19 percent of taxable payroll, we can see that these incremental measures are at least useful.

Improving the Options on Medicare

Legislation to replace the current Medicare system with some sort of voucher design would not, at present, be responsible: there is little evidence that it would actually save money, and it might make Medicare much less adequate for poorer, less healthy enrollees.

Yet the current Medicare design is flawed, especially with regard to the gaps in the benefit package but in other ways as well. The 1997 Balanced Budget Act attempts to correct some of those flaws and thus allow more informed choice later about further reforms. That effort should be intensified.

Make the BBA-97 Work

The first step would be to aid in making BBA-97 work by helping HCFA do its job. Medicare experts of all political persuasions agree that HCFA needs more resources to fulfill the tasks it was given under the 1997 Balanced Budget Act (Butler et al. 1999). HCFA should be given the extra hundreds of millions of dollars, and perhaps the administrative flexibility, that it needs.

Maintain (Mostly) the BBA-97's Cost Controls

The interests whose income is being constrained by the BBA-97 have been very vocal in asserting that it is unfair and that Medicare beneficiaries are the real losers (Goldstein 1999b). In itself, this is not surprising: what else would you expect those interests to say? In a few cases, especially where a cost control was expected to be only a stop-gap and HCFA was supposed to develop an alternative, the complaints may be justified.[4] In other cases, however, the federal government is really being asked to subsidize providers' losses in the private markets, or to guarantee profits on Medicare services even if they are inefficient.

Given that savings since the enactment of BBA-97 have greatly exceeded the projections at the time, there was room for modest "givebacks." However, the analytic case for most of that legislation's measures, such as lower Prospective Payment System (PPS) hospital updates and tighter constraints on home health spending, was strong. Any retreat from the savings in the BBA-97 should be cautious and modest.

The complaints from managed-care companies have been loudest of all, because they can dramatize their pleas by withdrawing from the Medicare + Choice program.[5] But that is no reason to overpay plans. If they can provide the Medicare benefit package more efficiently than traditional Medicare, they should be able to win customers and make money; those that cannot compete on those terms should not be paid extra to participate.

Follow Through on, and Expand, Experiments to Improve Competition

We already have competing plans within Medicare, in the form of Medicare + Choice. Measures that would make Medicare + Choice work better would also improve any future system of competing plans. Thus, the BBA-97's "competitive pricing" demonstrations must be fully implemented. Although there are many reasons to worry about a system in which plans' premiums would in some sense depend on their bids, the only way to find out if those problems could be solved is by testing approaches.[6]

Although the BBA-97 mandated that the secretary of Health and Human Services "broadly disseminate information" about plans, HCFA was only able to pilot-test informational materials in 1998. Its proposals for performance measurement were highly controversial (Dallek 1998). We do not even know whether it is possible to develop measures that potential enrollees will find useful. All of these are good reasons to encourage further experiments with different approaches in different markets. All such efforts should be accompanied by rigorous evaluation, including surveys of Medicare enrollees that determine what they learn from and how they use any information that they receive as part of the efforts to "make the market work."

A further issue about competing plans is how individuals can address perceived problems with their care. Again, the BBA-97 required the creation of an appeals process; again, time spent testing alternatives would be time well spent. Where that requires specific legislation (as it would for placing malpractice liability upon plans), Congress and the president should be disposed to provide that authority, so long as it is in limited places for limited periods of time.

In all these cases, there is little chance that experiments or demonstrations could be developed and yield clear answers in less than five years. Fortunately, in view of the current conditions of both the federal budget and the HI trust fund, there is time to get the reforms right.

Remove Noninsurance Functions from Medicare

The difficulties of paying combination plans in Medicare + Choice or in a different competing-plans design are exacerbated by Medicare's noninsurance functions, such as funding medical education and medical capital development.

I recognize the political advantages of funding these policies through Medicare. Medicare provides entitlement budget authority, so these purposes do not require annual appropriation. To the extent that this spending can be defined as part of the "cost" of care, it can be justified as part of Medicare's purposes rather than as a new federal program requiring more debate. Hiding medical education and supply issues within the arcane world of Medicare payment formulas also protects the participants in these battles from much public scrutiny. Any shift of these expenses out of Medicare would require difficult political steps such as increases in the caps on discretionary spending or the creation of new entitlements with dedicated funding. Nevertheless, in each case the advantages of greater accountability for the individual functions and greater flexibility for future Medicare reform justify removing these noninsurance functions from Medicare.

Medical education could be financed through an academic health services trust fund, which would receive contributions from all health-care purchasers or from general revenues, or both (Commonwealth Fund 1997).[7] There are good reasons to suspect that Medicare pays more than its proportional share of education costs now, so it would save a little money from a sensible reform.[8] After that reform, there would be no need for arguments about whether medical education costs should be included in the premiums paid to combination plans.

Medicare's role in medical capital investment is equally complex and sensitive. Yet it does not make a whole lot of sense to see capital as a Medicare cost. If hospitals can sell enough services to justify an investment, fine; if they cannot, they should not make the investment. Medicare should be blind to whether a hospital provides services using new facilities or old. If the government wants to finance construction or rehabilitation of existing plant, it should do that as part of a separate program of aid to rural areas or urban areas or whatever.

Before social insurance or the government paid most of the bills for patients in almost all countries, poor people went to hospitals that received government (in the United States, usually city or county) subsidies. DSH payments are a way to maintain that old system, which is necessary in the United States because we do not have national health insurance. The central cities and counties can no longer afford to support hospitals because so much of their tax bases have moved to the suburbs and because medicine has become much more expensive.

Advocates for the poor (and the facilities that serve them) worry that if the subsidies are not hidden within Medicare, they will be far less generous. I am afraid of that too, but I am willing to take the risk. I do not think DSH would be abolished if taken out of Medicare; and once it was made separate, it would be harder to ignore the harsh policy choice that it represents. DSH is an acknowledgment that the United States has an early-twentieth-century healthcare finance system for a large part of its twenty-first-century population. Let us make that clear.

Moreover, so long as DSH is financed through Medicare, advocates for social insurance will face an unfair bind. If they strive to make the DSH safety net more adequate, then "Medicare" spending per beneficiary will rise and "government" will look less efficient compared to the private sector—even though the DSH money is going not for Medicare beneficiaries but for people who are not eligible for Medicare, who are supposed to be covered by the private sector. And again, having DSH within Medicare potentially complicates the payment of combination plans. On the whole, I would rather make DSH separate.

Merge Parts A and B

As former Medicare Trustee Marilyn Moon and many other analysts have noted, "it makes little sense to maintain two separate parts to the program . . . over time, they have become closely linked, and changes in Part A affect Part B and vice versa" (Moon and Mulvey 1995: 111). Many Washington budgeteers like having a separate HI trust fund, so that they can argue that "Medicare's" future bankruptcy requires change in both HI and SMI policies. But it is not an honest argument and does not work so well anyway, and its dubious merits are not worth the flaws in the current separate arrangements.

Merging Parts A and B would have no immediate effect on 94 percent of Medicare enrollees, who already have both HI and SMI coverage.[9] About 2 million, however, are enrolled in HI but not in SMI. They generally have other coverage, so by refusing SMI they avoid paying the Part B premium. A small proportion of enrollees are in SMI but not HI, or HI but not SMI, for more peculiar reasons.[10] In the vast majority of these cases, the employers who provide the alternative coverage could restructure it as more generous wraparound coverage or even reimburse Medicare enrollees for their premiums.

With Parts A and B merged, it would also make sense to replace the separate HI and SMI deductibles with a single deductible (probably around $400). That would eliminate one of the flaws in the current benefit package, the high deductible for hospitalizations.[11]

Income-Related Premiums

As previous chapters have argued, the current flat premium for SMI is too high for some people to pay and less than others could pay; thus it violates the basic social-insurance principle that people should contribute according to their ability to pay.

Instead, the Medicare premium should be a proportion of enrollees' income. That would pose measurement problems, and it might be unpopular with the millions of enrollees whose incomes are low enough that they do not file tax returns now. But because many would benefit from paying lower premiums, the hassle of filing Form 1040 EZ seems fair.

On balance, a percentage-of-income Medicare premium would be fairer and more flexible than the alternatives. Many questions would still have to be answered. How large should it be? At a minimum it should raise the same percentage of Medicare costs as the current premium schedule (about 12% after the switch of home health–care costs to SMI is fully implemented).[12] Would a fairly low percentage raise enough money to justify abolishing the separate subsidies for the poor through the Qualified Medicare Beneficiary (QMB) and the Specified Low-Income Beneficiary (SLMB) programs? How should covered income be calculated? It would take some time to develop the answers to those questions. Nevertheless, a percentage-of-income premium is much more consistent with the ideals of social insurance than the current flat premium is, and it has practical advantages compared to either means-testing the premiums or instituting specific subsidies for the poor.

Medium-Term Spending Targets

Many analysts of health-care cost-control issues believe that total spending can and should be set in legislation.[13] It is tempting, then, to suggest that legislation should establish that Medicare spending may grow by no more than the standard that I have suggested, enrollment plus the growth of per capita income plus 1 percent per year.

I do not recommend that, for a few reasons. First, it can be perverse in times of recession and recovery. In addition, global caps are meaningless without detailed enforcement. Detailed enforcement involves controlling the components of costs, such as hospital and physician and home health services. It would be too easy to misjudge future trends in technology or demand and therefore plan for too much spending in one service and too little in another. It would be especially difficult to enforce specific targets fairly if healthier people are selecting themselves into combination plans, thus driving up the average utilization of other services in traditional Medicare.

Therefore, rather than suggest that Medicare spending targets be enacted for the ten years from 2002–12, I recommend only that policymakers plan to enact legislation in 2002 designed to restrain costs per enrollee to the 1 percent standard for the following five years.[14] But Medicare commentators should also make it clear that this is a responsible and attainable standard. If Medicare spending grows by 1 percent a year above the growth of both enrollment and per capita GDP, there will be extra money each year for the medical establishment and for extra services. This is not a draconian standard at all.

Medicare Summary

Some of the structural reforms that I recommend could be used to improve Medicare's financial balances. For example, restructured premiums could raise some extra money; if other payers contribute some of the graduate medical education funds that are presently paid by Medicare, that would represent a spending savings for the government.

The point of the structural reforms and experiments that I have suggested is not, however, to save money. My goals instead are to resolve some nagging problems and to bring Medicare to a point at which it will be possible to make better-informed decisions about moving to a different kind of basic program design, which might rely more on competing plans. If we chose not to do so, these reforms would still have improved the program.

Collecting More Money

The simplest way to address the future costs of Social Security and Medicare would be to raise the OASDI and HI payroll taxes however much is necessary to cover those programs' expenses. I have argued that the potential burden of such tax increases on future workers has been greatly overstated. Moreover, if we think of income and health-care support for the elderly as a good thing that is best guaranteed by government, then the aging of America's population means there is more need for that good thing. If voters like it, they may choose to pay for it.

Politicians today, including President Clinton, seem to be especially loath to increase payroll taxes. But the fact is that Social Security and Medicare payroll taxes have been increased frequently—certainly more often, and more significantly, than benefits to enrollees have been reduced. And although payroll tax increases are unpopular in principle, they are by no means less popular than benefit cuts. In the specific case of Social Security, public opinion expert Ben Page of Northwestern University reports, "When forced to choose between benefit cuts and tax increases, a large majority of Americans—63 percent to 32 percent in one 1997 survey—choose payroll tax increases" (1999: 20).

It will be easier to justify higher taxes to pay for higher per-enrollee costs for Medicare if we know that all sensible measures to control those costs have been taken. But unless eligibility is greatly restricted, it is obvious that some increased revenues will be needed to finance Medicare. As Lynn Etheredge writes, "a constant 1.45 percent (employer/employee) tax rate can hardly be expected to finance coverage for doubling the number of [HI] enrollees" (1999: 82). The benefit cuts needed to finance Social Security entirely at current tax rates would be draconian. Therefore, some increase in revenues must be on the table for reform.

Yet there are good distributional reasons not to rely on payroll tax increases to finance all future increases in Medicare and Social Security costs. The HI tax favors people who earn from investments over workers of all types, and the OASDI contributions take a larger share of income from workers below than above the cap. Because the payroll tax base is projected to shrink relative to national income, it will become somewhat less fair than it is today. Taxes on income in particular may also, at the margin, discourage work and employment, compared to alternatives such as consumption taxes. Thus, distributional arguments may favor raising income taxes instead, whereas economic arguments may favor financing increased costs through consumption taxes.

A sensible response to these concerns would be to plan to raise other taxes to finance some of the future increased costs of Medicare and Social Security. That is the implication of current law for Part B anyway and, as chapter 2 explained, it is also a misunderstood aspect of any use of trust-fund interest or balances to pay OASDI benefits.

But what would those future general revenues be? Higher income taxes? Distributed how? A new national Value Added Tax? If any decision ought to be left to voters in twenty or thirty years, it would be what *general* taxes they would choose to raise, if any.

Long-term legislation of payroll tax increases is much less problematic, as is shown by the fact it has been part of Social Security since the program's inception. Current policymakers, therefore, should seek the most justified set of payroll tax increases, covering a portion of future cost increases.

Paying for an Aging Society

Consider first the argument about raising the age of eligibility. Longer retirements will cost more. Proponents of raising the age of eligibility believe that the right response is to shorten retirements. Voters seem to disagree. Benjamin Page reports that "at least eighteen different surveys during the last two decades have asked about increasing the retirement age for Social Security, and all but two have found majorities opposed—usually very large majorities." The two exceptions had quite leading question wording (1999: 15). Voters may prefer to pay a larger share of their income while working, in order to maintain a social contract in which later workers do the same and each group gets to live a larger portion of their lives in retirement.

Some adjustment to reflect increased life expectancy after the baby boom retires is appropriate, but it should be more complex than simply raising the Normal Retirement Age and the Early Eligibility Age (see chapter 10). A balanced mix of measures—both payroll tax increases and a change in the terms of eligibility—might both be the best policy and seem the fairest to citizens. Devising such a package would require very complex choices. Fortunately, policymakers have time to study the issue and consider the choices.

Congress and the president, therefore, should appoint a new advisory council. That council may be asked to look at other issues as well, such as whether survivors' benefits should be increased and the extra payment to couples reduced.[15] But its major charge should be to devise a set of options to cope with the financial impact of longer life spans.

The options should not be expected to provide any extra savings or revenues until the already-scheduled increase in the retirement age is fully implemented, in 2022. Congress and the president should include in the legislation that creates this advisory council a target level of improvement in trust-fund finances. I would set a target of 1.5 percent of payroll, phased in by 2040.[16] It would be perfectly legitimate for the package to raise payroll taxes somewhat more early in the period and then lower them later, as the effects of eligibility changes are phased in. The advisory council should be instructed to prepare a legislative proposal and two alternatives, and the legislation that creates the council should include provisions for guaranteed and expedited consideration of the proposals on the House and Senate floors. Similar "fast track" devices have been used for measures such as trade agreements and legislation to close military bases.

Medicare Payroll Taxes

Raising Medicare payroll taxes is less problematic and requires fewer trade-offs. Because it applies to all wages, the HI payroll tax is less regressive than the OASDI levies. If the HI tax is replaced with a dedicated Medicare contribution, as HI and SMI are merged, then we need not worry about precisely covering current "HI" costs. But that does not mean the dedicated contribution should be left at the same level forever. In 1999 the Medicare actuaries forecast that HI costs will rise to 3.6 percent of payroll in 2015 and 4.0 percent in 2020. If anything, costs may rise more quickly. So, at a minimum, it would be fair to schedule an HI/Medicare payroll tax increase of 0.1 percent of payroll each year from 2015 through 2019, resulting in a steady 3.4 percent from 2019 on.

Raising the OASDI Income Threshold

Another particularly strong case for payroll tax increases involves the proportion of wage income that is subject to the OASDI payroll taxes. The fact that a disproportionate share of wage increases in the 1980s and 1990s went to the workers with the highest wages means that the proportion of wage income subject to payroll tax has declined. At one time, the base for OASDI contributions included 90 percent of total wages in covered employment. That figure is now projected to fall to under 85 percent of wages (Ball 1998: 24).

If the wage threshold was raised by somewhat more than average wage increases for a number of years, that increase would eventually require higher benefit payments as well. Yet raising the threshold would raise benefits by significantly less than revenues. Robert Ball and Thomas Bethel (Ball 1998: 244) have proposed raising the threshold an extra 2 percent beyond wage growth each year from 2000 to 2009, which would eventually cover 87.3 percent of wage income and reduce the projected long-term OASDI deficit by 0.27 percent of payroll.

The downside of raising the OASDI threshold for covered wages is that it would lower the rate of return for higher-income enrollees. Moreover, it would target the higher taxes particularly on what we might call lower-income higher-income people: people in that category today have incomes between $70,000 and $110,000 per year.

So the effect of raising the OASDI thresholds should be muted in comparison to Ball's plan, perhaps by both raising them less and slightly increasing the resulting benefits. I propose instead that the financial goal be less than half of that in Ball's plan. Alternatively, policies to raise the payroll cap and increase the taxation of benefits might be considered together, so as to calibrate the overall distributional impacts. I suggest that reforms aim for a total savings, from the two measures, of about 0.45 percent of payroll, compared to the 0.35 percent that has been estimated for taxation of benefits alone.

Diversifying the Social Security Trust Funds

There would be advantages in diversifying the portfolios of the Social Security trust funds by allowing some investment of the money in equities (see chapter 8). Critics fear that the accumulation of investments would give the government too much power, but in my view these concerns are excessive. They can also be limited by limiting the size of the fund that is created.

The amount that President Clinton proposed to invest as of early 1999, about $600 billion over the following fifteen years, was large enough to help but small enough to limit to a manageable level the risks that critics fear. My version of this proposal differs from the rather amorphous descriptions of the president's that were available in May of 1999. I suggest a specific schedule of investments: $40 billion in each year from 2004 through 2008 and $50 billion in each year from 2009 through 2016. I also would use the fund the way universities use endowments. Rather than to let the money accumulate and then draw down the balance, I would allow withdrawals from the fund, to fund Social Security benefits, at a rate that would allow the fund to maintain a constant size relative to the economy. In the specific scenario that I calculate in chapter 12, the privately invested trust-fund balance would reach just below 9 percent of GDP in 2028. Then the policy goal would be to maintain the balance at that level; excess earnings could then be used to finance Social Security benefits. These earnings would, in the calculations described in chapter 12, be about 0.45 percent of GDP.

The size of this fund should not be worrisome except to those who are already worried about existing private and government-managed investments. For example, Fidelity managed $522 billion as of September 30, 1997. Unless the market slumps severely, Fidelity will already be managing over $600 billion at the time the SSA would begin a thirteen-year period of investing $600 billion. At the same time, state and local pension plans already held a larger share of the economy in equities than the federal government would at the final level of my proposal, and the former assets would likely grow much larger in the future.[17]

During periods when returns were low, such that withdrawing the normal amount would dangerously deplete the fund, that amount could be made up by government borrowing with only minimal effects on the economy.[18] Therefore, neither the government's incentive to interfere with markets nor its vulnerability would be great. Economic events raise or lower deficits by more than half a percent of GDP frequently.

The benefits from trust-fund diversification depend, of course, on the return that would be received on the equities. I have assumed that the return would be three percentage points above the rate of interest on federal debt. This seems a moderate position. It is well below the actuaries' assumption and slightly below the General Accounting Office's low-return scenario, which was 3.295 percent above the assumed interest rate on Treasury Securities (GAO 1998a). However, it is not quite as pessimistic an assumption as might be derived from entirely accepting Dean Baker's critique. An income stream after 2028 of about 0.45 percent of GDP would be more than 1 percent of taxable payroll. It would make other, more painful, measures unnecessary. It is a limited and responsible measure that would make the partial prefunding of benefits more effective.[19]

Other Options

The federal government's efforts to aid seniors are not limited to Medicare and Social Security. In addition to programs that help elderly poor people (such as Medicaid, Meals on Wheels, SSI, and Food Stamps), the government provides tax breaks meant to either enable the elderly to keep more of their income or encourage retirement saving. Unlike Social Security and Medicare, other pension arrangements in many ways favor higher-income at the expense of lower-income workers. Lynn Etheredge comments that "if cutbacks are on the table for basic benefits . . . taxpayer support for supplemental pension benefits should be subjected to new scrutiny" (1999: 90, 91). Another possibility is to restrain tax breaks specifically for seniors. Although there are some countervailing ways that the tax code favors young people, on balance it seems to favor the elderly, and it would not make much sense to ignore that while claiming that Social Security and Medicare put horrible burdens on workers.[20]

When I began writing this book, therefore, I expected to recommend some of these nonentitlement reforms, on the grounds that they would address the real problem, overall federal finance, but do less damage to social insurance. Given the 1999 forecasts of surpluses, however, it was not clear what the federal government would do with extra savings. It makes more sense either to keep these options in reserve in case budgetary conditions worsen significantly or to use them to finance policy initiatives that otherwise would increase future budgetary risks.[21]

In this chapter I suggest moderate reforms to Social Security that, though hardly noncontroversial or painless, would qualify as incremental changes and have relatively broad support. I also identify an ambitious agenda of structural reforms for Medicare. These could be expected to yield modest savings at best, but they involve both issues that would have to be addressed in any shift to a voucher approach and attributes of Medicare that fit poorly with a social insurance scheme. So there is good reason to address these matters first; events to come will provide better guidance about the best approach for future Medicare cost control.

Both public opinion and common sense suggest that there should be some role for increased revenues in financing a larger population of Medicare and Social Security beneficiaries. I propose a small Medicare payroll tax increase from 2015 to 2019 and argue that higher contributions should be considered as part of a response to the effects of increased life expectancy on Social Security finance.

Finally, I endorse a modest amount of Social Security trust-fund diversification, in order to improve the prefunding of benefits.

In chapter 12 I fit these proposals into the case for moderate reform in two ways: I estimate how they would improve the underlying budget situation, leaving room for future voters to make their own decisions, and I suggest a path for debating and implementing the reforms.

TWELVE

Real Responsibility

Social Security and Medicare are two of the most important institutions of American life. They guarantee a basic level of income and medical care for Americans who, because of age or disability, should not be expected to gain that income and medical care from employment. They do so through an approach, social insurance, that balances individual responsibility and adequate security. Both programs provide individual security in return for contributing to society.

If current demographic and health-care-cost trends persist, Social Security and Medicare will become even more important in the future. Their share of GDP may nearly double over the next seventy years. Such forecasts have been used to create alarm and support for drastic reforms. At their worst, those reforms would destroy Social Security and Medicare in the name of "saving" them.

Social Security and Medicare will become more expensive because they will be more necessary. The antientitlement hysteria that has become conventional wisdom among journalists and politicians too often ignores the functions that social insurance programs for the elderly serve, while greatly exaggerating the economic consequences and inequities of their financing. Such arguments substitute a cartoon version of responsibility for reality. The cartoon version says that "planning for the future" by worrying about it a lot and taking drastic action is responsible. Real responsibility requires not just worrying about the future but carefully assessing the risks and benefits of action.

This book offers a careful assessment of the various entitlement "crises" and proposed reforms. I have made three points that differ greatly from standard discussions.

First, there are no crises. Radical reform is justified neither by the benefits of extra national savings nor by a sensible view of the risks of budgetary meltdown. Medical care costs per person need not grow as quickly as in some of the estimates; and the increases that do occur might be a perfectly acceptable use of the benefits of economic growth. Claims that "greedy geezer" baby boomers will be exploiting their children and grandchildren are badly misconceived.

Second, it is unreasonable to expect policy to make Social Security and Medicare "solvent" for seventy-five years into the future. We do not insist on establishing policy for anything else for such a long time, for the same reason we should not do so for pensions and health care for elderly persons: we do not know what the situations will be, what trade-offs will be possible and what future voters will desire.

In the case of Social Security, the forecast funding gap could and should be narrowed. Yet it is reasonable to leave room for voters in 2020 or 2040 to make some choices, especially if we can reduce their challenge significantly. In the case of Medicare, there are huge uncertainties about future developments in both medical capacity and methods of cost control. So the object of prudent reformers should be to maximize our ability to address cost issues in the future, rather than to pretend to solve them now.

Third, the "affordability" of Social Security and Medicare should be considered in terms of the federal government's fiscal capacity. Dedicated financing of OASI, DI, and HI is nice, but what really counts is how much money the government can collect for all its programs and what the total spending for all programs will amount to. The standard calculations of "long-term actuarial balance" that assume that money put into the trust funds now can be spent later do not accurately reflect the federal government's fiscal capacity. Yet, using Social Security or budget surpluses to reduce federal borrowing does offer a small benefit from extra economic growth and a more significant benefit from reducing future interest costs.

There is something for everyone to dislike in these three points. Conservatives want to believe there are crises that require drastic reforms. Liberals would like to believe that balances recorded in the trust funds can be spent on benefits with no effect on the ability of the federal government to pay for other programs. Virtually everyone would like social insurance programs to be clearly solvent for seventy-five years into the future.

Instead, the future of Social Security and Medicare depends above all on public understanding of why they are good programs and public support for the intergenerational compact according to which workers pay for benefits for elderly and disabled members of society, in return for themselves being supported later. It has worked since 1935 and can work as much longer as we want it to work.

Two Views of Planning for the Future

The antientitlement hysteria is wrong not only because it turns challenges into crises but also because it exaggerates what can be done about any problem. The future is unknowable; it is just as difficult to predict future citizens' values as it is to predict more material conditions; and therefore the demand that Americans "fix" Social Security and Medicare for decades to come just is not realistic.

Why Fairness Does Not Require Cutting Programs Now

Advocates for radical reform of Social Security and Medicare frequently argue that radical reform is necessary to improve future citizens' choices. In one version, continuing the intergenerational contract to pay for these programs would unfairly bind future voters to spending that they might not prefer over other uses of their incomes.[1] The difficulty with this argument is that radical reform also forecloses choices. Privatization of Social Security or creating Medicare vouchers would make it virtually impossible for future voters to choose programs more like what we have today. The interests created by wealthier individuals' having private accounts or by allowing insurance companies to sell voucher plans would make restoring the current forms of social sharing exceedingly hard. As we discussed in chapter 8, there is good reason to believe that in a system with private accounts and a residual, highly redistributive, public scheme, even that latter system may be in severe political danger.

A second argument that reform would improve future citizens' choices may be even more broadly believed than the "entitlement crisis" itself. It asserts that future retirees need to know now about any benefit cuts, so they can begin planning to compensate for those cuts (Board of Trustees 1998a: 5; Aaron and Bosworth 1997: 271). On its face, this argument may seem obvious. On reflection, however, one may notice a few flaws.

Some changes, if they are to be made at all, do need to be phased in over time, for reasons of practical administration or fairness. The benefits of either personal retirement accounts or a diversified trust fund depend on accumulation of earnings over time; such changes would therefore have to be adopted far in advance of their intended benefits. Some changes need to be adopted far in advance in order to seem fair to people: thus, raising the retirement age by three years effective immediately would seem outrageous, whereas creating a new system of eligibility based on a mix of age and time in the workforce, with the changes spread over a period of three decades, would be merely controversial.

Yet the idea that future retirees need plenty of warning in order to adjust their retirement plans to take account of changes is unrealistic or even biased in a lot of ways. First of all, it presumes that the changes will be benefit cuts. If instead revenues were raised in, say, 2040, retirees would not need to do anything beforehand.

Second, many people could do little to adjust to policy changes even if given warning. What are the alternatives to Social Security? An important one is private pensions, but the average worker cannot say, "Now that my Social Security has been cut, I'll demand a higher pension from my employer." More precisely, she can say that, but it may not get her anywhere except, perhaps, unemployed. If anything, employers are becoming less generous in their pension policies.[2] Individuals would have more opportunity to increase their private savings, but there are reasons why individuals with low incomes, in particular, tend not to save much. Absent the compulsion that is present in some privatization plans, many would not save.[3] And if they were compelled to save, that would not be a matter of their planning to compensate for cuts. It would just be the government changing the rules of its compulsory program.

Arguments that people need forewarning of changes in order to adjust their behavior are especially implausible if applied to Medicare. The advocates of voucher approaches claim that such approaches will not hurt anybody, that they could even improve benefits. Therefore, either because they believe it or in order to win political support, they are telling citizens that no adjustment will be necessary. If savings were realized through other measures, such as direct constraints on payments to medical care providers, the consequences for future senior citizens would also be ambiguous. So far there is scant evidence that such measures have affected available services. And even if they did—for instance, if there was less investment in medical technology because hospitals had lower incomes, and therefore there was less high-tech equipment in some distant year such as 2030—it is hard to see what any individual could do about that.

Third, the evidence that the average person actually behaves in the way that forewarning is supposed to help them behave is, to put it mildly, meager. Economists and public-opinion experts who study retirement saving and expectations continually report that people do not save "enough," do not know how much they need to save, do not know what their Social Security benefits will be or what Medicare will cover, and so on.[4] If these reports are true, how would some benefit cuts change them? The very fact that the Normal Retirement Age for Social Security was raised in 1983 and voters paid so little attention indicates that voters did not focus on such a long-term effect.

In short, the idea that it is only fair to current workers to cut their future benefits now is less than compelling. Most workers might consider it much more fair not to cut their benefits at all.

A Practical Approach to Future Challenges

Even though there are no crises, the aging of the population will make paying for necessary entitlements for retired persons more of a challenge, so modest improvements in prospects can be appropriate. These could include not only savings but also measures that improve the programs or would make it easier to make choices in the future.

In addition, some improvements must, by their very nature, be adopted far in advance of their intended benefits. Therefore, the absence of crisis does not mean there should be no debate about reforms nor that there should be no long-term changes. It does mean that voters should not allow themselves to be panicked into supporting politicians who proclaim that drastic change is the only option.

"Planning for the future" should not mean pretending that problems far in the future can be fixed for all time. It should mean taking those steps that seem likely to do more good than harm and trying to create situations that will make it easier for future citizens to make successful decisions.

Following these principles, I have argued against some reforms and for others. Chapter 11 provides an agenda for legislation that includes some significant changes in both programs. In addition to more traditional savings, I suggested diversification of the portfolio in the Social Security trust funds and alteration of the basis of eligibility from age alone to a mix of age and years in the workforce. For Medicare, I suggested transferring noninsurance functions out of the program, merging Parts A and B, and creating a proportion-of-income premium for beneficiaries. These reforms all would require substantial debate and careful design.

Part of planning for the future, then, should include considering in what order such reforms might be adopted. Another part is to forecast, recognizing the great uncertainties of such estimates, the budgetary position that would result from those reforms. We turn now to those two tasks.

A Schedule for Reform

I will assume that this book is being read in 2001. The following measures are all discussed in chapter 11.

The 107th Congress: 2001–2002

Perhaps Congress and President Clinton will have concluded during the budget fights of the year 2000 that the unrealistic discretionary caps, described in chapter 5, had to go, and they may have replaced them with something more reasonable. Perhaps they will have adopted sensible procedures to "protect the Social Security surpluses." But if they have not, the first order of business should be to get basic budget policy, separate from Social Security, straight.

The next step would be to enact incremental Social Security savings. The inclusion of state and local employees, raising the number of years of earnings included in the benefit calculation from 35 to 38, changes in the taxation of benefits to make it more similar to the treatment of private pensions, and an increase in the total amount of wages subject to the Social Security payroll taxes could and should be adopted quickly, preferably in 2001. The same legislation could establish the advisory council that would report back options for altering eligibility or raising revenues so as to improve Social Security financing, on a pay-as-you-go basis, by 1.5 percent of taxable payroll in 2040. That report could be scheduled for January 1, 2004.

The 107th Congress should also be expected to set the standard for the growth of Medicare costs per enrollee after 2002, perhaps for a five-year period, at no more than 1 percent per year above the growth of per capita GDP. That presumably would include detailed policies about the same issues addressed in BBA-97, such as setting the rates for the various old and new prospective payment systems. The legislation might also address a wide variety of issues about implementation of BBA-97 provisions, so long as it keeps spending within the targets.

Last, it would be desirable to enact legislation to diversify investment of the Social Security trust funds either in 2002 or 2003, so as to enable implementation beginning in 2005.

The 108th Congress, 2003–2004

The succeeding Congress could be expected to debate and enact the more substantial structural reforms in Medicare. These include alternatives to the current disproportionate share hospital (DSH), graduate medical education (GME), and capital finance policies; combining Parts A and B; and the creation of a percentage-of-income premium system. The eventual increase in the Medicare payroll tax that I have suggested can wait until this time, when Parts A and B are combined, and it can be compared to the percentage of income that is charged as a premium to beneficiaries (perhaps the two figures should be equal, if that is practical).

The controversies associated with creating new funding for graduate medical education and other functions will be daunting. That is reason enough to do them first, rather than to combine those difficulties with the challenges involved in transforming traditional Medicare into a voucher design. As a practical matter, implementation of whatever measures are adopted may well take until around 2008. That is not to say policymakers could not try to move more quickly. But since the budget situation seems not to require hasty action, they should not feel compelled to rush.

This Congress would also receive, and vote on, the advisory council's recommendations about how to address the long-term aging of the population. Those recommendations, as I have described, ought to include a mix of some payroll tax increase and a change in the basis of eligibility from age alone to a mix of age and years in the workforce. It is so fundamental a change, yet so logical, that it deserves separate debate. Ideally, structural Medicare reform could be addressed in 2003 and Social Security eligibility in 2004.

Subsequent Congresses

Policymaking for Social Security and Medicare would, naturally, extend far beyond this tentative schedule. And measures taken up in the 107th and 108th Congresses would not necessarily be confined to these limits.

I have emphasized, for example, the value of experimenting with measures that would improve competition among plans within Medicare. Not only should the experiments contemplated by BBA-97 be implemented, but also alternatives should be authorized wherever practical. It may even seem sensible to implement some significant changes in competition within Medicare + Choice without waiting for conclusive results. Such measures are fine so long as they do not threaten the viability of the basic Medicare insurance pool.

Depending on experience with both Medicare + Choice and the results of BBA-97's cost controls, policymakers might well conclude, by 2005 or shortly thereafter, that they know enough to implement a voucher system properly, and that is desirable. We cannot predict that and should not foreclose it.

Similarly, the budget situation may change, either for the worse or for the better. If so, further legislation also may seem desirable, either seeking new savings or expanding benefits, such as for Medicare prescription drugs.

The measures that I have suggested here, however, seem reasonable even with some changes in conditions and knowledge. If the stock market were to slump, for example, it still would be reasonable to diversify some of the trust funds' holdings, slowly. The market is unlikely to decline forever. As I wrote final revisions of this manuscript in July of 2000, there was some prospect that a prescription drug benefit would be enacted before this book's publication.

But the forecast budget surpluses improved by far more than the cost of any of the programs being proposed. And the proposals all were modest enough that there might still be pressures for further expansions. So it seems reasonably conservative to write as if the baseline for decision is the budget situation and Medicare program as of the time of my analysis. If the budget situation worsened significantly, the proposed Social Security measures still would be helpful, and Congress would not be likely to adopt much more stringent targets for Medicare spending. Getting programs like GME out of Medicare would still make sense. Vouchers still would not.

Budgetary Prospects with Responsible Reform

Throughout this book I have argued that, although crises have been exaggerated, there is reason to pay some attention to long-term forecasts of costs. Moreover, I have emphasized, contrary to the implications of focusing on Social Security trust funds alone, that the right question is program costs in pay-as-you-go terms, because that is what affects the federal government's overall fiscal position.

I have also emphasized that the economic benefits of fairly small—1 or 2 percent of GDP—alterations in the government's fiscal balance are extremely small compared to other effects on the economy. Therefore, the important goal is to give future voters room to protect themselves from the "doomsday scenario," in which deficits are feeding on themselves as a result of high interest costs and the process has accelerated to a point where only drastic action will stop it. Given reasonable modesty about predicting the future and how significantly long-term forecasts changed during the 1990s, it is not reasonable to try to protect voters fifty or sixty years from now. But it is appropriate to worry if forecasts project spiraling deficits within twenty or even thirty years.

Given the assumptions made by standard forecasts in 1999 and 2000, it is not yet time to worry (see chapter 5). But perhaps assumptions should be somewhat more conservative. Then how much better would the budget future seem if Congress and the president agreed on the measures that I have recommended?

Any answer to such questions must be rough and uncertain, given the difficulties of projecting future costs and revenues. I would much prefer to see CBO or GAO or other high-powered analytic agencies estimate the effects of a moderate package of reforms such as my own, rather than to expect readers to rely on my own efforts. But the figures I present here should be a reasonably conservative set of estimates.

Methodological Issues

I developed these estimates by working off the 1999 long-term estimates kindly provided by the General Accounting Office, as reported in chapter 5.[5] The baseline scenario therefore is less favorable than the economic assumptions in effect during either budget debate or the election campaign in the year 2000. I asked GAO to alter their baseline to include my assumption that discretionary spending would decline significantly more slowly as a share of GDP than in the GAO model. I had Medicare spending actually growing somewhat more quickly than in GAO's baseline, but at the basic standard for which I argue in chapter 7, until 2012. Based on those data, as supplied by GAO, I did a series of spreadsheet calculations, in which changes in one variable were used to adjust totals. The spreadsheet approach naturally is not as accurate as re-running the entire model would be. Yet the major difference is that by GAO's economic logic there should be positive economic feedbacks from the lower deficits that my suggestions produce in most years; thus, the spreadsheet figures, by excluding those feedbacks, if anything should underestimate the budgetary benefits of my proposals.[6]

In order to calculate overall budgetary effects, I also had to have figures for the effects of individual measures. Here, too, there are data issues, and I can claim only that I tried to be conservative.

Briefly, in estimating the effects of trust-fund diversification, I made the conservative assumptions described in chapter 11. The private investments accumulate to just under 9 percent of GDP in 2028; withdrawals then are 0.42 percent of GDP in 2029; they rise to 0.46 percent of GDP by 2045, and I then assume they would be stable at that level.

The Social Security Administration actuaries provided me with the runs that they had prepared to predict the annual effects of the state-local and 35–

38 reforms. I translated those into the calculations below by expressing the spending and revenue changes as percentages of GDP and then applying each year's change in the SSA model to the GDP in the GAO model.[7]

The state-local provision increases revenues first and spending later, so this combination of measures has more positive effects in the first thirty years than later. This is an example of where pay-as-you-go calculations are more revealing than the standard approach.

Estimation of the effects of increasing the HI payroll tax from 2015 to 2019 were straightforward, though I calculated them a bit conservatively.[8] Similarly, because I defined the savings to be reported by the new advisory council on responses to longer life expectancies in pay-as-you-go terms, rather than the usual "long-term percent of payroll," I could calculate the results on the assumption that the measures adopted meet the standard. That path would be 0.05 percent of payroll savings each year from 2022 to 2029 (thus, 0.4 percent in 2029), then increases of 0.1 percent each year from 2030 through 2040 (thus, from 0.5 percent in 2030 to 1.5 percent in 2040 and thereafter).

Unfortunately, I could not obtain pay-as-you-go savings figures for either taxation of benefits or raising the payroll tax threshold.[9] Here I had to simply invent a savings path, and I chose one that is meant to be conservative.[10]

Social Security Finance and General Revenues

The main focus of this analysis is the finance of the federal government as a whole. For readers who are interested in effects on the Social Security trust funds, however, I can provide some indications. The benefits of the measures dedicated to Social Security alone would peak around 2040. The trustees report that Social Security spending will be nearly a stable share of GDP from 2035 through 2060, as the large baby-boom cohorts pass away. In 2040 the savings, extra tax revenues, and receipts from diversification of the trust funds would be about 1.3 percent of GDP. The SSA actuaries estimate that, if no changes are made, in 2040 the program's spending will exceed its tax revenues by 1.90 percent of GDP. So my suggestions do leave a balance to be financed from general revenue.

That seems perfectly fine policy to me. As I explain in chapter 3, even Social Security's founders expected some use of general revenues to finance the program after 1980, since demographics would require payroll taxes above 10 percent. The balance that I am suggesting here, about 0.6 percent of GDP in 2040, is less than a tenth of total Social Security spending. *It also is less than the proportion of Social Security spending that standard estimates have assumed would be financed from general revenues while the trust funds are being depleted.* In the 1999 estimates, for example, the amount of interest and principal from the trust fund used to pay for benefits would have grown from 0.7 percent of GDP in 2019 to 1.9 percent of GDP in 2033.[11] That is general revenue.

In short, though I am making the use of some general revenue to finance Social Security in the future explicit, I am not really changing budget policy. There would have to be a technical change in budget law, because legislation would be needed that automatically appropriates the necessary extra general revenues.[12] But the vast majority of Social Security benefits would still also be financed from contributions directly devoted to Social Security, either payroll taxes or the prefunding of the equity component of the trust funds. Social Security benefits in 2040 would still be justified by workers' contributions.

Congress and the president might instead decide to seek further revenue increases or benefit cuts. Sometime in the years before 2040, if the economy does no better than projected, they are likely to be considering modest measures to maintain budgetary stability anyway, and Social Security could be part of the mix. But as a matter of Social Security policy alone, it would be reasonable policy to use general revenues to provide the extra financing needed after 2040.[13]

Budget Model Results

Figures 12.1 and 12.2 provide the fiscal results of the set of changes that I am proposing. Figure 12.1 shows the trend of annual deficits or surpluses, and figure 12.2 shows totals for the national debt or (for lack of a better word) accumulation. Each shows three scenarios: GAO's 1999 baseline scenario, the results of GAO's model when the discretionary spending and Medicare spending assumptions match my less favorable suggestions ("Revised Baseline"), and my calculations of how those results are altered by my further savings suggestions ("Moderate Reform").

Compared to the 1999 GAO baseline, my higher discretionary and Medicare spending does cause the deficit and the debt to return to worrisome levels more quickly. But the figures for the Moderate scenario tell a different story.

It produces lower surpluses than the GAO 1999 baseline and therefore also produces a smaller positive balance (though that is partly because the positive balance in the diversified Social Security trust funds is not counted within the general budget figures). But under the Moderate Reform scenario, the deficit returns only four years earlier than in the GAO baseline, in 2025 instead of 2029. In the model, deficits then are actually lower than the GAO baseline from 2032 through 2048.[14]

In the moderate scenario, we would not expect the deficit to reach worrisome dimensions until around 2050. There would certainly be time, in the 2030s, to consider the measures that would be needed to prevent it from spiraling out of control. The difference between doing more now and making decisions then is that voters in 2035 or so will have a much better idea of what good policy will be for them than we could possibly have today.

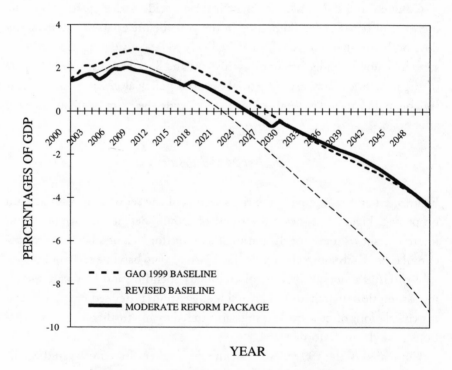

YEAR

Fig. 12.1. Federal surplus or deficit with moderate reforms

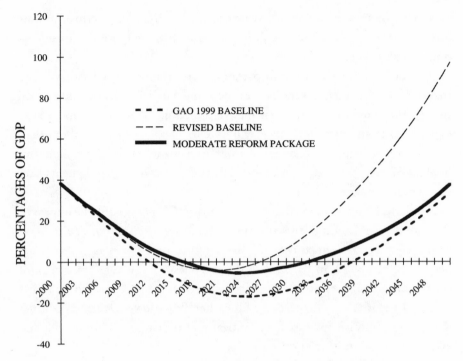

Fig. 12.2. National debt owed to the public with moderate reforms

Policymakers today might instead decide to have somewhat less stringent budgetary policies. For example, they might bring discretionary spending down more slowly. So long as they adopt sensible medium-term Social Security and Medicare policies, however, the budget should be reasonably controllable through 2050.[15]

Uncertainty and Responsibility

I do not mean for a minute to suggest that anyone, including me, knows what the budget situation *will* be in 2035, or 2020, or even 2005. Bad news could mean that the budget situation would be substantially worse much more quickly. But we need only look to the change in long-term forecasts through the 1990s, as displayed in chapter 5, to realize that good news could mean there is even less of a problem than I have projected. The basic long-term economic projections used in the forecasts I discuss here presume quite mediocre economic performance. It could be better.

Economic performance is only part of the uncertainty. Perhaps we will find that the HCFA actuaries were right in 1999, and Medicare costs could be held to their projected trend. Or voters may find even my alternative standard too draconian. Then the policymakers will have to decide what to do about that: to raise more revenues or change the program. For the reasons I explain in this book, however, they will be in a better position to make such judgments later than we are in now.

Similarly, I have assumed that Social Security's financing could be improved through diversification of the trust funds, building up a fund of equities that would yield extra, nontax, revenue. If the return on equities is as low as has been projected by Dean Baker, then the revenues from private investment of the trust fund will be lower, and budget adjustments to help pay for the costs of Social Security may be needed a bit earlier. But a lower return on equities also would diminish any case for privatization, so that possibility provides no extra reason for drastic reform.

The possible uncertainties are endless, but none of them threaten the basic argument of this book. Perhaps medical advances will greatly increase the demand for spending; but then, perhaps we will want to spend the money. Perhaps income inequalities will widen; but slashing Social Security and Medicare do not seem like an answer to that problem. Perhaps the private health-insurance market will deteriorate so badly that Congress and the president will enact national health insurance, putting Medicare policy into an entirely new context; but that hardly suggests that making Medicare more like the current private insurance system is a good idea. Perhaps, instead, the private insurance market will develop far superior methods of cost containment and medical service delivery; if so, we can make Medicare more like the private sector then, when we know what to imitate.

The most likely negative scenario based on my analysis here is that, in a decade or so, bad news might mean that the federal budget reaches the position I define in chapter 5: one in which a severe interest-cost spiral seems possible within twenty years. But that will be less likely if we adopt the incremental measures that I suggest in this book.

Another negative scenario is also, however, unfortunately likely. That is the possibility that, in a mistaken quest for "responsibility," policymakers will adopt partial privatizations of Social Security and Medicare or significant changes in the entitlements to the programs. Those too represent threats to the public from mistaken entitlement policy: threats that people who live so long will face a miserable old age.

The risks of radical reform must be balanced against the risks of incrementalism. I have shown that the risks of incrementalism can be managed. The honest case for radicalism therefore reduces to two assumptions. The first is that we really do owe it to "our grandchildren" to "ensure" that Medicare and Social Security are fully financed seventy-five years into the future. This is a very strange view of how the world could possibly work. Even if desirable, it is not possible, and to the extent that it involves our deciding in advance what they should sacrifice, it is not desirable.

The second argument for radicalism is that Medicare and Social Security are not in fact worth preserving. Some people believe that a voucherized Medicare would be better than the current program. Others (some the same, some not) believe a privatized, defined-contribution pension would be better than a social-insurance, defined-benefit one.

In this book I have given the reasons why I do not agree with either of the last two propositions. But at least they can be maintained as part of an honest debate. My main purpose here has been to show that the context of debate about entitlements for the elderly in recent years has been misleading and biased.

Radical reform of Social Security and Medicare has been promoted as necessary for the economy, when it is nothing of the sort. Radical reform of Social Security and Medicare has been promoted as a means to "fairness" between generations, which is no more true. Worst of all, radical reform has been promoted as a way to "save" Social Security and Medicare. That is nonsense at best, a lie at worst.

There is no need for hysteria about entitlements for elderly persons. The commentators who judge politicians' responsibility by whether those politicians strive to slay the entitlement "monster" have confused a nightmare with reality. When it comes to social insurance, the words of Franklin D. Roosevelt ring true. He said it in a different context, but it is right for this one: the only thing we have to fear is fear itself.

Afterword: Markets, Budgets, and Politics in the Second Bush Administration

There is no need to fear entitlements but need to fear for the survival of American social insurance programs. President George W. Bush clearly wants, under the guise of "saving" Social Security and Medicare, to transform them into, at best, programs that finance forms of casualty health insurance and individual pension savings, rather than programs of contributory social insurance.

As 2002 came to an end, there had been no legislation that directly advanced this transformative agenda. In the two years of the Bush Administration, however, there had been a series of events that could be relevant to future decisions. They can be summarized under three headings: markets, budgets, and politics.

Markets

The attractiveness of major proposals for radical reform of Social Security and Medicare, private accounts and Medicare vouchers, depends on the plausibility of arguments that "market mechanisms" can be used to better pursue goals currently sought through "bureaucratic government programs." Events have not been kind to those beliefs.

Stock Prices

On the Social Security front, private accounts likely were made attractive to many people by the stock market boom of the 1990s. The more responsible advocates of privatization would not have predicted that boom would continue, but did project that equities would earn their historic average long-term return in the future. As I discussed in chapter 8, as of 1999 there was very good reason to believe that, if the economy did no better than the Trustees' forecasts projected, stock market returns should not be as high as they had been in the past. At best, as Peter Diamond argued, there might be a decade or so of stagnation, followed by a return to the historic pattern (see pp. 147–49).

For most of 2000, both the Dow Jones Industrials and Standard & Poor's 500 indexes hovered at historically high levels. The S&P index, for example, grew by more than 50 percent from the beginning of 1998 to its peak during 2000. Just before the election, however, equity prices began a slow slide. The attacks on the United States on September 11, 2001, appear to have had a minor influence on equity prices. Those attacks were followed by a sharp drop in prices, but stocks recovered to their pre–September 11 levels within a few weeks. In October, however, the pattern of decline resumed. As a result, at this writing (December 2002), the S&P 500 index had lost more than one-third of its peak value, falling to about 10 percent below its level five years before (Bloomberg 2002).

The cycle of boom and bust within less traditional businesses than the bulk of the S&P 500 was even more extreme. The NASDAQ index tripled in value between the beginning of 1998 and March 2000; it gave back half those gains by the summer of 2001, recovered somewhat, and then began a devastating slide that, at this writing, left it at about 20 percent below its level five years before (Bloomberg 2002). And individual businesses, epitomized by Enron and WorldCom, rocketed upward and then crashed into spectacular bankruptcies. These latter developments were accompanied by accounting scandals that raised doubts about the reliability of corporate financial statements and charges that brokerage firms skewed their research to make corporate finances look better than they really were. Among the consequences of these scandals were the collapse of the Arthur Andersen accounting firm and massive fines paid by many major brokerage houses.

As many older workers who lost money in the stock market slump began to consider postponing retirement ("Bumpy Market" 2002), reliance on the stock market for financial security appeared to be a less attractive idea. Individuals wondered both about the general trends of the market and about whether they could manage their own investments successfully, given the difficulty of getting reliable information. As the *New York Times* reported, "the $7 trillion in losses that investors have suffered since 2000, along with revelations that some research analysts had recommended stocks while privately warning their big clients against them, have made small shareholders deeply suspicious that the markets are rigged against them" (Berenson and Sorkin 2002). By December 2002, a *Los Angeles Times* poll was reporting that only 38 percent of those polled supported "allowing workers to divert part of their Social Security payroll taxes into individual accounts" and "nearly four in ten of the supporters say they wouldn't back the idea if it required a reduction in the guaranteed Social Security benefit" (Brownstein 2002).

From a point of view that is concerned with only average rates of return, the stock market collapse could be said to make *future* privatization *more* attractive in 2002 than it should have been in 2000. Then values were inflated; now they have come down; it is more reasonable to expect future increases now that the first part of Peter Diamond's scenario has begun to come true. But a normally cautious person might prefer to wait on the private investments until things look up again. Moreover, the declines also highlighted the great risks associated with relying on the stock market for a decent retirement. People who invested in stocks that were recommended by many of the "experts" could go bust. People who retired at the end of 2002 could expect much lower annuity payments than people who followed the same investment strategy but retired at the beginning of 2000 (just as in Gary Burtless's description of the 1973–74 slide; see p. 150). In short, the events of the past three years dramatized all the economic risks of privatization.

Health Care Costs

The case for Medicare vouchers was battered by two developments: accelerating costs for private health insurance and a near collapse of the "Medicare + Choice" system that had been intended, by its sponsors, to be the forerunner of a voucher system. The best available estimates reported that premiums for employment-based insurance rose by 8.3 percent in 2000, 11.0 percent in 2001, and 12.5 percent in 2002 (Strunk et al. 2002: W306). The increases in 2002, if anything, understated the trend, as employers reduced the coverage available in the plans they offered. In actuality, "taking account of the sizable amount of 'benefit buy-down' in 2002, the true increase in the cost of health insurance for employers and employees was about 15 percent" (Strunk et al. 2002: W299).

As private premiums rose, Medicare costs per enrollee grew much more slowly. Congress enacted Medicare "givebacks" in 2000 that caused spending per enrollee to grow almost as quickly in 2001 (9.6%) as average premiums for employment-based insurance (11.0%). But in the absence of further legislation, and given the fact that prescription drugs are not covered by Medicare and the tough underlying payment rules for physician and other services, Medicare costs were expected to grow quite slowly in 2002 and even more slowly in 2003 (Board of Trustees 2002b: Table IV.B1; Strunk et al. 2002: W306; CMS 2002b). To summarize, premiums for private employers rose about 47 percent in the five years from 1998 through 2002, while Medicare costs per enrollee rose by about 15 percent.[1]

This difference likely is no better guide to the cost-control potential of Medicare's traditional methods as compared to the private sector than was the brief period of private sector superiority during the mid-1990s. Short-term effects are likely to have driven both trends; the difference is that many of the unsystematic trends of the 1992–96 period reversed afterward. There was a retreat from "managed care" as employers, in a tight labor market, responded to employee backlash against restrictive networks and practices. The underwriting cycle switched over, with insurers getting out of markets and concentrating where they could raise their prices, instead of lowering prices to get into markets. In the earlier period, providers panicked and accepted discounts; in the later period they consolidated, decided they had the market power, and demanded higher prices. While the publicity about the coming world of managed care in the earlier period had encouraged concessions, the more recent political backlash against "managed care" encouraged defiance. And, while Medicare did worse in the earlier period because of its failure to control home health costs that it covered more substantially than did employment-based plans, the employment-based plans suffered later because of their better coverage for prescription drugs (while traditional Medicare cracked down on home health through BBA-97 and the campaign against "fraud and abuse"). Of course any of these trends could shift, and so we might expect the private sector cost control performance to improve and the recent gap to narrow again. (For a similar discussion, focusing on private insurance alone, see Strunk et al. 2002.)

Hence, there are lots of excuses, even reasons, for the recent difference between costs of traditional Medicare and private insurance premiums. Yet that difference makes it harder than ever to credit the theory that vouchers could "save" Medicare by making medical care more efficient. Developments within Medicare make the case for vouchers even weaker.

As I argued in the original text, experience after the creation of Medicare + Choice did not live up to voucher proponents' hopes. But it got worse. In 1998 about 74 percent of beneficiaries had access to any Medicare + Choice plan; by 2002 only 60.5 percent had such access. In 1999 61 percent had access to a Medicare + Choice plan with no extra premium; by 2002 only 32 percent did. Coverage for prescription drugs continued to decline (figures from CMS 2002c; see also Adams 2002). As a result, enrollment in M+C plans, which peaked in 1999 at about 6.35 million (MedPAC 2002: 82), fell to "nearly five million seniors and disabled Americans" (CMS 2002a). The Bush Administration advocated this program so strongly that it reorganized the Health Care Financing Administration (HCFA), renaming it the Centers for Medicare and Medicaid Services (CMS), and made administration of Medicare + Choice a separate "center" at the same level of administration as the much larger traditional Medicare and Medicaid programs (Thompson 2001). But, by September 2002, CMS administrator Tom Scully was reduced to declaring that "a continued goal of the Bush Administration is to stabilize the Medicare + Choice participation. . . . There is bipartisan support for saving Medicare + Choice" (CMS 2002a).

Gee, I thought the idea was to save Medicare.

Readers should still remember that health care cost control is really, really difficult, and nobody knows what will work far into the future. My analysis in previous chapters emphasized that all options should be held open, that serious efforts should be made to find ways to make vouchers a more viable option. That's just the prudent thing to do. But it would be worse than imprudent to pretend now that vouchers represent a way to "save" Medicare.

Budgets and Forecasts

At the end of the second Bush year, trends were not a whole lot better for government finances than for investors and purchasers of private health insurance.

The Trustees' Forecasts

The most standard forecast measure of Social Security and Medicare solvency actually marginally improved. In the 2002 reports of the programs' Trustees, the HI trust fund was not projected to be exhausted until 2030 (compared to 2026 in Table 1.1) and the OASDI trust funds until 2041 (compared to 2036). Nevertheless, the underlying dynamic projected for Medicare worsened dramatically. Compared to the 2000 reports, the 2001 reports raised projected total Medicare spending in 2030 from 4.36 percent of GDP to 4.51 percent; in 2050 from 4.79 percent to 6.01 percent; and in 2070 from 5.19 percent to 7.94 percent (Board of Trustees 2002a; Board of Trustees 2001b: Table III.B1; Board of Trustees 2000c: Table III.B1).

The difference is entirely explained by a decision to adopt a less optimistic assumption about the long-term trend for Medicare spending per enrollee. Instead of assuming that costs per enrollee would grow at the same rate as per capita GDP after 2020, the Trustees decided it is more realistic to assume that costs per enrollee will grow one percentage point per year faster than per capita GDP. When it is compounded over fifty years, 1 percent turns into a huge difference in spending. CBO adopted a similar assumption that, in turn, must alter long-term budget forecasts.

In adopting this assumption, the Trustees followed the recommendations of an advisory panel that was convened in the summer of 2000. This panel argued that health care expenditures grow because of "the fundamental . . . pressure from advances in medical technology" (Technical Review Panel 2000: 33) and that the growth of health care costs due to medical technology alone was likely to be that 1 percent per year (Technical Review Panel 2000: 35). Although I am less convinced of the inevitable effects of technology, in this book I have already argued that, other things being equal, a good estimate of the default trend of medical costs per person is that same 1 percent per year above the growth of per capita GDP.[2]

Unlike voucher advocates, however, the Technical Review Panel argued that this level of growth should apply to the health care system as a whole—regardless of any differences between traditional Medicare and private insurance. In fact, they were explicitly projecting long-term National Health Expenditures, not Medicare spending. They therefore suggested that, while Medicare costs in 2075 would rise to more than 8 percent of GDP, *total na-*

tional health costs would rise to 38 percent of GDP (Technical Review Panel 2000: 30). They also argued that this level of spending might even be acceptable—"recognition that technological advances are associated with health care expenditure growth is not intended to imply that expenditure growth is too high" (Technical Review Panel 2000: 35).

Maybe yes, maybe no. What should be clear is that the basis for the large increase in projected Medicare costs is an assumption that simply cannot be viewed as a programmatic Medicare problem. Any "fix" would have to involve the health care system as a whole; if Medicare at 8 percent of GDP becomes unaffordable, what would that say about the 30 percent of GDP devoted to all other health care? How would everybody else's insurance be financed? The changed projections, therefore, whether sensible or not, provide no rationale for reforming Medicare alone. And the panel's logic could be interpreted as suggesting that nothing could be done about the supposed problem.

The changed Medicare projection, therefore, tells us only that a smart and experienced review panel made some interesting judgments about future American health care costs. It does not tell us what will happen or what if anything to do about it. So long-term budget projections look worse, but the underlying conditions have not changed.

Short-Term and Long-Term Budget Trends

The most obvious reason for this Afterword is that the budget forecasts in chapters 5 and 12 are clearly out of date. That does not change the possible benefits of the measures modeled in chapter 12, and it does not change the reasons to beware of budget forecasts discussed in chapter 5. But it does call for some updating, so readers might not imagine that the budget situation in fact was as positive in 2003 as the book previously described.

The Congressional Budget Office adopted its own version of a more pessimistic long-term Medicare cost growth assumption in its October 2000 long-term budget projections (CBO 2000a). CBO assumed that after 2020 costs per enrollee would grow by 1.1 percent per year on top of the growth of per capita GDP. CBO also adopted somewhat more reasonable (meaning pessimistic) discretionary spending projections than it had before, and projected that revenues would be cut and held steady. Even with those changes, CBO was projecting large surpluses for many years due to positive short-term budget trends through mid-2000. But the new forecast suggested the budget could begin spiraling out of control in 2040. (For a more thorough discussion, see White 2002.)

Potential trouble in 2040 was not enough to spark much concern, but then the short-term budget trends turned sour at stunning speed. In January 2001, CBO was projecting cumulative federal budget surpluses of $5.6 trillion dollars for 2002–11. By the summer of 2002, those projected surpluses had virtually disappeared. CBO was projecting deficits through 2005, with large surpluses recurring only in 2011 (Kogan and Greenstein 2002; CBO 2002a).

Four major factors explain the deteriorating short-term forecasts. First, an overall economic slowdown reduced revenues and increased some mandatory spending. But, second, revenues fell far more than could have been expected from the slowdown in economic growth alone (just as they had grown more quickly than expected in the late 1990s). So about 15 percent of the budget deterioration over a ten-year period was due to the general economy and 29 percent due to re-estimates of "technical" factors such as the relationship of revenues to GDP. The third and largest part, 31 percent, could be attributed to the effects of the tax cut that President Bush pushed through Congress early in his term, before Senator Jim Jeffords of Vermont bolted the Republican party and temporarily cost the administration control of the Senate. Fourth, increased spending for defense, homeland security, and international programs—partly due to the Bush Administration's preferences, but also due to the horrifying attacks of September 11, 2001—accounted for about 16 percent of the budget deterioration (Kogan and Greenstein 2002).

The budget situation as I wrote this Afterword seemed likely to be worse than these projections, because some of the underlying trends could be understated. In particular, the tax cut had been designed with some very strange timing. First, much of it was "backloaded"—many of the cuts were scheduled to take effect not immediately but in 2004 and beyond. These included most of the reductions in rates for higher earners and repeal of the estate tax, that is, the provisions that most excited Republicans and most depressed Democrats. Because of this backloading, the figure for the tax cut's effect on the budget over the full ten-year period greatly understates its effect toward the end of the period, when it would be fully phased in. But, second, all of the bill's provisions—including those that did not take effect until 2010—were scheduled to terminate or "sunset" on January 1, 2011. (For a summary of provisions, see Allred 2001.) This makes the effect in the final year of the ten-year forecast seem much smaller than it would be if the tax cut's provisions were extended.

Congressional negotiators agreed to the sunset provision so that they could enact more, different cuts while fitting them within the total revenue loss for ten years that was allowed under the Budget Resolution they had adopted earlier in 2001. The lead negotiators clearly expected that Congress would not allow the bill to expire, because that would create an automatic, very large tax hike in 2011. They in fact began politicking for an extension of the provisions as soon as the bill was signed (Parks and Swindell 2001; Nitschke and Swindell 2001). Analysts who had preferred the previous budget policies (such as were described in this book) wanted to repeal many of the tax cut's provisions, but even they believed that a few of the revenue losses, particularly relief for the "Alternative Minimum Tax," would have to be extended (Orszag et al. 2002: 3; see also Kogan and Greenstein 2002). So it is very unlikely that the entire effect of the tax cut will disappear in 2011, which means revenues are likely to be lower from 2011 on than the standard forecasts at the end of 2002 suggested.

In addition, the normal ten-year forecasts were assuming a level of restraint in domestic spending that remained unlikely, especially given the pressures for spending on "homeland security." It is true that the Bush Administration took a very hard line in favor of spending restraint, in essence arguing that homeland security expenses should be paid for by cutting other programs. The administration even proposed creating the new Department of Homeland Security while suggesting no extra appropriations for transition costs—a totally implausible position. But CBO's baseline assumption for discretionary spending remained too low, even if not quite so unrealistic as in the forecasts discussed earlier in this book. (For CBO's own report of the effect of changing its baseline assumptions, see CBO 2002a.)

What, then, was the long-term budget outlook as of the end of 2002? It was foggy, of course, given the difficulty projecting even a year in advance. But the most recent CBO forecast, in July 2002, projected that deficits would reach 4.8 percent of GDP in 2040 and then spiral upward (CBO 2002b: Table 3). In February 2002, GAO projected that, if discretionary spending grew with GDP and the entire tax cut were extended, deficits would reach about 5 percent of GDP and then spiral upward in the middle of the 2020s (GAO 2002: 6–7 and Figure 2). In chapter 5, I argued that policy makers should take action to reduce forecast long-term deficits when it is reasonably projected that deficits will reach 10 percent of GDP within two decades. Even GAO's most

pessimistic scenario in February 2002 did not reach that standard. But updated forecasts may bring that date closer, and the situation as I wrote this
analysis at least merited close attention, and action where the merits of action
are pretty clear.

A reasonable set of actions would include repealing most of the planned
future tax cut as soon as possible. One reason it was possible to enact the tax
cuts is that Federal Reserve Chairman Alan Greenspan testified that the
prospect of paying off the national debt required that measures be taken to
slow the pace of surpluses, thereby preventing a large economic shock when
the elimination of the debt made it necessary to eliminate the surpluses
quickly (Norton 2001).[3] He testified to this effect because the budget forecasts at the beginning of 2001 were so phenomenally favorable—though, as
it happened, wrong. He did add at the time, as the *National Journal* reported,
that perhaps Congress should include in any legislation a "mechanism to sus-
pend tax cuts if surplus projections turn out to be too optimistic" (Norton
2001). Since the legislation was not written with such a mechanism, acting
soon to repeal most of the future installments of the tax cuts seems appropriate. Those measures give the vast majority of benefits to a small fraction of the
population. Some provisions (such as relief for the Alternative Minimum Tax,
and increases in the child credit) could remain in place, but the cuts in the
highest marginal tax rates, and the elimination of the estate tax, should certainly be repealed.[4]

I would also recommend taking the other steps that I proposed in part IV
of this book. Combined with repeal of part of the tax cut, those steps ought
to improve long-term budget prospects significantly. Such action would not
cause projections to be quite so comforting as they seemed when I did the
analysis for chapter 12. The improvement, however, ought to move the projected time of serious budget problems far enough into the future to allow for
a period of watching and waiting. Given recent experience with budget forecasts, the reasons not to base radical change on such forecasts appear stronger
than ever—as perhaps Chairman Greenspan could attest.

Politics

There is absolutely no chance that the 108th Congress and President Bush
would enact these recommendations. Indeed, the postelection issue of *Con-*

gressional Quarterly reported that, with the Republican takeover of the Senate, "Tax Cut Becomes Top Priority" and that the "permanent extension of the [2002] tax cut . . . is expected to move as a stand-alone bill early next year" (Ota 2002: 2895). Republican leaders were expected to try to grease the wheels for tax cuts by appointing new budget process referees—the directors of the Congressional Budget Office and Joint Committee on Taxation—who would adopt procedures that would reduce the estimated costs of those cuts (Taylor and Ota 2002).[5]

The Bush Administration so thoroughly opposes taxes that, as part of its main statement about policies for homeland security, it argued that higher taxes to pay for homeland security efforts would hurt the economy. A $38 billion bill for homeland security efforts, it reported, would cost the economy not only $24 billion in foregone personal consumption, and $14 billion from reduced private sector investment, but a further 27 cents for every dollar spent because "under any tax system, every dollar collected in taxes results in distortions that reduce the efficiency of the economy and lower national income" (Office of Homeland Security 2002: 65). It is fair to say that any increase in federal revenues, whether for the budget in general or for Social Security and Medicare in particular, is off the table until some other government takes office.

Given the events in the financial and health care markets and the questionable popularity of both privatization and vouchers, one might expect most politicians to proceed cautiously. But President Bush is not such a typical politician. His view of the presidency, as revealed by his own behavior and comments, is much more aggressive. "Most presidents have high hopes," Bob Woodward reports in his book on *Bush at War*. "Some have grandiose visions of what they will achieve, and he was firmly in that camp" (339). After the 2002 election, *Congressional Quarterly* noted that "much of Bush's presidency has been about proving wrong the conventional wisdom on the danger of acting too boldly. When he took office in 2001, facing a divided Congress after losing the popular vote, lawmakers advised him to start cautiously; he responded by pushing through the biggest tax cut in two decades" (Nather with Cochran 2002: 2891). Where his father famously derided the "vision thing," George W. Bush insists that "the vision thing matters" (Woodward 2002: 341). "I will seize the opportunity to achieve big goals," he told Woodward (339), and Bush in fact has pursued a clear set of goals from his campaign through the first two years of his administration, with very little wavering.

Social Security privatization and Medicare vouchers have been two of those goals. Not so much was done in the first two years of the Bush Administration on the Medicare front, for two reasons. First, Medicare "reform" has become tangled up with the issue of a prescription drug benefit, which costs money and on which it has been relatively easy for Senate Democrats to oppose the administration's position. (For an overview, see "Special Report" 2002.) Second, the obvious approach to a controversial issue—appoint a "bipartisan" commission that can be expected to propose the solution you want—was not possible because the National Bipartisan Commission on the Future of Medicare had reported too recently.

Nevertheless, President Bush has publicly identified the administration with the position of Senator Breaux, Representative Thomas, and the majority of that commission. His administration endorsed legislation sponsored by Breaux, Thomas, and Senator Bill Frist (R-TN), and the president argued for "modernizing" Medicare by giving Medicare enrollees "the power to choose" insurance plans that would "compete with each other," with the government contribution to seniors' costs related to the "average cost of all Medicare plans" (Bush 2001). The stunning ascension of Senator Frist to the position of Senate Majority Leader in December 2002 makes efforts to pass such legislation more likely.

The major obstacles to the administration's position are that many Americans do not appear to have favorable opinions of "managed care" plans; that in a voucher system it is hard to devise a payment scheme that would actually save money but also maintain equity (for an extensive discussion, see White 1995a); and that current seniors might feel especially threatened by reform. For all these reasons, Democrats in the Senate might have the backbone to mount a filibuster and a few Republicans might defect from the administration's position. Bush (2001) addressed those fears by promising that "no senior will see any change that he or she does not want or does not seek. If you like things the way they are, that's just the way they'll stay." But making that substantively credible will be difficult.

The administration made a more concerted effort to push its Social Security agenda. On May 2, 2001, the president appointed the President's Commission to Strengthen Social Security. President Bush charged the commission with proposing reforms that met several principles, most significantly that "Social Security payroll taxes must not be increased," "government must not invest Social Security funds in the stock market," and "modernization must include individually controlled, voluntary personal retirement accounts" (President's Commission 2001b: 10). The membership of the commission showed the administration's penchant for combining bipartisan symbolism with largely partisan substance. The co-chairs were a former Democratic Senator, Pat Moynihan, and a black business entrepreneur, Richard Parsons, co-chief operation officer of AOL Time Warner; but White House Press Secretary Ari Fleisher reported that all members shared "the president's view that personal retirement accounts are the way to save Social Security" (Campaign for America's Future 2001).

Congressional Republican leaders worried that it would take "something of a marketing miracle to sell private accounts to the public" (Goldreich 2001), but that did not stop the administration from forging ahead. The commission issued an interim report that attempted to set the stage for creating personal retirement accounts by making the underlying financing of Social Security look as negative as possible. For example, it emphasized that "Social Security Cash Deficits Are Projected to Begin in 2016," seeking therefore to make the crisis seem quite close at hand (President's Commission 2001a: 15). Its rationale was that any payment of benefits from interest earnings on the trust funds is really a subsidy from general revenues. It claimed that, to find those revenues, the government would have to cut all sorts of important programs for poor people. Chapter 4 of this book explains what was wrong with the commission's position, and in particular why some use of general revenues to finance benefits, when the revenues are available because previous program surpluses reduced federal interest costs, is entirely sensible (see also Greenstein and Kogan 2001). The fact that its accounting for the existing Social Security program was mainly an attempt to sell the privatization position became obvious when the commission was quite willing to use general revenues to finance personal accounts. (For an extensive discussion of faulty analysis in the commission's work, see Diamond and Orszag 2002.)

In spite of these tactics, when the commission issued its report in December 2001 it landed "with a thud," and the president "let the moment pass without comment" (Nather with McQueen 2001: 2982). Clearly, many Republican politicians, whatever their personal preferences, did not feel the time was ripe to take a political risk on Social Security. One has to suspect that the market developments discussed earlier in this chapter explain much of that fear. By the time of the 2002 campaign, the National Republican Congressional

Committee advised candidates that they had to fight against the "label" of privatization, and candidates accordingly insisted that personal accounts were not "privatization," and they would never allow cuts or otherwise risk Social Security benefits (for documentation of this approach, see Campaign for America's Future 2002; Hickey et al. 2002).

Nevertheless, many candidates did support "personal accounts," even as they described those accounts in terms that readers of this book might find implausible. Many in the Bush Administration, conservative interest groups, and even candidates interpreted their election victory as "a mandate for changes to Social Security that President Bush has long sought" (Goldstein 2002). The available evidence does not suggest that the election was a shift in public sentiment toward Republican issue positions on this or much of anything else. Republicans gained some seats because of redistricting and a small shift in the margins of the popular vote, caused largely by discouraged Democrats not going to the polls. It was a personal victory for the president only in that he succeeded in mobilizing his partisan base slightly more (half a percentage point) than in 1998, while Democratic turnout fell by an estimated 1.3 percentage points—enough to swing a number of close races (Nather with Cochran 2002: 2892–93). But the fact remains that the Republican tactics to avoid blame for Social Security "privatization" did work and did elect a group of legislators who largely favor "personal accounts" if not "privatization."

Moreover, the administration can still call on the rhetoric of "crisis" to support its position. Its strategy, like that of conservative critics of Social Security and Medicare for the past decade, has been to make the programs seem "unsustainable" so that radical reform, which promises (rightly or not) less pain than any other method that would also promise solvency immediately, will seem the only alternative. That strategy might work because conventional wisdom remains that the programs are unsustainable and should be "fixed" immediately.

Thus, the General Accounting Office (GAO 2002) and the Social Security and Medicare Board of Trustees (2002a: 1, 15) are still issuing warnings and calling for quick action to solve the coming fiscal crisis. As the year came to an end, the most informed of journalists are still writing that "Hard Truths Are Avoided On Social Security," as "Democrats cannot face the fact that this crown jewel of the New Deal . . . will begin running out of money during the lifetime of most of today's workers" (Rosenbaum 2002). David Broder (2002) reported, in an approving tone, that ex-President Clinton seemed to be contemplating private accounts.[6]

Hence, this Afterword must end where the book began. Alarm about Social Security and Medicare remains endemic; that alarm is being used to support an agenda that could destroy the programs in the name of saving them. So long as ordinary citizens imagine it is possible for any government to guarantee the funding of programs seventy-five years in advance, that alarm will seem credible. It will seem especially credible given that voters generally do not accept tax increases until they seem necessary compared to a worse alternative—and the arguments for privatization and vouchers assert that they offer a free lunch of better pensions and health benefits.

Modest, incremental measures would be sufficient for the times and better policy. They will not happen during the 108th Congress. Readers who agree with the analysis in this book should hope only for gridlock in 2003 and 2004, and a different president and Congress in 2005.

NOTES

Preface to the Paperback Edition

1. Governor George W. Bush, "Saving Social Security and Medicare," fact sheet prepared by the Bush campaign, May 15, 2000, p. 1.

2. Quotes from Bush speech, "A Defining American Promise," Rancho Cuca-monga Senior Center, Rancho Cucamonga, Calif., May 15, 2000.

3. For instance, on one hand, a Gore campaign press release on the day of Bush's major campaign speech denounced the Bush initiative as a "Lose-Lose-Lose Social Se-curity Privatization Proposal" that "Could Cost a Trillion Dollars, Eliminate Guar-antee of Retirement Security, and Result in Massive Government Bail Outs." On the other hand, economist Paul Krugman criticized Bush for making statements that "a politician can't honestly say" but noted quite nastily that "he'd never be able to get away with it if Al Gore were still alive" (2000).

One: Introduction

1. The examples given in the text include some of the nation's best-known re-porters, writing for establishment journals (the *Wall Street Journal*'s news columns should not be confused with its editorial page). For good examples from political an-alysts, see Schneider 1997, Ornstein 1997, and Cook 1996.

2. Education has been and remains the larger expense, though it should be expected to become smaller eventually. For comparative figures, see Bixby 1997, tables 1 and 2.

3. See Aaron and Reischauer 1998a, Baker and Weisbrot 1999, Ball 1998, and Leone and Anrig 1999. Kingson and Schulz 1997a is an excellent overview of Social Security issues. A discussion that goes beyond Social Security is Marmor, Mashaw, and Har-vey 1992. The work that comes closest to the purpose of this book is Moon and Mul-vey 1995.

4. I will argue later that the conventional projections do not exactly show the affordability of the programs, but that is irrelevant to the point about volatility that is made by the table.

5. Spending totals were higher in intermediate years.

Two: Why Americans Trust Social Insurance
and Distrust Entitlements

1. If a parent "misbehaves," society may not want to help the parent, but most peo-ple may feel queasy about saying that the sins of the mothers and fathers should be

visited on the children. That, of course, is why the program benefits depended on the children—it was Aid to Dependent Children and, later, Aid to Families with Dependent Children.

2. For example, Peter G. Peterson (1996) calls for an "affluence test," but it is called a means test in his index!

3. As discussed in later chapters, replacement rates alone do not measure return on contributions. On average, higher earners live longer, and so collect more payments, than workers with lower wages. Thus, total collections are much more proportional to contributions than are the monthly pensions.

4. For figures on earnings, see *Economic Report of the President* 1997, tables B-31, B-45.

5. See Board of Trustees 2000a: 191–92. Taxable payroll was projected to decline to 37.4 percent of GDP in 2040 and 35.0 percent in 2075. The reasons were that average earnings were expected to grow more slowly than productivity (thus, more slowly than return on capital); wages (which are taxable) to grow more slowly than fringe benefits (which are not); and earnings to grow more quickly for individuals who earned more than the maximum amount for payroll tax than for people who earned less.

6. For discussions of entitlements within the broader context of budgeting, see White 1998b, 1999a.

7. The figures are for federal fiscal years, and the 1997 figure is not final. See table 8.3, "Percentage Distribution of Outlays by Budget Enforcement Act Category: 1962–2002," in *Historical Tables: Budget of the United States Government, Fiscal Year 1998* (Washington, D.C.: GPO, 1997). Not all of the rest of spending was technically entitlements: thus, net interest is not, and there are some small items such as payments to foreign governments and repayment of loans and loan guarantees. For a further discussion of definitional issues, see Gist 1996.

8. See White and Wildavsky 1991 on deficit politics. The evolution of the use of the term *entitlements* can be traced in Congressional Budget Office reports over the 1980s. For example, see CBO 1980, 1983. See also Weaver 1984 and Shuman 1984: 105–6.

9. The 1972 increases, dramatic as they seemed at the time, may be argued to have only returned benefits to the level planned when the program was created.

10. Gist (1996) concludes from the 1980s figures that entitlements did not cause the deficits; Minarik and Penner (1990) argue, as I do here, that blame for the deficit depends on the year chosen as a baseline.

11. Federal outlays rose from 21.7 percent of GDP to 22.1 percent from 1980 to 1990, or 0.4 percent. Medicaid rose from 0.5 percent to 0.7 percent, and Medicare from 1.2 percent to 1.9 percent, an increase of 0.9 percent. However, interest costs rose from 1.9 percent of GDP to 3.2 percent, as the Reagan-era deficits fed on themselves. See tables F-5, F-8, and F-13 in CBO 1997c.

12. Some Medicaid cost increases had as much to do with intergovernmental cost-shifting games as with higher health-care costs; see Holahan and Liska 1996.

13. These figures involve a different way of counting from that in column 5. Column 5 counts anticipated actual workers, a few of whom will be under 20 or over 64, whereas some people in that age bracket will not be working. Similarly, some people age 65 and over will not be beneficiaries, and some under age 65 will be. So columns 3 and 4 measure the actual demographic trends, and column 5 pertains to the exact rules of the Social Security program.

14. Author's calculation from data in table 2.1. Cutler et al. 1990 reported that the dependency burden would not have exceeded its peak during the baby boom's childhood until even later.

15. The economic burden on workers could also be calculated including the workers themselves, an approach that would reduce projected increases in burdens even more.

16. There are four main categories of Medicaid spending: for elderly persons, which means mainly nursing home care and some supplements to Medicare, such as support for SMI premiums; for blind and disabled persons; for younger families; and separate "disproportionate share hospital" (DSH) payments to hospitals that treat a relatively high number of uninsured patients. The DSH payments cannot easily be attributed to any group. Holahan and Liska (1996) report that in 1966, of the $80.8 billion in federal spending on the other three categories, $25.7 billion went to elderly persons and $29.2 billion to blind and disabled persons.

17. My opinion, explained in White 1995a, is that all Americans should and could have decent health insurance, obviating the need for a separate means-tested program like Medicaid. But I can see reasons to means-test a long-term care benefit for elderly persons.

18. For a powerful critique of the worldview that treats politics as the sum of the actions of isolated individuals, see Stone 1997. People are born into, raised in, and live in communities; what matters most to people, as Aaron Wildavsky told me, is other people; they form their preferences in communication with and influenced by other people; and the social processes that generate belief in social insurance are just as much part of human life as is isolated cogitation.

Three: Social Security

1. For a good summary of the program, send for a copy of *Social Security: The Basics* (New York: Century Foundation, 1999 or later). For more detail, see U.S. House, Committee on Ways and Means 1998, or more recent updates. A good statistical summary is SSA/ORES 1997; figures here not otherwise attributed come from that source.

2. Self-employed individuals can deduct the employer half of their OASDI payroll taxes from their net earnings before computing their Social Security tax and may also deduct half of their Social Security tax as a business expense for income tax purposes. The goal of these provisions is to ensure that, as both employee and employer,

self-employed individuals receive the same tax treatment overall as separate employers and employees do (U.S. House, Committee on Ways and Means 1996: 5–6).

3. Estimates for 1997 from U.S. House, Committee on Ways and Means 1996: 42. The exact rules are that up to 50 percent of benefits are subject to income tax, to the extent that the benefits raise income for an individual above $25,000, or for a couple above $32,000. The revenue from this taxation of benefits is deposited in the OASDI trust funds. A further 35 percent of benefits is subject to income tax if those benefits raise the income for an individual over $34,000 or for joint filers over $44,000. This revenue then is deposited in the HI trust fund.

4. In 1983, when the Democrats wanted to raise taxes rather than cut benefits and the Republicans wanted to do the opposite, the former counted the imposition of taxes on 50 percent of benefits as a tax increase, and the Reagan administration claimed it was a benefit cut. In 1993, when the Democrats wanted to claim that their deficit-reduction bill was a balanced package and the Republicans wanted to claim that it was a huge tax hike, the Democrats counted taxing up to 85 percent of benefits as a spending cut, and the Republicans called it a tax increase.

5. The minimum earnings in 1998 were $700 per quarter (*Social Security Bulletin* 61, no. 4 [1998]: back page).

6. For simplicity's sake, the figures assume that a worker's wages in all years bear the same relation to the population earning distribution. So an "average" earner earns the average wage in all years, not just the final year of work. For an example of results with various different (and more realistic) assumptions, see Bosworth, Burtless, and Steuerle 1999.

7. The formula is that monthly payments are reduced by $5/9$ percent for each month of early retirement; thus, retiring 36 months early creates a reduction of $36 \times 5/9 = 20$ percent.

8. On trust funds in general, see Patashnik 1997.

9. For examples of discussion in these terms, see the papers in Aaron 1990; "Four Reasons Not to Cut Taxes" 1990; and National Economic Commission 1989.

10. For an overview of the whole period, see Hager and Pianin 1997. Other good accounts of the primacy of deficit politics include Makin and Ornstein 1994, Haas 1990, Woodward 1994, Maraniss and Weisskopf 1996, and White and Wildavsky 1991.

11. There were a number of efforts to make the problem seem bigger, such as exaggerating its consequences or using the 1987 stock market crash as an excuse for action. They did not work. For a similar discussion of the general question of the effect of Social Security surpluses during the era of high deficits, see Peter Diamond's comments in note 20, question 3, of NASI 1998.

12. Appendix, "Statement of the Council on the use of the trust funds," adopted unanimously on April 29, 1938, in Committee on Economic Security 1985.

13. Quotes from Concord Coalition 1997: Jan. 28, April 28, 1997.

Four: Medicare's Structure, Benefits, and Financing

1. Sheila Burke was top aide to Senator Robert Dole (R-Kan.) when he was Senate Majority Leader.

2. For instance, the premium to buy into HI in 1997 was $311.00 per month. The SMI premium of $43.80 per month was supposed to represent 25 percent of costs, so the total would have been $175.20 per month. Adding the HI and SMI figures together gives a total of $486.20 per month, or $11,668.80 per year for a couple.

3. See the "View" of Celinda Lake as well as those of Karlyn Bowman and Robert Blendon in Reischauer, Butler, and Lave 1997.

4. HI does cover services provided by physicians who are essentially hospital employees, such as residents and pathologists. But independent physicians, such as the admitting physician, bill through SMI.

5. Examples include immunosuppressive drugs following an organ transplant and some oral cancer drugs, as well as some vaccines.

6. Background data supplied by Office of the Actuary, HCFA, on June 4, 1998.

7. Estimate from Aaron and Reischauer 1995: 11. Ken Thorpe (1998: 11) reports that unpublished contract work done in 1992 for the Department of Health and Human Services estimated that 10 percent of plans provided less financial protection and 90 percent provided more.

8. The average employment-based plan has not only less onerous individual cost-sharing provisions but also some cap on total out-of-pocket expenses. Those caps averaged about $1,250 per person in a 1996 survey (PPRC 1997: 197).

9. The dispute influences even the language used. To providers, their preferred fee is the right amount, and the difference between Medicare's schedule and their fee is the "balance" left over. To many policymakers, the difference between the Medicare fee and what providers want to charge is "extra." Under current law, physicians can charge no more than 109.25 percent of the fee schedule amount, and they have other incentives not to extra-bill, which explains why they do so so rarely. For discussions, see Mason and Nohlgren 1989: 14–28; PPRC 1997: 313–14; U.S. House, Committee on Ways and Means 1996: 183–84; and Culbertson and Lee 1996.

10. When that act does not pass separately, the appropriation is provided in an omnibus "continuing resolution."

11. Author's calculations from data in Board of Trustees 1998c.

12. The "arms race" continues even in the current "competitive" environment; see Hilzenrath 1998.

13. GME payment rates vary among hospitals for many reasons, including that the payment formula includes actual costs in the past. In 1997 Medicare also paid about $300 million to train allied health providers. See MedPAC 1998d: 124–26.

14. Good examples of this focus on the whole system of coverage include Aaron

and Reischauer 1995 and Wilensky and Newhouse 1999. A classic example of the political maneuvering created by efforts to combine entitlement constraint ("saving" Medicare) and expansion (a drug benefit) was the dispute over whether reforms promoted by the National Bipartisan Commission on the Future of Medicare would expand coverage; see Altman and Tyson 1999; Goldstein 1999a; Pear 1999; and Vladeck 1999.

15. For estimates of participation in these types of program, see PPRC 1997: 318.

16. Only 14 percent of Medigap enrollees choose one of the three standard plans that include pharmaceutical benefits. Each of those has a $250 deductible and pays only half of subsequent costs up to a maximum; that cap in two plans is $1,250 in benefits and in the third is $3,000. See Davis et al. 1999; U.S. House, Committee on Ways and Means 1998: 216–17; Health Care Financing and Organization, *Findings Brief* 1, no. 2 (1997).

17. Thus, Marilyn Moon and Karen Davis report, "The current method of paying HMOs for Medicare patients is seriously flawed" (1995: 42). The editor of *Health Affairs* notes in the prologue to Newhouse, Buntin, and Chapman 1997 that "almost from the first day that Medicare began contracting with . . . (HMOs), . . . policy analysts have criticized the payment methodology used." See also PPRC 1997: 21–76, 177–200; ProPAC 1997b: 36–39; Feldman and Dowd 1997; Robinson and Powers 1997; Marmor and Oberlander 1998.

18. For examples of such claims from around the world, see McPherson 1990; Roos and Roos 1994; and Wennberg 1984.

19. PPRC reported that for the six months before enrolling in Medicare Risk plans, beneficiaries' costs were 37 percent below those of a fee-for-service comparison group. "In the six months after disenrolling, beneficiaries costs were 60 percent above the fee-for-service average" (1997: 79).

20. Eighty-two percent of beneficiaries reported that they had prescription drug coverage; see MedPAC 1998b: 134–35.

21. For instance, a quality difference within the small proportion of seriously ill people over two years might, out of the whole population, be so small as to be statistically insignificant. Yet cumulated over twenty years, it might be important. Worse, if data are from satisfaction surveys, people who have the most reason to be dissatisfied, being dead, cannot respond to the survey.

22. Much of the literature focuses on traditional group- or staff-model HMOs, such as Kaiser-Permanente, and so tells us nothing about, say, an Independent Practice Association model in Miami.

23. For a review of measurement issues and a few research citations, see MedPAC 1998b: chap. 3.

24. For coverage in other countries, see White 1995a.

Five: Why All the Fuss?

1. In the pages that follow, I cite the work of many scholars, most of whom I know personally and greatly respect. I do not intend to suggest that they should be viewed as partisans in all they do—only that, because they have records of being appointed by one party or the other (and other related associations as well, such as advising campaigns), they are identified with parties by journalists and other observers. For example, Robert Reischauer was appointed director of the Congressional Budget Office by the Democratic leaders of Congress. Barry Bosworth served in the Carter administration, Henry J. Aaron in the Johnson administration, and Charles L. Schultze in both. Rudy Penner served in the Ford administration and was appointed CBO director when the control of Congress was split and it seemed the Republicans' turn. Eugene Steuerle served in the Reagan administration. Edward M. Gramlich was appointed chair of the 1994–96 Advisory Council on Social Security when the Democrats controlled the presidency and Congress, and he was appointed to the Federal Reserve Board by President Clinton.

2. For a superb overview of deficit politics more generally, see Savage 1988.

3. For a more extensive account of the change in view by economists associated with the Democratic party in particular, see White and Wildavsky 1991. Some economists still emphasize demand management rather than savings; see in particular Eisner 1986; Galbraith 1998. Their criticisms justify further doubt about the conventional wisdom, but the more important point is that even the numbers based on conventional wisdom do not justify significant cuts in Social Security and Medicare.

4. There are exceptions to the rule that monetary policy is more flexible and easily implemented. In a serious recession, loosening the money supply may be "pushing on a string" because nobody wants to borrow to invest anyway, and direct public employment may be more effective. The "automatic stabilizers" in budget policy, such as the ways unemployment benefits rise and taxes fall in a recession, influence the economy more quickly than monetary policy could. But as a matter of discretionary, purposive response to most economic swings, monetary policy is a quicker and more flexible tool.

5. Author's calculations from *Economic Report of the President* 1996, tables B-27, B-45.

6. One more alternative, less emphasis on free trade, was anathema and would not even get serious consideration. No mainstream economic model would show benefits from more protection. See Schultze 1997.

7. Aside from the sources cited in the text and notes, a reader interested in a nicely balanced, longer treatment of the issues about savings and Social Security might consult Penner 1989.

8. In an earlier work, CBO (1993: 74) estimated a 30 percent offset from the decline in private savings.

9. Estimates should also be difficult, and could be overstated, because of a fourth problem, diminishing returns. If you assume investors are rational, then each extra dollar of investment should gain a lower yield than the average to date. But there is no way to guess the rate at which returns would diminish.

10. Author's calculations from economic and budget estimates in CBO 1999.

11. All of Aaron 1990 illustrates how closely the campaigns for higher national savings have been linked to some economists' *defenses* of Social Security.

12. Among the other Democratic signers of this statement were the president of the AFL-CIO, Lane Kirkland, and the chair of the House Budget Committee, William Gray (D-Pa.).

13. In 1999 the high-cost forecast's GDP was 6.4 percent lower than that of the intermediate forecast in 2008. The low-cost scenario's GDP in 2008 was 7.9 percent higher than in the intermediate scenario. The gaps would, of course, widen substantially in subsequent years. See Board of Trustees 1999a: 58–59, table II.D1.

14. Even if the estimated calculation was changed by 0.2 percentage points per year, real wages would, over a thirty-year period, become about 6 percent larger than in the intermediate scenario.

15. *Analytical Perspectives* 1997: 23–30; see also CBO's critique in CBO 1997b: 17.

16. For background on discretionary spending caps, see Schick 1995: esp. 8–10, 39–41, 135, 188–92.

17. For another discussion, see *Analytical Perspectives* 1999: 30–31. OMB's assessment that an inflation adjustment nevertheless is a reasonable baseline is unconvincing.

18. Retirement of the debt is made even more difficult by the fact that at some point all that will be left will be thirty-year bonds whose owners will not be willing to sell them to the government "at prices that the government would be willing to pay" (CBO 2000: 19). But that just means the question of what to do with surpluses, other than to retire debt, would be faced even when some debt is still outstanding.

19. The GAO staff very kindly reran their full model with the different discretionary spending assumption, and I then used spreadsheet calculations to estimate further changes. The very busy people at GAO are under no obligation at all to provide such assistance to outside scholars, and I am sincerely grateful for their generosity. Their assistance in no way indicates any endorsement of any of the arguments in this book. My discretionary figures begin with spending of 6.6 percent of GDP in fiscal year 1999, declining by 0.1 percent of GDP per year to 5.7 percent in 2008. So my spending trends to about 0.4 percent of GDP higher than in the GAO 1999 baseline in figure 5.1. I also raised Medicare spending a bit above GAO's 1999 assumption (which was more optimistic in the long run than CBO's but did not include the shocking short-term restraint that CBO had to incorporate in its 2000 figures). My only

change in a more "optimistic" direction was to assume that increases in Part B premiums over time would constitute extra revenues. By holding revenues constant, GAO and CBO had projected that taxes would be cut as Part B premiums rose, which seems nonsensical.

20. The proposal was also explained (well, sort of) in a press briefing before the State of the Union Address by Gene Sperling, a transcript of which I obtained from the White House Web site.

21. Readers can find discussion of these two sequesters as part of an appendix in each year's version of CBO's *The Economic and Budget Outlook* volume.

22. Many Democrats argue that any controls should be defined in a way that does not allow projected Social Security surpluses to be used for any other purpose, such as finance of a privatization scheme. Republican "lockbox" proposals, naturally, usually leave an out for just such a scheme. Although I share the Democrats' preferences, I believe there is a big difference between using potential Social Security surpluses to reform Social Security (even in a way with which I disagree) and using those surpluses for other budgetary goals. Budget process restrictions should apply to only the latter.

23. For example, a report by the McKinsey Global Institute in June 1996 suggested that capital investment is more productive, per dollar invested, in the United States than in Germany or Japan. Moreover, the McKinsey analysts argued, a focus on net national savings, which were much lower in the United States, was misplaced; the most important factor was gross business investment, which was only modestly lower in the United States. See Lewis 1996; Zachary 1996; Samuelson 1996a.

Six: Can Americans Afford to Grow Old and Sick?

1. Further elaboration of some points in this chapter may be found in White 1999b,c. The Medicare spending trends for 1990–95 reported here correct data errors in White 1999b.

2. I discuss this briefly in White 1999b, based on conversation with CBO staff members who desire and deserve to remain anonymous.

3. As discussed in chapter 7, some benefit cuts are already legislated. Moreover, pension benefits during retirement grow more slowly than per capita GDP except during recession.

4. See also Gornick, McMillan, and Lubitz 1993. Nursing home costs that Medicare does not cover may rise with longevity, but that is not relevant to Medicare cost estimates.

5. Medicare cost control laws often have provisions that are expected to expire, which means that everyone expects them to be renewed. This point was actually made by Republicans to show that the cuts they proposed in 1995 were not as big as they seemed. See Kahn and Kuttner 1999: 40.

6. Author's calculations from Medicare annual spending projections provided by

the HCFA Office of the Actuary, May 26, 1999. I, of course, am not privy to debates within HCFA; I can report only what I have been told about the basis for the much more optimistic 2002–12 estimates.

7. I provide more detail on the assumptions in this analysis in White 1999b.

8. Enrollment changes alone would still, by 2070, raise Medicare to only about 34 percent of total health-services costs. I calculated this figure by comparing the costs of Medicare and the total national health-care costs, excluding government public-health activities and research and construction activities for 1995, as reported in Levit et al. 1998a, exhibits 2, 4. I then adjusted these figures for the population shares as of 1995 that I report in table 7.2, and applied that ratio to the shares projected for 2070. Actual total costs for the Medicare population will rise more than Medicare costs because of all the services that Medicare does not reimburse. It would be nice to have an update to Waldo et al. 1989, but reasonable extrapolations from those data still suggest that total costs for the Medicare population would be less than half of the national total, and much of the Medicare population's non-Medicare spending will be paid by those beneficiaries, not future workers.

9. This estimate is based on the average family premium in KPMG Peat Marwick's 1996 Health Benefits Survey, $5,188. Median family money income was $42,300, so premiums were 12.26 percent of the median, which, doubled, would be 24.52 percent. That figure, however, is based on employer-purchased insurance; premiums if people had to purchase insurance on their own would be at least 20 percent higher. See Gabel, Hunt, and Kim 1998; *Economic Report of the President* 1998: 320, table B-33.

10. As described in White 1995a, Australia tried the voluntary route with government subsidies through 1984 and still had a substantial uninsured population. For a nice statement of the situation in the United States, see Broder 1999a.

11. Actually, national systems that allow physicians to charge more in "private" practice for services that are covered by the public system do encourage physicians to create longer-than-necessary "waiting lists" within the public system. For critiques of this effect within the British National Health Service, see Yates 1987; Light 1997.

Seven: Exploiting Our Grandchildren?

1. One may argue, however, that we should be concerned only with people who lose. From this perspective, only the "doomsday" generation, the one that pays but gets no benefits at all, has a real complaint. And assuming that the program continues, there is no doomsday generation.

2. Because it is conventional to compare cohorts of equal numbers of years, these five-year groupings are used in all the available analyses. Although that means the cohorts do not match the conventional definition of the baby-boom generation, they are close enough to assess claimed inequities.

3. Author's calculation from Board of Trustees 1998a, table II.D1, using interme-

diate assumptions, exact figures for the real-wage differential from 1998 to 2007, and an increase of 0.9 percent per year afterward.

4. Author's calculation from data in Board of Trustees 1998a: 169, table III.A2. I have assumed pure pay-as-you-go finance, so benefits in 2035 would be paid entirely from higher taxes, with no earnings from the trust funds. This would be the maximum estimate of the burden on workers.

5. The same logic is unlikely to apply to housing, because it is easier to continually add to a stock portfolio than to continually trade upward in housing value. Stocks do not have maintenance and property-tax costs, and houses do.

6. As Sylvester J. Schieber points out, quoting Adam Smith, concepts of minimal need are relative. Hence "necessaries" are "not only the commodities which are indispensably necessary for the support of life, but whatever the custom of the country renders it indecent for creditable people, even of the lowest order, to be without" (1997: 271).

7. Weaver 1999, p. 191 and table 5.1. For example, the normal retirement age in the United States was either higher or scheduled to become higher than those in 13 of the 15 countries as of 1995, and benefit adjustments to inflation or wage increases were more generous in more countries than they were less generous. For this and other details, see SSA/ORES 1995; also OECD 1996: 31.

8. Author's calculations, from Board of Trustees 1999a: background table III.B5, at <www.ssa.gov/OACT/TR/TR99/lr3B5-1.html>.

9. I am deeply indebted to a wide range of scholars for responding to my plaintive appeals on the Internet for guidance in analyzing poverty rates and family budgets. Among those who helped, and who deserve credit for the virtues but no blame for the demerits of my analysis that follows, were John Myles, Ken Oliver, Sheila Shaver, Robert Stephens, John Veit-Wilson, and especially Gordon Fisher, who dipped into his vast fund of knowledge to provide many citations and warnings. Thank you, all.

10. For a history of the official poverty threshold, see Fisher 1997. As early as the 1960s, the "moderate living standard" for a retired couple as developed by the Bureau of Labor Statistics was well above the official poverty threshold. See Orshansky 1968; Brackett 1968. For discussion of new "experimental" poverty thresholds, all much higher than the official one, see Olsen 1999.

11. An individual who contributed at the maximum level for the entire computation period and retired at age 65 in 1996 with a spousal supplement would have had a benefit of $22,480 per year. The right combination of inflation adjustments and birth year might allow some earlier retirees to have higher benefits, but the simpler explanations for the couples above this level are that either the wife's benefits from her own earnings were more than 50 percent of the husband's or one or both spouses worked past age 65. See Social Security Bulletin (1997), annual statistical supplement, vol. 71, table 2.A28.

12. I will provide further information about the rationale and data sources for this analysis upon request.

13. As one example, I am assuming only $600 per year for automobile insurance, which is way too low in some communities.

14. The calculations assume that promised benefits will be financed by raising payroll taxes as necessary, that is, on a pay-as-you-go basis. The description and analysis is in Goss 1997: 177–80, app. 2; 199–216, tables and charts.

15. I am being imprecise because the data are reported only on charts (Goss 1997: 206–14). The only exceptions, again, involve maximum earners.

16. For good reviews of the arguments, see Galbraith 1998; Mishel, Bernstein, and Schmitt 1997. For information on education levels, though the data may not be quite representative, see Paulin and Riordon 1998.

17. For explanations of his methods, see Baker 1998: 8–10, 18. Briefly, he projected that wages would grow by the OASDI trustees' intermediate scenario as of 1998. He then assumed that payroll taxes would be raised to cover the demographically driven portion of increased costs; so the employer and employee contributions to OASDI would each be raised by 0.05 percent per year from 2010 to 2046, for a total increase of 3.6 percentage points. He deducted the employer contributions from before-tax wages (on the assumption that employers would pay lower wages as they paid more taxes) and the employee contributions from after-tax wages, so both effects are in the after-tax figures. The way he estimated Medicare costs is likely to understate future burdens. If we assume instead that Medicare costs will increase by as much as 2 percent of GDP more through 2070, thus by about 5 percent of payroll, then, as a very rough approximation, readers might expect the baseline net wages to be 1 percent lower than the table in 2010, 4 percent lower in 2030, 5 percent lower in 2050, and 6 percent lower in 2070. The effects of income inequality, as reported in the bottom half of the table, remain far more dramatic.

Eight: Privatizing Security?

1. Some readers may wonder why supposedly antigovernment conservatives would support government compulsion. The logical political answer is that once Social Security already exists as a mandatory program, mandatory private accounts seem preferable to mandatory participation in social insurance. For another discussion of the rationales for government involvement, see World Bank 1994.

2. A less-prominent argument says that workers as fund-holders would have a sense of ownership of the economy that they do not have today. See, for example, Kerrey 1998. Robert Kuttner is among those who have argued, in response, that the government could open accounts at birth (say, with payments of $1,000 per year for five years) and make those a supplement to the existing Social Security program.

3. Among plans that cut basic benefits without guaranteeing their replacement

were the Personal Security Accounts plan recommended by five of the thirteen members of the 1994–96 Advisory Council on Social Security and the Individual Accounts option proposed by that council's chair, Edward M. Gramlich, and council member Marc Twinney. Both plans are described in detail in Advisory Council on Social Security 1997a. Also in this category were a proposal developed by the self-appointed National Commission on Retirement Policy (NCRP), S. 2313, whose prime political sponsors were conservative Democrats Senator John Breaux (D-La.) and Representative Charles Stenholm (D-Tex.) and Republicans Senator Judd Gregg (R-N.H.) and Representative Jim Kolbe (R-Ariz.); and the "Social Security Solvency Act of 1998," S. 1792, cosponsored by Senators Daniel Patrick Moynihan (D-N.Y.) and Bob Kerrey (D-Nebr.). All are described in U.S. Senate Committee on Finance 1999.

4. Examples include plans promoted by Martin Feldstein, as in CBO 1998c; Feldstein 1998b; and Feldstein and Samwick 1998, as well as the plan sponsored by Representatives Bill Archer (R-Tex.) and E. Clay Shaw (R-Fla.), which is described in Copeland, VanDerHei, and Salisbury 1999: 23.

5. In the Moynihan-Kerrey proposal as of late 1998, the payroll tax would have been cut by one percentage point for employers and one point for employees; contributions to personal accounts would then have been voluntary, and if employees chose to invest their 1 percent in individual accounts, employers would have been required to match the contributions. Gramlich's plan required workers to invest an extra 1.6 percent of covered payroll in individual accounts.

6. The estimated minimum administrative costs were $25 to $50 per year; with mean taxable earnings of $23,000, a 2 percent contribution yields the 5–11 percent estimate. See NASI 1998: 9, executive summary. Assuming more choice among funds, thus more marketing and other expenses, the NASI panel concluded that "the estimate of the Advisory Council on Social Security—of an annual charge of 1 percent of the account balance, for Personal Security Accounts, funded by 5 percent of the payroll tax—is roughly correct on average once the system is mature" (5, question 5). See also Olsen and Salisbury 1998.

7. So long as there is competition among insurers to sell annuities, however, there would still be some selection effects. Individual insurers, as in other markets, would compete to sell their products to potentially less costly individuals and try to avoid selling to others. Presumably some regulation of prices and marketing would be required.

8. Poterba and Warshawsky's figures are averages for "nonqualified" annuities offered by commercial insurers in June 1998, calculated using the estimated mortality of the annuitants instead of the general population. The lower costs are for men, and the higher are for women. I am using their riskier portfolio, which consists of BAA corporate bonds, as the closest comparison to the stock-bond mix assumed by privatizers. See also Mitchell, Poterba, and Warshawsky 1997; Poterba 1997.

9. I am grateful to Gary Burtless and Barry Bosworth for explaining objections to

the Baker argument. They, of course, are not responsible for my summary or conclusions.

10. Although the CIEBA and GAO reports were oriented toward issues of trust-fund diversification, the rate-of-return question is identical. The analyses for the CIEBA report were performed by Goldman, Sachs, and Co., Morgan Stanley Dean Witter, J. P. Morgan Investment Management, and INVESCO Global Strategies.

11. A third effect of a defined-contribution scheme is that the uncertain benefits make the program's value to any beneficiary less than the projected benefit, because that amount should be discounted for the risk. For an attempt to "risk-adjust" benefits, see Olsen et al. 1998.

12. Investments made by the entity that pays an annuity must be much more conservative than investments by people saving for retirement in the far future. The reason is that a person earlier in her career may rely on stock market slumps to average out over time, for she does not have to use any proceeds for a long time. But the seller of an annuity must begin paying out immediately. Consider what would have happened to a seller that invested the purchase price of an annuity in an index fund based on the Standard and Poor's 500 in 1965. The investment would have lost 4.65 percent annually for ten years (Wessel 1997a), making paying benefits at the end of that period quite difficult. Better experience after 1975 would not help the annuity company.

13. Some people suspect that the government would compensate retirees after such a slump, but then it would hardly be a truly privatized pension. And should the government tax pensions more when stocks go up more than usual? See Heller 1998: 14.

14. Imagine two people, one investing $3,000 per year and the other $1,000. Whatever portfolio the latter chose, the former could do exactly the same thing with his first $1,000 and then invest the other $2,000 more speculatively. He therefore would have as much security and a much higher average return. Richer, as Aaron Wildavsky wrote in another context, is safer.

15. The earnings of the second earner are sometimes misrepresented as being "wasted" if they produce a benefit lower than the spousal benefit, but that is at best a question of perspective. The woman (usually) simply gets the higher of two amounts, what would be merited by her own earnings or by her husband's; it is not as if the spousal benefit pays her less than she would get if she were unmarried.

16. Larin and Greenstein show that when the NCRP plan "took full effect, the Social Security disability benefits provided to an individual who had earned average wages before becoming disabled would be reduced nearly 20 percent, as compared to current law" (1998: 3). The PSA plan also required significant disability benefits cuts, as its sponsors acknowledged (Advisory Council on Social Security 1997a: 124–25).

17. For example, the difference between the median white worker and the median black worker should be greater than the difference between average white and black workers, which is what is reported by the Social Security actuaries' approach. See Beach and Davis 1998c: 5–7.

18. The Heritage analysts calculated average rate of return by comparing benefits to contributions for a person with average life expectancy. But everybody who lives longer collects more, and everybody who dies earlier pays less. Since the average African American lived to age 67, the Heritage calculations exaggerate contributions by assuming that even dead people paid to the Normal Retirement Age, and the calculations depressed benefits by assuming that nobody collected past age 67. The point was explained by Robert J. Myers, former chief actuary of the Social Security Administration, in a draft letter to the editor of the *Wall Street Journal,* April 13, 1998.

19. The error was that they gave survivors' benefits the same life insurance value for both blacks and whites and netted it out of the comparison. But because of shorter life expectancies, life insurance actually would be worth more to blacks than to whites.

20. Statistics are for December 1996 from the *Social Security Bulletin* (1997), annual statistical supplement, 183, 190, table 5.A1.

21. Feldstein dismissed the required savings as only 4 percent of the federal budget and thus "not an impossible task" (1998b: 14). Hardly simple, either, if you remember that that would be equivalent to a $69 billion spending cut in 1999.

22. CBO makes the same criticism without being so pointed, by citing Feldstein and Pellechio 1979. For further discussion of the issue, see CBO 1998d.

23. This is quite a new argument; I had not seen it until 1998 and could cite lots of eminent commentators, including Alan Greenspan, saying that privatization per se would not increase savings. There is little basis for estimating the size of the effect, and it would have to be very long-term. For further discussion of savings issues, see NASI 1998, questions 1, 2.

24. For instance, the Archer-Shaw plan "pays for itself by 2047" (testimony of Representatives Bill Archer and Clay Shaw before the House Budget Committee Task Force on Social Security, June 29, 1999, 106th Cong., 1st sess., p. 4).

25. For more on British pensions, see Daniel 1998. It may not be a coincidence that British experience is rarely cited in any detail by advocates of privatization.

26. I focus on "Public Law Paygo," which was defined as maintaining existing benefits and raising taxes whenever necessary to keep reserves in the trust fund equal to the next year's expected expenses. See Advisory Council on Social Security 1997a for the analyses, e.g., p. 168.

27. Among the more significant differences in modeling choices, the EBRI analysis includes a feedback loop from reform choices to economic performance and back to pension funding and benefits. The EBRI reports focus on OASI alone, whereas the Advisory Council figures include Disability Insurance contributions and benefits. The EBRI methodology allows analysis of risk in ways that the Advisory Council methods do not. Also, the EBRI reports provide results only for single individuals, whereas the Advisory Council data consider other family structures, and the two sets of data analyze results with different ranges of birth years. The Advisory Council analyses assume that workers earn the same proportion of average wages throughout their work-

ing lives, and EBRI assumes that workers earn more as they age. So EBRI, with a more realistic contribution pattern, should project earnings on individual accounts more accurately (and more conservatively, since the lower contributions will accumulate earnings over longer periods and the higher contributions over shorter periods). However, EBRI assumes that a larger share of contributions will be invested in equities earlier in individuals' careers (100% for workers in their twenties), whereas the Social Security actuaries assume investment of 55 percent in equities for all workers under age 40 and a smaller share toward the end of working years (23% for workers age 60 and over, compared to 43% in the Advisory Council assumptions). This pattern will offset the difference in assumed earnings patterns, since EBRI will have younger people earning higher rates on lower contributions and older people earning lower rates on higher contributions. EBRI, as noted earlier, also assumes a lower rate of return on equities than the Advisory Council does. I should add that the EBRI model was being adjusted over time, so the model used for the March 1998 report was not the same as that used for the June 1999 report.

28. Returns would be 41 percent higher for women and 17 percent higher for men from "raising taxes only" (see Olsen et al. 1998: 13, table 3).

29. For the PSA plan, see Advisory Council on Social Security 1997a: 210, chart 5, for comparisons for total composite workers. For Moynihan-Kerrey, see Copeland, VanDerHei, and Salisbury 1999: 9, table 3.

30. The most prominent supporter of diversification, at least for a while, was President Clinton, who proposed it in his 1999 State of the Union address. See "The Text" 1999. The first major recent statement of the case for investing some portion of the trust-fund balance in equities was as part of the "Maintain Benefits" plan supported by six of the thirteen members of the 1994–96 Advisory Council on Social Security. See Advisory Council on Social Security 1997a: 59–101. Aaron and Reischauer (1998a) provide one of the best briefs for diversification; see also Robert Ball's comments in "Taking Stock" 1999.

31. Aaron and Reischauer suggest that the government could also decline to exercise voting rights; the problem with that is that it might be seen as giving one side or the other an advantage in any internal battle that requires a set percentage of total shares to change policy. But that may be a rare situation. All of these concerns are discussed in the citations in the previous note.

32. Thus, in a year when there were no earnings at all, the extra borrowing, at 1 percent of GDP, would have only weak macroeconomic effects.

Nine: Medicare Vouchers

1. For an extensive discussion of those merits, including my own take, see the special issue of the *Journal of Health Politics, Policy, and Law* 24, no. 5 (1999).

2. A nice example is a letter sent by Aetna, under the name of its former chair-

man, Richard L. Huber, to assorted people interested in health policy (such as myself) on January 20, 1999, explaining that the proposed merger with Prudential HealthCare offered "greater choice."

3. Different surveys in 1999 gave different results. The employee benefits consulting group Towers Perrin reported that large employers' health-benefits costs would increase by about 7 percent, compared to 4 percent in 1998 (*BNA Health Policy Report,* Jan. 11, 1999, pp. 81, 63). The William M. Mercer Inc. survey estimated 1998 cost increases at 6 percent, significantly higher than in the other studies, and reported that increases in 1999 could be about 9 percent (*BNA Health Policy Report,* Feb. 1, 1999, p. 222). The lowest estimates of premium increases in 1999 were about 5 percent, from the Kaiser Family Fund–Hospital Research and Educational Trust and the Hay Benefits Report, cited in CSHSC 1999.

4. For the reasons why the usual economic case against price controls applies poorly to health care, see White 1994.

5. I explain the possibilities at length in White 1999d, but I do not have truly determinative evidence, either.

6. The analysis that follows is based largely on two sources: Moon, Gage, and Evans 1997; and O'Sullivan et al. 1997. Readers might also consult Board of Trustees 1998c: 19–24; MedPAC 1998b. Where I use numbers, they are estimates as of when BBA-97 passed; actual results may be quite different.

7. The new PPS for outpatient care was also an attempt to reduce the extremely high cost-sharing for those services, though it would do so only very slowly. See MedPAC 1998a: 77–88.

8. The home health transfer was phased in over six years and the effect on the Part B premium over seven, from 1998 to 2004. See O'Sullivan et al. 1997: 34, 43, 45; Moon, Gage, and Evans 1997: 17.

9. Since states would not have federal funding for all eligible beneficiaries, the law said they should accept qualifying applicants in the order in which they applied. See U.S. Senate Committee on Finance 1997, sec. 93.

10. The actual level in each county would depend on other provisions, but the basic idea was to raise the payment in each county not by the local increase in FFS (fee-for-service) costs but by that figure minus 0.8 percent in 1998 and minus 0.5 percent in each of 1999, 2000, 2001, and 2002 (U.S. Senate Committee on Finance 1997: 3).

11. There were a few other escape hatches, such as that a group-or-staff HMO based in clinics could not be required to accept more members than its facilities could handle. See also O'Sullivan et al. 1997: 53.

12. *BNA Health Policy Report,* Jan. 25, 1999, pp. 142–43.

13. I provide the basic objections to MSAs in White 1995b.

14. Individuals who already have costs in excess of the deductible for uncovered services, such as pharmaceuticals, and who have not been able to find insurance that provided the extra coverage at a lower premium than their out-of-pocket cost, would

be one group with high expected costs who would seek out MSAs—assuming that MSA insurers did not manage to avoid signing them up. But that group has to be a minority of the chronically ill.

15. As emphasized by Moon, Gage, and Evans 1997: 7, quoting the conference report on the bill. Kahn and Kuttner (1999) describe the budget limits in the 1995 legislation as something more required by CBO score-keeping than desired by the bill's drafters, but they protest too much. The House proposal clearly was designed to cap total federal spending, and contributions to premiums in each area were to be "budgeted" and "grow each year under rates of growth that are consistent with our plan of growth through the year 2002." The quotation is from a document distributed by the House leadership to explain the bill: "Summary of the Medicare Preservation Act: The Comprehensive Plan for a Better Medicare" (undated; available from the author), p. 13.

16. HCFA provides monthly figures in a report that is posted on its Web site. See HCFA 2000.

17. In one reporter's summary, "HMOs said Wednesday that they are simply the agents in the middle, passing along the ever-rising price of a high-technology medical system" (Rosenblatt 1999; see also Pear 2000). Not the best evidence for their cost-control prospects.

Ten: Too Young or Too Rich for Social Insurance?

1. For this reason, raising the retirement age is especially superior to any reduction of cost-of-living adjustments. See Valdivia 1997.

2. This figure is based on estimates for age-adjusted premiums if either all or only 40 percent of eligible 65-to-66-year-olds had purchased insurance in 1997, from McDevitt 1998: 16–17.

3. I should note that I was one of the other panelists, and the moderator, Meryl Comer, remarked that this might be the first time Dr. Lesher and I agreed on something!

4. This argument was made by Gail Wilensky on "It's Your Business" 1997.

5. The original program name was Aid to Dependent Children; the replacement in 1996 was Temporary Assistance to Needy Families (TANF).

6. Calculation by Curtis S. Florence from the March 1997 Current Population Survey. For further information on uninsured children, see Thorpe and Florence 1998.

7. Yet Peterson himself must consider the affluence test a form of means-testing. Otherwise, in the index to his book, the entry for "affluence tests" would not read, "See means tests" (1996).

8. Among the merits, by focusing on total income it does not risk taking more from moderate-income people who rely largely on federal benefits than from people with the same income from largely private sources. Any direct benefit reduction would

target the former group. Of course, a plain old progressive income tax would also meet the goal of "horizontal equity"—treating people with like incomes alike. Among the obvious practical issues are why the same threshold would apply to couples and single people, public distrust of taxing any noncash benefits, and how to monetize such in-kind benefits. For instance, would the calculated "value" of Medicare be the same for everyone or lower for younger beneficiaries and higher for older ones? For further discussion, see Downey 1995: 111–14.

9. Among the problems, the original proposal would have charged sick people more than healthy people and would have required that private Medicare carriers and intermediaries have tax return information about individuals.

10. Address by Senator John Breaux to the annual meeting of the National Academy of Social Insurance, Washington, D.C., National Press Club, Jan. 28, 1999 (author's recollection).

11. "Number of Enrollees Affected by the Senate Finance Bill for the Income Related Premium," a table prepared by the Division of Medicare and Medicaid Cost Estimates, Actuarial and Health Cost Analysis Group, Health Care Financing Administration, July 17, 1997; kindly supplied to the author by John Gist of the American Association of Retired Persons Public Policy Institute.

12. Author's calculation from projections of OASDI beneficiaries' income separated by tax filing status (married, single, nonfilers) and income group, kindly provided by the Office of the Actuary, Social Security Administration, July 24, 1997. OASDI beneficiaries are an imperfect surrogate for SMI beneficiaries but of course are a quite similar group. Neither SSA nor HCFA has good data by which to project future income distributions, because nobody does. But the SSA data seem roughly similar to estimates for 1998 from the Barents Group Individual Income Tax Model, which were provided to me by the AARP Public Policy Institute. Projections of the future in the SSA data are very simple: in essence, income at all points in the distribution as of one year is assumed to grow at the same rate. The Office of the Actuary cautioned me that nobody should put great reliance on these numbers. But they were the only ones available with which to estimate long-term effects of the means-test proposal.

13. Board of Trustees 1998d gives an estimated annual cost per SMI enrollee, which presumably represents the premium, of $5,803 in 2008.

14. Author's calculations of numbers of affected enrollees from the SSA data generated on July 24, 1997, and cited in note 12 above. The estimated premium amount is from background CBO data provided in June 1998. Estimates with data as of the year 2000 presumably would differ, yet my basic point, that both savings and political risk would be much greater in the future, remains true.

15. Clinton proposed a similar income-related premium for Medicare in his 1993 Health Security Act. The other major difference between the administration and congressional negotiators involved whether the IRS would administer and collect the new

premium provisions. Although the Concord Coalition called that a "dispute without substance," it became the ostensible reason the president and congressional Republicans failed to agree. See Concord Coalition 1997; Pear 1997c; Mitchell 1997.

16. For a useful analysis of this issue, see McClellan and Skinner 1999.

17. German retirees pay the same percentage of their basic pensions as workers pay from their salaries; French retirees pay significantly less. There are proposals to expand the base for contributions in Germany to more fully include other sources of income; see Advisory Council for the Concerted Action 1998: 55.

18. For instance, it would be impossible to know a person's income at the time he was making contributions. It would even be difficult in year Y (say, 2001) to know his income in year Y-1 (2000), because the tax return for 2000 would not be filed until April 15, 2001, and would have to be processed after that. It should be possible, however, to charge people based on an estimated rate and then adjust each year with a correction factor based on over- or undercharges in previous years.

19. This analysis was written before Moynihan (2000) changed his position to reducing COLAs by 0.8 percentage points a year. That does not affect the basic argument here.

20. We should remember that even a full inflation adjustment, so long as real wages are rising, leaves pensioners falling behind the trend in the national standard of living.

21. There are actually multiple CPIs; the CPI-W measures expenses for certain wage-earners and is used for Social Security indexing, but the CPI-U measures price changes for urban consumers and is used for most other purposes. See Abraham 1995.

22. Remember that payroll taxes rise with nominal wages (that is, including inflation), but benefits (after retirement) only with measured inflation. If measured inflation is lower, the spread between total wage increases (thus, revenue increases) and inflation (benefit increases) each year will be larger; put differently, the real-wage differential will grow.

23. Moynihan proposed that a cost-of-living board could scale back the adjustment if it believed BLS had made appropriate changes. But it might not be disposed to do so. See S. 1792 (105th Cong., 2d sess.), pp. 26–37.

24. See Boskin 1996; Boskin Commission 1996.

25. Boskin (1996) estimates that productivity growth would have been ¾ percent higher per year. He does not draw the logical conclusion that he and other economists have been wrong about economic fundamentals.

26. Senator Moynihan claimed that "most" of the BLS changes "were already anticipated when the Boskin Commission issued its report" (1998: 10). The total adjustment by the BLS was 0.69 percentage points; see *Economic Report of the President* 1998: 79.

27. CBO listed effects that might cause the CPI to be upwardly biased but had not been analyzed empirically; its discussion, however, seems a lot more cautious than the Boskin Commission's.

28. For a variety of analyses, see Abraham, Greenlees, and Moulton 1998; Deaton 1998; Diewert 1998; Nordhaus 1998. For a further report on what the BLS was already doing to change its measurements at the time of the Boskin report, see Greenlees and Mason 1996. For a very detailed critique of the Boskin Commission report, see Baker 1997b.

29. See Diewert 1998; Nordhaus 1998. I should add that one of the major examples given of the CPI being overstated because of quality improvement is medical care; the logical conclusion would be that spending more for medical care is not such a bad idea, reducing the Medicare "crisis."

30. See Stewart and Pavalone 1996. They report that the CPI-W (on which Social Security COLAs are calculated) increased by 14.1 percent from December 1990 through December 1995, but the experimental CPI-E increased by 15.9 percent. This would be an annual difference in rate of 0.3 percent.

Eleven: Moderate, Though Hardly Modest, Reforms

1. State and local governments have long had the right to voluntarily include workers in the system. The 1983 Social Security bailout legislation banned governments that had included workers voluntarily from withdrawing from the program, "which effectively made coverage mandatory" for those employees. In 1990 Congress required coverage if the state or local government did not provide an alternative pension plan. See GAO 1998b: 4–5.

2. That proposal is slightly different from the one that I include in chapter 12.

3. It would favor higher-income beneficiaries because they have, on average, lower rates of return; so the 85 percent figure may have been high for them. These 1997 estimates are from Ball 1998: 9; and I provide them because the Social Security Advisory Board did not list the options separately in its 1998 report. Members of the Advisory Council also supported transferring back into the OASDI funds the proportion of benefits taxation that currently is dedicated to the HI trust fund. I do not suggest that because, from the perspective of the overall federal budget, it is irrelevant.

4. An example is the BBA-97's $1,500 annual caps on reimbursements for forms of therapy. See Hilzenrath 1999.

5. Or, as HCFA official Robert A. Berenson put it, HMOs complained more than hospital and doctor representatives because the latter "had little choice in the matter"—they could not do without Medicare's business (quoted in Iglehart 1999: 146).

6. Ken Thorpe (1999) argues that though experiments would be useful, a competitive-pricing approach is very likely to be an improvement, and recommendations by Medicare's Competitive Pricing Advisory Committee are steps in the right direction. So perhaps Congress should just enact a competitive bidding system for all of Medicare + Choice and address problems as they arise. For a detailed discussion of the practical issues in competitive bidding from a Medicare perspective, see Feldman

and Dowd 1997; for supplementary discussion of similar issues in the context of the 1993–94 health reform debate, see White 1995a, esp. chap. 8 and the appendix.

7. This should not be a partisan issue; something similar was proposed by House Republicans in 1995 in HR 2491, as subtitle E of the Medicare Preservation Act. The rationale was described in summary documents released by the House Republican Leadership in September 1995.

8. Academic health centers are so complex that allocating costs among functions (e.g., education and treatment) is very hard. Nevertheless, it appears that Medicare's Indirect Medical Education payments are greater than the extra costs that teaching hospitals incur for treating Medicare patients. See, for example, Anderson, Greenberg, and Lisk 1999: 158, 164. Direct Medical Education payments may also be more adequate than the hospitals claim. Skeptics have long suspected that residents are awfully cheap labor and that when Medicare pays for the direct costs of residencies, teaching hospitals are being paid up front for services that, if provided by different kinds of staff in different institutions, would have to be paid out of regular billings. Reports of New York hospitals discovering that even being paid for residents they did not train was not as good a deal as having residents work at their standard compensation rates seem to fit that suspicion.

9. Author's calculation for 1997, from enrollment tables available on the HCFA Web site.

10. Some really poor people may choose not to pay the SMI premium but instead to rely on other sources for care. My suggested premium reform would require much smaller contributions from them, in return for their having full coverage. Some of the people with SMI but not HI coverage may have some form of Medicaid or other benefits.

11. My thanks to Ken Thorpe for this point.

12. In 1996 the annual Part B premium was $510. Based on median incomes reported by SSA/ORES (1998b: table III.1), a tax rate of 4.1 percent would have yielded the same amount. But that figure must be high for two reasons: mean incomes are higher than median incomes, and the federal government should not be trying, in a reformed system, to collect all the money it was previously paying itself through QMB and SLMB.

13. For the argument applied to Medicare alone, see Marmor and Oberlander 1998; more generally, see Altman and Cohen 1993; Aaron and Schwartz 1993. For a very informative discussion, see Glaser 1993.

14. Somewhat higher targets might be justified if the extraordinary spending constraint in 1999, which I was not including in my calculations as I drafted this book, is not reversed and is seen to have endangered necessary services. That is a judgment, however, that could be made only in 2002, when we know what does happen to Medicare spending and have some sense of the consequences of the trend. The reasons to be cautious about planning rates of growth after 2002 are just another exam-

ple of why it would be absurd to pretend we really know what rates would be appropriate in 2030.

15. I do not mean to imply any criticism of the current Social Security Advisory Board, which might even provide the core of a new advisory council. But I think that if some nongovernmental study group is to be given a very specific task and the authority to report draft legislative language that would be considered on a fast track, it should be a separate organization, without other responsibilities.

16. In my modeling, I assume that the savings will be 0.05 percent of payroll in 2022, will grow by 0.05 percent annually through 2029 and then by 0.1 percent each year after, and so will reach 0.5 percent of payroll in 2030, 1 percent of payroll in 2035, and 1.5 percent of payroll in 2040.

17. For instance, in Munnell and Balduzzi's (1998) calculation, state and local equity holdings were about 12 percent of GDP in 1996. GAO reported that state and local pension funds in the third quarter of 1997 had $2 trillion in assets, of which 61 percent (about $1.2 trillion) was invested in stocks. That would translate into 15 percent of GDP (GAO 1998a: 21; *Economic Report of the President* 1999: 326, table B-1). At least until the retirement of the baby boom really hits, possibly causing other funds to decline, then so long as the return on stocks is higher than economic growth, these shares of the economy held by Fidelity or state and local funds could only get bigger.

18. The question of what to do about varying returns is actually complicated. The policy could be that the equity fund would contribute earnings to pay for benefits only if that left the fund balance at the target share of GDP, here about 9 percent. So if there were losses, or if growth were slower than the growth of GDP, there would be no payments. And if earnings were higher, all of the excess would be used. The advantage of this policy is that it would prevent the fund from ever exceeding the target balance at the end of a year. It would also, on average, lead to *higher* savings to the government from having the equity investments. (The reason for that is that if the years with losses are covered out of general revenues, then general revenues, which are paid for by the interest rate on the federal debt, are used to finance equities, which earn the equity premium. This is a much more modest and defensible version of the trick behind the PSA plan's returns.) The catch is that this policy would require the fund to sell a substantial portion of its assets after a year of very high earnings (say, 25%), a sell-off that might marginally affect the equity markets. Policymakers might choose, instead, to allow some small variation of the fund balance up or down (say, 8–11% of GDP), to smooth out such effects.

19. Other things being equal, the benefits of diversification, in terms of the earnings on the assets, should be compared to the costs. The cost is that the money invested in equities would not be used to retire federal debt, so the federal government would be paying more in interest. In the peculiar case of the 2000 budget estimates, however, there was not going to be any federal debt by 2028, even with diversification. It seems unlikely that the federal government would be allowed to accumulate

private assets for any purpose other than prefunding Social Security; thus, it seems fair to say that virtually all the earnings on the private investments would be extra income for the government. From the standpoint of Social Security trust-fund accounting, it would certainly be fair to credit all those earnings to the program.

20. For more discussion of the Internal Revenue Code and elderly persons, see Moon and Mulvey 1995: 24–28. The most obvious way to favor elderly persons is to tax capital gains at a lower rate than wage income. The fact that conservatives tend to favor that balance in taxation, while bemoaning the future burden of public pension and health programs on workers, is one indication that the argument really is not about burdens. It is really about government-sponsored benefits versus market-based income, with the former, to conservatives, being bad and unnatural and therefore a burden that should be reduced and the latter being good and therefore not a burden at all.

21. Expansion of Medicare benefits to include some prescription drug coverage is one possibility. Providing health coverage to uninsured persons is another. But such trade-offs are beyond the scope of this book.

Twelve: Real Responsibility

1. As I write this, I am thinking especially of an exchange I had with C. Eugene Steuerle, one of the fairest-minded advocates of radical Social Security and Medicare reform, on a panel at the annual research conference of the Association for Public Policy Analysis and Management, Washington, D.C., Nov. 4, 1999.

2. The percentage of employees with private pensions through employment has not grown for two decades; some analysts believe it has begun to decline; and the form of coverage has shifted markedly from more secure defined-benefit plans to less certain defined-contribution plans. For good discussions of private pensions, see American Academy of Actuaries 1998a; Schieber and Shoven 1997a.

3. Asset earnings are 18 percent of income for aged persons, compared to Social Security at 40 percent. Asset earnings are a much lower share of income for most elderly persons: 3 percent for the lowest quintile, 6 percent for the second quintile, and 9 percent for the middle quintile of the income distribution (see SSA/ORES 1998b: 15–16).

4. For just a few examples of claims that savings are currently insufficient, see American Academy of Actuaries 1998a: 17; Schieber 1997; Bernheim 1991; and Burtless 1996b. For examples of public (lack of) knowledge about Medicare, see Bernstein and Stevens 1999: 183–85; and, for an example in which public ignorance was especially significant, see Rovner 1995.

5. A more detailed explanation of my calculations is posted on the Social Security Network Web site of the Century Foundation, <www.tcf.org>. The favor done for me by GAO, especially Paul Posner, Ph.D., and Rick Krashevski, Ph.D., in providing

me the basic information from their model is so substantial that it deserves a second expression of gratitude. Not only am I grateful, but also I want to reiterate, as in chapter 5, that neither GAO nor any of its staff bear any responsibility for any of my interpretations, misinterpretations, or arguments.

6. As mentioned in chapter 5, I did assume that higher Medicare premiums would increase federal revenues, which would improve budget conditions relative to the standard CBO and GAO assumption that higher premiums would somehow be offset by tax cuts. Whether you think of premiums as a benefit reduction or taxes, the standard assumption seems bizarre policy.

7. I thank Stephen C. Goss, Alice Wade, and Daniel Wallace for providing me with these figures. They and the SSA as an institution bear no responsibility for the use I have made of the numbers. The tables are Catalog nos. 99–50T and 99–65T. I compared the figures in those tables to baseline spending and revenue figures from Board of Trustees 1999a, table III.B4, and translated the differences into percentages of taxable payroll and of GDP using table III.B1. Both of these tables are among the long-range tables at the SSA Web site, <http://www.ssa.gov/OACT/TR/TR99>. The alternative approach would have been to translate the changes in Social Security financing into percentages of SSA's baseline Social Security spending and then apply those percentages to GAO's baseline. I did not do the calculation that way because GAO's baseline Social Security spending was higher than SSA's; the way I did it was the more conservative choice. However, the proposals used here had all new hires by state and local governments included in Social Security beginning with the year 2001, and the benefit computation period increased from 35 to 38 years by raising it by one year each in 2006, 2010, and 2014. Since I am assuming that my proposal could not be implemented in fact until 2002, I excluded the savings in 2001 from the calculation, but I am still marginally overstating the benefits of the state and local provision.

8. The question was what amount of HI taxable payroll to assume, given that only OASDI taxable payroll is reported by the OASDI actuaries. Robert Ball projects that under current law OASDI taxable payroll will be 84.5 percent of total payroll after 2006. So I adopted for this calculation an 86 percent figure, which means that I multiplied the OASDI payroll base by $\frac{1}{0.86}$ instead of $\frac{1}{0.845}$, so by a smaller figure.

9. The Social Security actuaries provided me with Catalog no. 99–30T, which provides the effects of a much larger increase in the thresholds than I would recommend. I did not want to risk inferences from those figures.

10. I assumed that savings would grow from 0.01 percent of payroll in 2005, in increments of 0.015 percent, to 0.1 percent of payroll in 2011. Then savings would rise by increments of 0.01 percent of payroll per year to 0.22 percent of payroll in 2023, would stay at that level through 2040, would decline to 0.17 percent by 2045, and then would stay at 0.17 percent of payroll through 2075. The value of changes in the taxation of benefits should decline over time, since, under current law, the value of the $25,000 and $32,000 income exclusions would be inflated away anyway.

11. Author's calculation from detailed long-term tables III.C1 and III.C2 associated with Board of Trustees 1999a, posted at <http://www/ssa.gov/OACT/TR/TR99>.

12. To preserve some of the disciplinary effects of relying on the payroll tax and trust-fund finance, the percentage of GDP that could be automatically appropriated as needed might be limited by statute, for instance, to 1 percent of GDP. The right figure would be the sum of the amount that would normally be anticipated as necessary, plus the earnings from the private investments of the trust fund, to allow for a market slump in which it would be best not to take any earnings from the fund.

13. The general revenues required in my scenario would grow after 2040 for a few reasons. First, I have built in a decline in the value of my savings, for instance, because inclusion of all state and local workers eventually no longer saves money. This totals 0.2 percent of GDP. Second, the trustees' assumptions include that taxable payroll will decline as a share of GDP, from 37.9 percent in 2040 to 35.8 percent in 2070. This translates into a decline of a further 0.2 to 0.3 percent of GDP in payroll tax revenues. We could argue that this is a good reason for further general revenue financing or for a slightly higher payroll tax rate. Finally, Social Security spending is projected by the trustees to grow by 0.14 percent of GDP from 2040 to 2070. So, assuming no economic feedbacks or other policy changes, the amount of general revenues needed for Social Security could increase to 1.2 percent of GDP. This still would be barely a sixth of total spending and would be justified in part by the decline in taxable payroll's share of GDP; thus it would be reasonable policy. But it would also be reasonable, over the period from 2040 to 2070, to improve Social Security's dedicated financing by most of the difference between the projected need for general revenues in 2040 (0.6 percent of GDP) and in 2070 (1.2 percent). Another decision that can be made by future voters.

14. As noted in the text, my spreadsheet calculation should produce a more pessimistic forecast than the same measures would if they were modeled with economic feedbacks. For example, it produces deficits fairly similar to those in the original GAO baseline. But it is calculated from the "revised baseline," which has an economy that is about 4 percent smaller in 2040 than in the original GAO baseline. If the economy instead were as large as in the original baseline, revenues would be higher, reducing deficits below the figure in the spreadsheet calculation.

15. In an alternative calculation, I started with the recommended package here and then increased discretionary spending by between $20 and $30 billion from 2000 to 2011. I kept discretionary spending $30 billion higher from 2011 on, which means I allowed inflation slowly to eat away at the value of the extra spending. This is a slower, longer-term, decline in spending. The resulting estimates brought the federal debt down to zero in 2021 but with little accumulation of a positive balance. Deficits were just over 5 percent of GDP in 2050.

Afterword: Markets, Budgets, and Politics in the Second Bush Administration

1. Author's calculation from Strunk et al. 2002: Exhibit 5; Board of Trustees 2002b: Table IV.B1.

2. I would emphasize, however, that the high current level of U.S. health care costs relative to the value of care delivered, as appears to be revealed by comparisons to other countries, and the relatively high prices of individual services in the United States, suggests that substantial efficiencies could be realized through policy choices, which could offset some of the cost growth that the Technical Review Panel assumed.

3. Greenspan, as discussed in chapter 8, devoutly opposed any federal government investment in the markets, so his position was that once the debt disappeared the federal government would have to increase spending or cut taxes by that year's projected surplus—which could have been as much as half-a-trillion dollars. Such measures, by standard neoclassical economic theory, could be highly inflationary.

4. The scheduled cuts would lower the top marginal tax rate from 38.6 percent in 2003 to 35 percent in 2006; the next highest rate from 35 percent to 33 percent; the next level from 30 percent to 28 percent; and the next from 27 percent to 25 percent. The estate tax is scheduled to be entirely repealed in 2010. This is not the place for a disquisition on tax policy, so I do not make the case in more detail. It clearly is mostly a matter of values: personal beliefs about who should bear how much tax burden. But the country was doing just fine with the pre-2001 tax code, and any argument that high rates on higher-income earners are bad for the economy must explain why the economy did so well in the years after rates were raised in 1993.

5. The concept in question, "dynamic scoring," has been promoted by many congressional Republicans but resisted by mainstream Republican economists, including Chairman Greenspan, as either wrong in principle or impossible to implement with any accuracy.

6. Whether Clinton in fact did so, or meant to do so, remains a matter of some dispute.

REFERENCES

Aaron, Henry J., ed. 1990. *Social Security and the Budget.* Proceedings of the First Conference of the National Academy of Social Insurance, December 15–16, 1988. Lanham, Md.: University Press of America.

Aaron, Henry J., and Barry P. Bosworth. 1997. "Preparing for the Baby Boomers' Retirement." In Reischauer 1997b.

Aaron, Henry J., Barry P. Bosworth, and Gary Burtless. 1989. *Can America Afford to Grow Old?* Washington, D.C.: Brookings Institution.

Aaron, Henry J., and Robert D. Reischauer. 1995. "The Medicare Reform Debate: What Is the Next Step?" *Health Affairs* 14, no. 4.

———. 1998a. *Countdown to Reform: The Great Social Security Debate.* New York: Century Foundation Press.

———. 1998b. "Perspective: 'Rethinking Medicare Reform' Needs Rethinking." *Health Affairs* 17, no. 1.

Aaron, Henry J., and William B. Schwartz. 1993. "Managed Competition: Little Cost Containment without Budget Limits." *Health Affairs* 12, suppl.

Aaron, Henry J., and Lawrence H. Thompson. 1987. "Social Security and the Economists." In Edward D. Berkowitz, ed., *Social Security after Fifty: Successes and Failures.* Westport, Conn.: Greenwood Press.

AARP. *See* American Association of Retired Persons.

Abraham, Katherine G. 1995. "The Consumer Price Index: What Does It Measure?" *Challenge,* May–June, pp. 59–62.

Abraham, Katherine G., John S. Greenlees, and Brent R. Moulton. 1998. "Working to Improve the Consumer Price Index." *Journal of Economic Perspectives* 12, no. 1.

Adams, Rebecca. 2002. "GOP Pushes Private Coverage." *Congressional Quarterly Weekly Report,* November 23, pp. 3070–71.

Advisory Council for the Concerted Action in Health Care. 1998. "The Health Care System in Germany: Cost Factor and Branch of the Future." Vol. 2, "Progress and Growth Markets, Finance and Remuneration." Advisory Council for the Concerted Action, Bonn, Germany.

Advisory Council on Social Security. 1997a. *Report of the 1994–1996 Advisory Council on Social Security.* Vol. 1, *Findings and Recommendations.* Washington, D.C.: GPO.

———. 1997b. *Report of the 1994–1995 Advisory Council on Social Security.* Vol. 2, *Reports of the Technical Panel on Assumptions and Methods, Technical Panel on Trends and Issues in Retirement Savings and Presentations to the Council.* Washington, D.C.: GPO.

Allred, Victoria. 2001. "Tax Package's Timetable." *Congressional Quarterly Weekly Report,* June 2, pp. 1306–7.

Altman, Stuart H., and Alan B. Cohen. 1993. "Commentary: The Need for a National Global Budget." *Health Affairs* 12, suppl.

Altman, Stuart H., and Laura D'Andrea Tyson. 1999. "Medicare: Why We Said No." *Washington Post,* March 29, p. A19.

American Academy of Actuaries. 1998a. "Financing the Retirement of Future Generations: The Problem and Options for Change." American Academy of Actuaries, Washington, D.C.

————. 1998b. "Social Security Privatization: Trust Fund Investment." American Academy of Actuaries, Washington, D.C.

American Association of Retired Persons, Public Policy Institute, and the Lewin Group (AARP). 1997. "Out-of-Pocket Health Spending by Medicare Beneficiaries Age 65 and Older: 1997 Projections." AARP Public Policy Institute Report no. 9705. American Association of Retired Persons, Washington, D.C.

Analytical Perspectives: Budget of the United States Government, Fiscal Year 1998. 1997. Washington, D.C.: GPO.

Analytical Perspectives: Budget of the United States Government, Fiscal Year 1999. 1998. Washington, D.C.: GPO.

Analytical Perspectives: Budget of the United States Government, Fiscal Year 2000. 1999. Washington, D.C.: GPO.

Anderson, Gerard F., George Greenberg, and Craig K. Lisk. 1999. "Academic Health Centers: Exploring a Financial Paradox." *Health Affairs* 18, no. 2.

Baker, Dean. 1997a. "Saving Social Security with Stocks: The Promises Don't Add Up." A Twentieth Century Fund/Economic Policy Institute Report. Economic Policy Institute, Washington, D.C.

————. 1997b. "Does the CPI Overstate Inflation? An Analysis of the Boskin Commission's Report." Economic Policy Institute, Washington, D.C.

————. 1998. "Defusing the Baby Boomer Time Bomb." Economic Policy Institute, Washington, D.C.

Baker, Dean, and M. Weisbrot. 1999. *Social Security: The Phony Crisis.* Chicago: University of Chicago Press.

Baldauf, Scott. 1999. "Case Studies of Putting Public Funds in Stocks." *Christian Science Monitor,* February 2.

Ball, Robert M. 1985. "The 1939 Amendments to the Social Security Act and What Followed." In Committee on Economic Security 1985.

————. 1997. "Reflections on How Medicare Came About." In Reischauer, Butler, and Lave 1997.

Ball, Robert M., with Thomas Bethel. 1998. *Straight Talk about Social Security: An Analysis of the Issues in the Current Debate.* New York: Century Foundation Press.

Bauer, Gary. 1997. "Save Social Security, Save Our Families." *New York Times,* January 23, p. A23.

Beach, William W., and Gareth G. Davis. 1998a. "Social Security's Rate of Return." Heritage Foundation Center for Data Analysis Report no. CDA98-01. Heritage Foundation, Washington, D.C.

———. 1998b. "Social Security's Rate of Return for Hispanic Americans." Heritage Foundation Center for Data Analysis Report no. CDA98-02. Heritage Foundation, Washington, D.C.

———. 1998c. "Social Security's Rate of Return: A Reply to Our Critics." Heritage Foundation Center for Data Analysis Report no. CDA98-08. Heritage Foundation, Washington, D.C.

Berenson, Alex, and Andrew Ross Sorkin. 2002. "How Wall Street Was Tamed." *New York Times,* December 22, p. C1.

Berkowitz, Edward D. 1996. "Social Security and the Financing of the American State." In W. Elliot Brownlee, ed., *Funding the Modern American State, 1941–1995.* Washington, D.C.: Woodrow Wilson Center Press; Cambridge: Cambridge University Press.

Bernheim, Douglas. 1991. *The Vanishing Nest Egg: Reflections on Saving in America.* New York: Twentieth Century Fund.

Bernstein, Jill, and Rosemary Stevens. 1999. "Public Opinion, Knowledge, and Medicare Reform." *Health Affairs* 18, no. 1.

Berry, John M. 1996. "CPI Report Coming under Fire." *Washington Post,* December 19.

Bixby, Ann K. 1997. "Public Social Welfare Expenditures, Fiscal Year 1994." *Social Security Bulletin* 60, no. 3.

Bloomberg.com. 2002. Chart Center, 5-Year Graph of Dow Jones Industrial Average, S&P 500 index, and NASDAQ index. Accessed December 26, 2002.

Board of Trustees of the Social Security and Medicare Trust Funds. 1997a. *1997 Annual Report of the Board of Trustees of the Federal Hospital Insurance Trust Fund.* Washington, D.C.: GPO.

———. 1997b. *1997 Annual Report of the Board of Trustees of the Federal Supplementary Medical Insurance Trust Fund.* Washington, D.C.: GPO.

———. 1998a. *1998 Annual Report of the Board of Trustees of the Federal Old Age, Survivors and Disability Insurance Trust Funds.* Washington, D.C.: GPO.

———. 1998b. *Status of the Social Security and Medicare Programs: A Summary of the 1998 Annual Reports.* Washington, D.C.: GPO.

———. 1998c. *1998 Annual Report of the Board of Trustees of the Federal Hospital Insurance Trust Fund.* Washington, D.C.: GPO.

———. 1998d. *1998 Annual Report of the Board of Trustees of the Federal Supplementary Medical Insurance Trust Fund.* Washington, D.C.: GPO.

———. 1999a. *1999 Annual Report of the Board of Trustees of the Federal Old-Age and Survivors Insurance and Disability Insurance Trust Funds.* Washington, D.C.: GPO.

————. 1999b. *Status of the Social Security and Medicare Programs: A Summary of the 1999 Annual Reports.* Washington, D.C.: GPO.

————. 1999c. *1999 Annual Report of the Board of Trustees of the Federal Hospital Insurance Trust Fund.* Washington, D.C.: GPO.

————. 1999d. *1999 Annual Report of the Board of Trustees of the Federal Supplementary Medical Insurance Trust Fund.* Washington, D.C.: GPO.

————. 2000a. *2000 Annual Report of the Board of Trustees of the Federal Old-Age and Survivors Insurance and Disability Insurance Trust Funds.* Washington, D.C.: GPO.

————. 2000b. *Status of the Social Security and Medicare Programs: A Summary of the 2000 Annual Reports.* Washington, D.C.: GPO.

————. 2000c. *2000 Annual Report of the Board of Trustees of the Federal Hospital Insurance Trust Fund.* Washington, D.C.: GPO.

————. 2000d. *2000 Annual Report of the Board of Trustees of the Federal Supplementary Medical Insurance Trust Fund.* Washington, D.C.: GPO.

————. 2001a. *Status of the Social Security and Medicare Trust Funds: A Summary of the 2001 Annual Reports.* Washington, D.C.: GPO.

————. 2001b. *2001 Annual Report of the Trustees of the Federal Hospital Insurance Trust Fund.* Washington, D.C.: GPO.

————. 2002a. *Status of the Social Security and Medicare Trust Funds: A Summary of the 2002 Annual Reports.* Washington, D.C.: GPO. At <www.ssa.gov/OACT/TRSUM/trsummary.html>.

————. 2002b. *2002 Annual Report on the Status of the Federal Hospital Insurance Trust and Supplementary Insurance Trust Funds.* At <www.cmms.gov/publications/trusteesreport/2002>.

Boskin, Michael J. 1996. "Prisoners of Faulty Statistics." *Wall Street Journal,* December 5, p. A20.

Boskin Commission. *See* U.S. Senate Committee on Finance 1996.

Bosworth, Barry. 1986. "Fiscal Fitness: Deficit Reduction and the Economy." *Brookings Review* (winter–spring).

————. 1997. "What Economic Role for the Trust Funds?" In Kingson and Schulz 1997a.

Bosworth, Barry, Gary Burtless, and Eugene Steuerle. 1999. "Lifetime Earning Patterns, the Distribution of Future Social Security Benefits, and the Impact of Pension Reform." CRR WP 1999-06. Center for Retirement Research at Boston College, Chestnut Hill, Mass.

Bowman, Karlyn. 1997. "View." In Reischauer, Butler, and Lave 1997.

Brackett, Jean C. 1968. "A New Budget for a Retired Couple." *Monthly Labor Review* (June): 33–39.

Broder, David S. 1996. "The Party's Over: By 2000, the GOP or the Democrats Could Fade in Favor of a Third Party." *Washington Post,* August 11, p. C1.

————. 1999a. "Medical Outcasts: Does Anyone Care?" *Washington Post,* May 12, p. A27.

————. 1999b. "Charades on the Hill" *Washington Post,* August 4, p. A21.

————. 2002. "Still the Idea Man." *Washington Post,* December 15, p. B7.

Brownstein, Ronald. 2002. "Uncertainty on Bush Cure for Economy." *Los Angeles Times,* December 18.

Bryant, Ralph C. 1994. "Consequences of Reducing the U.S. Budget Deficits." Brookings Discussion Papers in International Economics, no. 104. Brookings Institution, Washington, D.C.

"Bumpy Market Has Many Delaying Retirement, Survey Finds." 2002. *New York Times.* December 17.

Burke, Sheila. 1997. "View." In Reischauer, Butler, and Lave 1997.

Burtless, Gary. 1996a. "The Folly of Means-Testing Social Security." In Diamond, Lindeman, and Young 1996.

————. 1996b. "Will American Workers Be Ready for Retirement?" Testimony for the Subcommittee on Aging, Committee on Labor and Human Resources, U.S. Senate, June 13. Draft copy in possession of the author.

————. 1998a. "The Role of Individual Personal Saving Accounts in Social Security Reform." Testimony for the Subcommittee on Social Security, Committee on Ways and Means, U.S. House of Representatives, June 18. Draft copy in possession of the author.

————. 1998b. "Increasing the Eligibility Age for Social Security Pensions." Testimony for the Special Committee on Aging, U.S. Senate, July 15. Draft copy in possession of the author.

Burtless, Gary, and Barry Bosworth. 1997. "Privatizing Social Security: The Troubling Trade-Offs." Brookings Policy Brief no. 14, March. Brookings Institution, Washington, D.C.

Burtless, Gary, R. Kent Weaver, and Joshua M. Wiener. 1997. "The Future of the Social Safety Net." In Reischauer 1997b.

Bush, George W. 2001. "Remarks by the President on Medicare." July 12. At <www .whitehouse.gov/news/releases/2001/07/print/20010712.html>.

Butler, Stuart M. 1998. "Medicare Price Controls: The Wrong Prescription." *Health Affairs* 17, no. 1:72–74.

Butler, Stuart M., and Robert E. Moffitt. 1995. "The FEHBP as a Model for a New Medicare Program." *Health Affairs* 14, no. 4.

Butler, Stuart M., et al. 1999. "Open Letter to Congress and the Executive: Crisis Facing HCFA and Millions of Americans." *Health Affairs* 18, no. 1.

Calmes, Jackie. 1997a. "Fiscal Fitness: Washington Wants Discipline in Budgets to Carry beyond 2002." *Wall Street Journal,* February 3, p. A1.

————. 1997b. "Fast Rise in Retirement Age Would Raise Money, Fury." *Wall Street Journal,* February 10, p. A20.

———. 2000. "Bush's Social Security Plan Has Democrats Wondering." *Wall Street Journal,* May 8.

Campaign for America's Future. 2001. "Bush Social Security Commission Members: Who Are They?" At <www.ourfuture.org/articles/20020116132652.pdf>.

———. 2002. "Candidates Mislead Voters about Private Accounts in 2002." At <www.ourfuture.org/articles/20021113072111.pdf>.

"Campaigning on Social Security." 2000. *New York Times,* May 29, p. A18.

CBO. *See* U.S. Congressional Budget Office.

Center for Studying Health System Change (CSHSC). 1996. "Policy Implications of Risk Selection in Medicare HMOs." Issue Brief 4. Center for Studying Health System Change, Washington, D.C.

———. 1997. "Health Care Costs: Will They Start Rising Rapidly Again?" Issue Brief 10. Center for Studying Health System Change, Washington, D.C.

———. 1999. "Tracking Health Care Costs: Long-Predicted Upturn Appears." Issue Brief 28. Center for Studying Health System Change, Washington, D.C.

Centers for Medicare and Medicaid Services (CMS). 2002a. "Statement of Tom Scully, Administrator, Centers for Medicare and Medicaid Services: Medicare + Choice Plan Renewals and Nonrenewals." September 25. At <www.cmms.gov/media/press/release.asp?Counter=490>.

———. 2002b. "Medicare Announces Physician Pay Changes for 2003." December 20. At <www.cmms.gov/media/press/release.asp?Counter=671>.

———. 2002c. "Medicare + Choice Changes in Access, Benefits and Premiums, 2001 to 2002." Charts from <www.cmms.gov/healthplans/mplusc_changes.pdf>.

The Century Foundation. 1999. *Social Security: The Basics.* New York: The Century Foundation.

Chait, Jonathan. 1999a. "Security Risk." *New Republic,* January 18.

———. 1999b. "Washington Diarist: Doubletalk." *New Republic,* February 22.

CIEBA. *See* Committee on Investment of Employee Benefit Assets.

Committee on Economic Security. 1985. *The Report of the Committee on Economic Security of 1935.* 50th anniversary ed. Washington, D.C.: National Conference on Social Welfare.

Committee on Investment of Employee Benefit Assets (CIEBA). 1999. "Implications of Investing Social Security Funds in Financial Markets." Committee on Investment of Employee Benefit Assets, Washington, D.C.

Commonwealth Fund. 1997. "Leveling the Playing Field: Financing the Missions of Academic Medical Centers." Commonwealth Fund, New York.

Community Action Board. 1993. "Report of the Community Action Board and Commission on Aging's Ad Hoc Committee to Construct a Minimum Standard of Need for Elderly Households in Montgomery County, Maryland." Montgomery County Commission on Aging, Rockville, Md.

Concord Coalition. 1997. "Facing Facts: The Truth about Entitlements and the Budget." Fax alert, January 28, April 28, July 16. Concord Coalition, Washington, D.C.

Cook, Charles E. 1996. "Changing the CPI Gives Both Parties a Social Security Fix." *Roll Call,* December 5, p. 8.

Copeland, Craig, Jack VanDerHei, and Dallas Salisbury. 1999. "Social Security Reform: Evaluating Current Proposals: Latest Results of the EBRI SSASIM2 Policy Simulation Model." *EBRI Issue Brief,* no. 210 (June).

Crystal, Stephen, and Richard W. Johnson. 1998. "The Changing Retirement Prospects of American Families: Impact of Labor Market Shifts on Economic Outcomes." AARP Public Policy Institute Report no. 9801. American Association of Retired Persons, Washington, D.C.

CSHSC. *See* Center for Studying Health System Change.

Culbertson, Richard A. 1996. "How Successfully Can Academic Faculty Practices Compete in Developing Managed Care Markets?" *Academic Medicine* 71, no. 8:858–70.

Culbertson, Richard A., and Philip R. Lee. 1996. "Medicare and Physician Autonomy." *Health Care Financing Review* 18, no. 2:115–30.

Cutler, David M., Mark McClellan, and Joseph Newhouse. 1997. "The Costs and Benefits of Intensive Treatment for Cardiovascular Disease." Paper presented at American Enterprise Institute/Brookings Institution conference, Measuring the Prices of Medical Treatments, Washington, D.C., December 12.

Cutler, David M., James M. Poterba, Louise M. Sheiner, and Lawrence H. Summers. 1990. "An Aging Society: Opportunity or Challenge?" *Brookings Papers on Economic Activity,* no. 1:1–73.

Dallek, Geraldine. 1998. "Consumer Protections in Medicare + Choice." Menlo Park, Calif.: Kaiser Family Foundation.

Daniel, Caroline. 1998. "Taxing Reforms for British Retirees." *Washington Post,* August 9, p. C3.

Davidson, Paul, and James K. Galbraith. 1999. "The Dangers of Debt Reduction." *Wall Street Journal,* March 3.

Davis, Margaret, et al. 1999. "Prescription Drug Coverage, Utilization, and Spending among Medicare Beneficiaries." *Health Affairs* 18, no. 1:231–43.

Deaton, Angus. 1998. "Getting Prices Right: What Should Be Done?" *Journal of Economic Perspectives* 12, no. 1.

Derthick, Martha. 1979. *Policymaking for Social Security.* Washington, D.C.: Brookings Institution.

———. 1990. *Agency under Stress.* Washington, D.C.: Brookings Institution.

Diamond, Peter A. 1999. "What Stock Market Returns to Expect for the Future?" Center for Retirement Research at Boston College Issue Brief 3. Center for Retirement Research, Chestnut Hill, Mass.

Diamond, Peter A., David C. Lindeman, and Howard Young, eds. 1996. *Social Secu-*

rity: What Role for the Future? Washington, D.C.: National Academy of Social Insurance.

Diamond, Peter A., and Peter R. Orszag. 2002. "A Response to the Executive Director of the President's Commission to Strengthen Social Security." Center on Budget and Policy Priorities Issue Brief, June 25. Center on Budget and Policy Priorities, Washington, D.C.

Diewert, W. Edwin. 1998. "Index Number Issues in the Consumer Price Index." *Journal of Economic Perspectives* 12, no. 1.

Dionne, E. J., Jr. 2000. "Social Security: We Need to Talk." *Washington Post,* May 19, p. A31.

Dowd, Bryan, Robert Coulam, and Roger Feldman. 2000. "A Tale of Four Cities: Medicare Reform and Competitive Pricing." *Health Affairs* 19, no. 5:9–29.

Downey, Thomas J. 1995. "Additional Views." In *Bipartisan Commission on Entitlement and Tax Reform Final Report to the President.* Washington, D.C.: GPO.

Easterlin, Richard A., Christine Macdonald, and Diane J. Macunovich. 1990. "Retirement Prospects of the Baby Boom Generation: A Different Perspective." *Gerontologist* 30, no. 6:776–83.

Easterlin, Richard A., Christine M. Schaeffer, and Diane J. Macunovich. 1993. "Will the Baby Boomers Be Less Well Off Than Their Parents? Income, Wealth, and Family Circumstances over the Life Cycle in the United States." *Population and Development Review* 19, no. 3.

Economic Report of the President. 1996–99. Washington, D.C.: GPO.

Eisner, Robert. 1986. *How Real Is the Federal Deficit?* New York: Free Press.

———. 1996. "What Social Security Crisis?" *Wall Street Journal,* August 30, p. A8.

———. 1998. *Social Security: More, Not Less.* New York: Century Foundation Press.

Escarce, Jose J., Judy A. Shea, and Wei Chen. 1997. "Segmentation of Hospital Markets: Where Do HMO Enrollees Get Care?" *Health Affairs* 16, no. 6:181–92.

Etheredge, Lynn. 1999. "Three Streams, One River: A Coordinated Approach to Financing Retirement." *Health Affairs* 18, no. 1.

"Feds Triple Health Fraud Cases." 1999. *USA Today,* February 23, p. 1A.

Feldman, Roger, and Bryan Dowd. 1997. "Structuring Choice under Medicare." In Reischauer, Butler, and Lave 1997.

Feldstein, Martin. 1997. "Don't Waste the Budget Surplus." *Wall Street Journal,* November 4.

———. 1998a. "Let's Really Save Social Security." *Wall Street Journal,* February 10.

———. 1998b. "Savings Grace." *New Republic,* April 6.

———. 1999. "Clinton's Social Security Sham." *Wall Street Journal,* February 1, p. A20.

Feldstein, Martin, and Anthony Pellechio. 1979. "Social Security and Household Wealth Accumulation: New Microeconometric Evidence." *Review of Economics and Statistics* 61, no. 3:361–68.

Feldstein, Martin, and Andrew Samwick. 1998. "Two Percent Personal Retirement Accounts: Their Potential Effects on Social Security Tax Rates and National Saving." *National Bureau of Economic Research Working Papers,* no. 6540.

Fenno, Richard E., Jr. 1966. *The Power of the Purse: Appropriations Politics in Congress.* Boston: Little, Brown & Co.

Fielding, Jonathan E., and Pierre-Jean Lancry. 1993. "Lessons from France—Vive la Difference." *Journal of the American Medical Association* 270, no. 6.

Fierst, Edith U. 1997. "Supplemental Statement." In Advisory Council on Social Security 1997a.

———. 1998. "Social Security Is Essential for Blacks." *Los Angeles Times,* January 14.

Fisher, Gordon M. 1997. "Disseminating the Administrative Version and Explaining the Administrative and Statistical Versions of the Federal Poverty Measure." *Clinical Sociology Review* 15:163–82.

Foerstel, Karen. 1999a. "Senate Braces for Managed Care Debate, with Lott Maneuvering to Derail Democratic Amendments." *Congressional Quarterly Weekly Report,* July 10, p. 1679.

———. 1999b. "Accentuating the Negative in Managed Care Overhaul." *Congressional Quarterly Weekly Report,* August 14, pp. 2007–8.

"Four Reasons Not to Cut Social Security Taxes." 1990. Symposium. *Brookings Review* (spring).

Francis, David R. 1998. "Keeping Social Security Out of the Gap." *Christian Science Monitor,* December 28.

Freedman, Audrey. 1996. "Presto Change-o! On the Consumer Price Index." *Challenge,* March–April.

Fuchs, Victor. 1999. "Health Care for the Elderly: How Much? Who Will Pay for It?" *Health Affairs* 18, no. 1.

Gabel, Jon, Kelly Hunt, and Jean Kim. 1998. "The Financial Burden of Self-Paid Health Insurance on the Poor and Near-Poor." The Commonwealth Fund Improving Health Care Coverage and Affordability Series. Commonwealth Fund, New York.

Galbraith, James K. 1998. *Created Unequal: The Crisis in American Pay.* New York: Free Press.

GAO. *See* U.S. General Accounting Office.

Georges, Christopher. 1997. "Senate Republicans, in a Shift, Propose Higher Medicare Premiums for the Rich." *Wall Street Journal,* June 24, p. A4.

Georges, Christopher, and Jackie Calmes. 1997. "Clinton Plan to Lift Medicare Premiums Draws a Lukewarm Response from GOP." *Wall Street Journal,* July 23, p. A4.

Gergen, David. 1996. "When the Baby Boomers Retire." *U.S. News and World Report,* October 28, p. 100.

Germond, J., and Witcover, J. 1997. "Much Ado about a Budget Nothing." *National Journal,* May 10, p. 947.

Gigot, Paul. 2000. "Why Bush Thinks He Can Win on Social Security." *Wall Street Journal,* April 28.

Gilmour, John B. 1990. *Reconcilable Differences?* Berkeley: University of California Press.

Ginsburg, Paul B. 1999. "Health Spending: Questioning the Assumptions." *Health Affairs* 18, no. 1:272–74.

Ginsburg, Paul B., and Jon R. Gabel. 1998. "Tracking Health Care Costs: What's New in 1998?" *Health Affairs* 17, no. 5.

Ginsburg, Paul B., and Jeremy Pickreign. 1997. "Tracking Health Care Costs: An Update." *Health Affairs* 16, no. 4.

Gist, John. 1996. "Entitlements and the Federal Budget: Facts, Folklore, and Future." *Milbank Quarterly* 74, no. 3:327–55.

Glaser, William A. 1991. *Health Insurance in Practice.* San Francisco: Jossey-Bass.

———. 1993. "How Expenditure Caps and Expenditure Targets Really Work." *Milbank Quarterly* 71, no. 1.

Gold, Marsha, Lyle Nelson, Randall Brown, Anne Ciemnecki, Anna Aizer, and Elizabeth Docteur. 1997. "Disabled Medicare Beneficiaries in HMOs." *Health Affairs* 17, no. 5:149–62.

Goldberg, Mark A., T. R. Marmor, and J. White. 1995. "The Relation between Universal Health Insurance and Cost Control." *New England Journal of Medicine* 332, no. 11:742–44.

Goldreich, Samuel. 2001. "Bush Names Social Security Panel as Politically Palatable Options for Overhaul Begin to Narrow." *Congressional Quarterly Weekly Report,* May 5, p. 1021.

Goldstein, Amy. 1999a. "Medicare Panel in Policy Deadlock." *Washington Post,* March 16, p. A1.

———. 1999b. "Health Lobby Seeks Ease on Government Caps." *Washington Post,* May 10, p. A1.

———. 2002. "Administration Considers Action on Social Security: Debate Centers on Timing, Political Risks." *Washington Post,* November 17, p. A4.

Goldstein, Amy, and George Hager. 1998. "Social Security Investment Plans Weighed." *Washington Post,* December 8.

Gornick, M., A. McMillan, and J. Lubitz. 1993. "A Longitudinal Perspective on Patterns of Medicare Payments." *Health Affairs* 12, no. 2:140–50.

Goss, Stephen C. 1997. "Comparison of Financial Effects of Advisory Council Plans to Modify the OASDI Program." In Advisory Council on Social Security 1997a.

Gramlich, Edward M. 1984. "How Bad Are the Large Deficits?" In Gregory B. Mills and John L. Palmer, eds., *Federal Budget Policy in the 1980s.* Washington, D.C.: Urban Institute.

———. 1996. "Different Approaches for Dealing with Social Security." *Journal of Economic Perspectives* 10, no. 3.

————. 1997. "How Does Social Security Affect the Economy?" In Kingson and Schulz 1997a.

Greenlees, John S., and Charles C. Mason. 1996. "Overview of the 1998 Revision of the Consumer Price Index." *Monthly Labor Review,* December.

Greenstein, Robert. 1999. "The Archer-Shaw Social Security Proposal." Center on Budget and Policy Priorities Issue Brief, May 5. Center on Budget and Policy Priorities, Washington, D.C.

Greenstein, Robert, and Richard Kogan. 2001. "Paying Social Security Benefits: Where Will the Money Come from after 2016?" Center on Budget and Policy Priorities Issue Brief, August 21. Center on Budget and Policy Priorities, Washington, D.C.

Greenstein, Robert, Wendell Primus, and Kilolo Kijakazi. 1998. "The Feldstein Social Security Plan." Center on Budget and Policy Priorities Report, December 15. Center on Budget and Policy Priorities, Washington, D.C.

Guterman, Stuart. 1998. "The Balanced Budget Act of 1997: Will Hospitals Take a Hit on Their PPS Margins?" *Health Affairs* 17, no. 1:159–66.

Haas, Lawrence J. 1990. *Running on Empty: Bush, Congress, and the Politics of Bankrupt Government.* Homewood, Ill.: Business One Irwin.

Hager, George. 1999a. "GOP Attacks New Social Security Plan." *Washington Post,* February 3, p. A4.

————. 1999b. "A Primer on Budget Surplus." *Washington Post,* August 5, p. A21.

Hager, George, and Eric Pianin. 1997. *Mirage: Why Neither Democrats nor Republicans Can Balance the Budget, End the Deficit, and Satisfy the Public.* New York: Random House.

Havemann, Judith. 1997a. "Senate Panel Backs Limited Means-Testing for Medicare Recipients." *Washington Post,* June 18, p. A4.

————. 1997b. "Senate Leaders Back Medicare Means Test." *Washington Post,* June 19, p. A1.

HCFA. *See* U.S. Department of Health and Human Services, Health Care Financing Administration.

Heller, Peter S. 1998. "Rethinking Public Pension Reform Initiatives." Working Paper of the International Monetary Fund, April. International Monetary Fund, Washington, D.C.

HHS Inspector General. *See* U.S. Department of Health and Human Services, Office of Inspector General.

Hickey, Roger, Hans Riemer, and Adam Luna. 2002. "Social Security in the 2002 Elections: Candidates Won by Renouncing Privatization." Campaign for America's Future, Washington, D.C., November 8. At <www.ourfuture.org/articles/20021113094926.pdf>.

Hilzenrath, David W. 1998. "GWU Plans to Build New Hospital." *Washington Post,* February 26, p. A1.

———. 1999. "Patients Are Caught Short as Benefits Wane." *Washington Post,* May 10, p. A1.

Hitt, Greg. 1999. "Surplus Converts Chief GOP Deficit Hawk." *Wall Street Journal,* February 1, p. A22.

Holahan, John, and David Liska 1996. "Where Is Medicaid Spending Headed?" Manuscript prepared for the Kaiser Commission on the Future of Medicaid, Washington, D.C.

Horney, James. 1999. "Spending a Non-Existent Surplus." Center on Budget and Policy Priorities Issue Brief, October 20. Center on Budget and Policy Priorities, Washington, D.C.

Iglehart, John K. 1998. "Interview: Physicians as Agents of Social Control: The Thoughts of Victor Fuchs." *Health Affairs* 17, no. 1.

———. 1999. "Bringing Forth Medicare + Choice: HCFA's Robert A. Berenson." *Health Affairs* 18, no. 1.

Ignagni, Karen. 1998. "Covering a Breaking Revolution: The Media and Managed Care." *Health Affairs* 17, no. 1.

"It's Your Business." 1997. Transcript of program no. 929, June 21–22. U.S. Chamber of Commerce, Washington, D.C.

Jones, Nora Super. 1999. "Medicare Competitive Pricing: Lessons Being Learned in Phoenix and Kansas City." National Health Policy Forum Issue Brief no. 750, November 8. National Health Policy Forum, George Washington University, Washington, D.C.

Kahn, Charles N., III, and Hanns Kuttner. 1999. "Budget Bills and Medicare Policy: The Politics of BBA." *Health Affairs* 18, no. 1.

Kendall, David B. 1995. "A New Deal for Medicare and Medicaid: Building a Buyer's Market for Health Care." Progressive Policy Institute Report no. 25. Progressive Policy Institute, Washington, D.C.

Kerrey, Robert J. 1998. "Testimony of Senator Bob Kerrey." In U.S. Senate Committee on Finance 1999.

Kijazaki, Kilolo. 1998. "African Americans, Hispanic Americans, and Social Security: The Shortcomings of the Heritage Foundation Reports." Center on Budget and Policy Priorities Issue Brief, October 5. Center on Budget and Policy Priorities, Washington, D.C.

Kingson, Eric R., and James R. Schulz, eds. 1997a. *Social Security in the Twenty-first Century.* New York: Oxford University Press.

Kingson, Eric R., and James R. Schulz. 1997b. "Should Social Security Be Means-Tested?" In Kingson and Schulz 1997a.

Kirchoff, Sue. 1999. "Social Security: Next Salvo." *Congressional Quarterly Weekly Report,* October 30.

Klein, Joe. 1996. "Pretty Close to Awful: Dole's Fading Campaign Makes It Less Likely the Next President Will Break the Entitlement State." *Newsweek,* September 16, p. 51.

Kleinke, J. D. 1998. "A Paradigm Lost: The Case for Columbia/HCA." *Health Affairs* 17, no. 2:7–39.

Kogan, Richard, and Robert Greenstein. 2002. "The New Congressional Budget Office Forecast and the Remarkable Deterioration of the Surplus." Center on Budget and Policy Priorities Issue Brief, September 3. Center on Budget and Policy Priorities, Washington, D.C.

Koitz, David. 1998. "Benefit Analysis of Three Social Security Reform Plans." *CRS Memorandum,* June 17.

Kosterlitz, Julie. 1996. "Do It Yourself." *National Journal,* November 23, pp. 2532–36.

———. 1997. "When We're 64." *National Journal,* September 27, pp. 1882–85.

———. 2001. "Economics: Taxing Questions about Life after Debt." *National Journal,* February 3. Accessed December 27, 2002.

Kritzer, Barbara E. 1996. "Privatizing Social Security: The Chilean Experience." *Social Security Bulletin* 59, no. 3.

Krugman, Paul. 2000. "Reckonings." *New York Times,* May 31.

Kuttner, Robert. 1998. "Toward Universal Coverage." *Washington Post,* July 14, p. A15.

———. 1999. "The Politics of Good Economics." *Boston Globe,* February 28.

Larin, Kathy, and Robert Greenstein. 1998. "Social Security Plans That Reduce Social Security Retirement Benefits Substantially Are Likely to Cut Disability and Survivor Benefits as Well." Center on Budget and Policy Priorities, December 15. Center on Budget and Policy Priorities, Washington, D.C.

Lee, Carole, and Deborah Rogal. 1997. "Risk Adjustment: A Key to Changing Incentives in the Health Insurance Market." Alpha Center Special Report. Alpha Center/Academy for Health Services Research and Policy, Washington, D.C.

Leone, Richard C., and G. Anrig, eds. 1999. *Social Security Reform: Beyond the Basics.* New York: Century Foundation Press.

Levit, Katharine R., and colleagues. 1996. "National Health Expenditures, 1994." *Health Care Financing Review* (spring): 205–42.

———. 1998a. "National Health Spending Trends in 1996." *Health Affairs* 17, no. 1.

———. 1998b. "National Health Expenditures in 1997: More Slow Growth." *Health Affairs* 17, no. 6.

Levitt, Arthur. 1998. "The SEC Perspective on Investing Social Security in the Stock Market." Speech to John F. Kennedy School of Government Forum, Harvard University, October 19.

Levy, Frank. 1987. *Dollars and Dreams: The Changing American Income Distribution.* New York: Russell Sage Foundation.

Lewis, Bill. 1996. "The Wealth of a Nation." *Wall Street Journal,* June 7, p. A12.

Light, Donald W. 1997. "The Real Ethics of Rationing." *British Medical Journal* 315 (July 12): 112–15.

Light, Paul C. 1985. *Artful Work: The Politics of Social Security Reform.* New York: Random House.

Lipson, Debra J., and Jeanne M. De Sa. 1996. "Impact of Purchasing Strategies on Local Health Care Systems." *Health Affairs* 15, no. 2.

Longrest, Beaufort B., Jr. 1998. *Health Policymaking in the United States.* 2d ed. Chicago: Health Administration Press.

Lubitz, J., J. Beebe, and Colin Baker. 1995. "Longevity and Medicare Expenditures." *New England Journal of Medicine* 332, no. 15:999–1003.

Makin, John M., and Norman J. Ornstein. 1994. *Debt and Taxes: How America Got into Its Budget Mess and What to Do about It.* New York: Random House.

Mankiw, N. Gregory, and David N. Weil. 1988. "The Baby Boom, the Baby Bust, and the Housing Market." *National Bureau of Economic Research Working Paper,* no. 2794 (December).

Mann, Thomas E., and Norman J. Ornstein, eds. 1995. *Intensive Care: How Congress Shapes Health Care Policy.* Washington, D.C.: American Enterprise Institute and Brookings Institution.

Maraniss, David, and Michael Weisskopf. 1996. *Tell Newt to Shut Up.* New York: Simon & Schuster.

Marmor, Theodore R., and Jacob Hacker. 1997. "Ends Don't Justify the Means Test." *Los Angeles Times,* July 14.

Marmor, Theodore R., with Jan S. Marmor. 1971. *The Politics of Medicare.* Chicago: Aldine Publishing.

Marmor, Theodore R., J. L. Mashaw, and Philip L. Harvey. 1992. *America's Misunderstood Welfare State: Persistent Myths, Enduring Realities.* New York: Basic Books.

Marmor, Theodore R., and Jonathan Oberlander. 1998. "Rethinking Medicare Reform." *Health Affairs* 17, no. 1:52–68.

Mason, Diane, and Stephen Nohlgren. 1989. *The Medicare Survival Guide.* New York: Signet Books.

"Maybe Not the Third Rail." 1999. *Washington Post,* November 23, p. A26.

McClellan, Mark, and Jonathan Skinner. 1999. "Medicare Reform: Who Pays and Who Benefits?" *Health Affairs* 18, no. 1.

McDevitt, Roland D. 1998. "A Medicare Buy-In: Examining the Costs for Two Populations." AARP Public Policy Institute Report no. 9804, April. American Association of Retired Persons, Washington, D.C.

McPherson, Kim. 1990. "International Differences in Medical Care Practices." In Organisation for Economic Cooperation and Development, *Health Care Systems in Transition.* Paris: OECD.

Medicare Payment Advisory Commission (MedPAC). 1998a. *Report to the Congress: Medicare Payment Policy.* Vol. 1, *Recommendations.* Washington, D.C.: Medicare Payment Advisory Commission.

———. 1998b. *Report to the Congress: Context for a Changing Medicare Program.* Washington, D.C.: Medicare Payment Advisory Commission.

————. 1998c. *Health Care Spending and the Medicare Program: A Data Book.* Washington, D.C.: Medicare Payment Advisory Commission.

————. 1998d. *Report to the Congress: Medicare Payment Policy.* Vol. 2, *Analytical Papers.* Washington, D.C.: Medicare Payment Advisory Commission.

————. 1999a. *Report to the Congress: Medicare Payment Policy.* Washington, D.C.: Medicare Payment Advisory Commission.

————. 1999b. *Report to the Congress: Rethinking Medicare's Payment Policies for Graduate Medical Education and Teaching Hospitals.* Washington, D.C.: Medicare Payment Advisory Commission.

————. 2002. *Report to the Congress: Assessing Medicare Benefits.* Washington, D.C.: Medicare Payment Advisory Commission.

MedPAC. *See* Medicare Payment Advisory Commission.

Merlis, Mark. 1999. "Medicare Restructuring: The FEHBP Model, A Summary." Henry J. Kaiser Family Foundation, Menlo Park, Calif.

Miller, Robert H., and Harold S. Luft. 1997. "Does Managed Care Lead to Better or Worse Quality of Care?" *Health Affairs* 16, no. 5:7–25.

Miller, Robert J. 1996. "Competition in the Health System: Good News and Bad News." *Health Affairs* 15, no. 2.

Minarik, Joseph J., and Rudolph G. Penner. 1990. "Fiscal Choices." In Isabel V. Sawhill, ed., *Challenge to Leadership.* Washington, D.C.: Urban Institute.

Mishel, Lawrence, Jared Bernstein, and John Schmitt. 1997. *The State of Working America, 1996–97.* Armonk, N.Y.: M. E. Sharpe.

Mitchell, Alison. 1997. "Clinton to Press Medicare Measure." *New York Times,* July 23, p. A1.

Mitchell, Daniel J. 1998. "Why the Government Should Not Invest Americans' Social Security Money." Heritage Foundation Backgrounder Executive Summary no. 1240. Heritage Foundation, Washington, D.C.

Mitchell, Olivia S., James M. Poterba, and Mark J. Warshawsky. 1997. "New Evidence on the Money's Worth of Individual Annuities." *National Bureau of Economic Research Working Papers,* no. 6002.

Moon, Marilyn. 1996. "Restructuring Medicare's Cost-Sharing." Commonwealth Fund Program on Medicare's Future. Commonwealth Fund, New York.

————. 1999. "Will the Care Be There? Vulnerable Beneficiaries and Medicare Reform." *Health Affairs* 18, no. 1.

Moon, Marilyn, and Karen Davis. 1995. "Preserving and Strengthening Medicare." *Health Affairs* 14, no. 4.

Moon, Marilyn, Barbara Gage, and Alison Evans. 1997. "An Examination of Key Medicare Provisions in the Balanced Budget Act of 1997." Commonwealth Fund Papers, September. Commonwealth Fund, New York.

Moon, Marilyn, and J. Mulvey. 1995. *Entitlements for the Elderly: Protecting Promises, Recognizing Realities.* Washington, D.C.: Urban Institute Press.

Morgensen, Gretchen. 1999. "With Stock Plan, the President Hopes to Keep the Bulls Charging." *New York Times,* January 20, p. A19.

Moss, Michael. 1997. "For Older Employees, On-the-Job Injuries Are More Often Deadly." *Wall Street Journal,* June 17, p. A1.

Moynihan, Daniel Patrick. 1998. "Social Security Saved! Address by Senator Daniel Patrick Moynihan." Spring Exercise on Social Security Reform, Institute of Politics, John F. Kennedy School of Government, Harvard University.

———. 2000. "Building Wealth for Everyone." *New York Times,* May 30.

Munnell, Alicia H. 1998. "Proposals to Preserve and Protect Social Security." In U.S. Senate Committee on Finance 1999.

Munnell, Alicia H., and Pierlugi Balduzzi. 1998. "Investing the Social Security Trust Funds in Equities." AARP Public Policy Institute Report no. 9802, March. American Association of Retired Persons, Washington, D.C.

Musgrave, Richard A. 1986a. "The Role of Social Insurance in an Overall Programme for Social Welfare." In *Public Finance in a Democratic Society: Collected Papers of Richard A. Musgrave,* vol. 2. New York: New York University Press.

———. 1986b. "A Reappraisal of Financing Social Security." In *Public Finance in a Democratic Society: Collected Papers of Richard A. Musgrave,* vol. 2. New York: New York University Press.

Myers, Robert J. 1993. *Social Security.* 4th ed. Philadelphia: University of Pennsylvania Press.

———. 1998. "Statement with Regard to Proposals to Preserve and Protect Social Security." In U.S. Senate Committee on Finance 1999.

NASI. *See* National Academy of Social Insurance.

Nather, David, with John Cochran. 2002. "Still-Thin Edge Leaves GOP with a Cautious Mandate." *Congressional Quarterly Weekly Report,* November 9, pp. 2888–93.

Nather, David, with Anjetta McQueen. 2001. "Social Security Overhaul Panel's Report Lands with a Thud." *Congressional Quarterly Weekly Report,* December 15, pp. 2982–83.

National Academy of Social Insurance. 1998. *Evaluating Issues in Privatizing Social Security: Report of the Panel on Privatization of Social Security.* Washington, D.C.: National Academy of Social Insurance.

———. 1999. *Medicare and the American Social Contract: Final Report of the Study Panel on Medicare's Larger Social Role.* Washington, D.C.: National Academy of Social Insurance.

National Commission on Retirement Policy. 1998. "The Twenty-first Century Retirement Security Plan," May 19, <http://www.csis.org/retire/fullplan.html#3>.

National Economic Commission. 1989. *Report of the National Economic Commission.* Washington, D.C.: GPO.

Neuman, Patricia, and Kathryn M. Langwell. 1999. "Medicare's Choice Explosion? Implications for Beneficiaries." *Health Affairs* 18, no. 1:150–60.

Newhouse, Joseph P., Melinda Beeuwkes Buntin, and John D. Chapman. 1997. "Risk Adjustment and Medicare: Taking a Closer Look." *Health Affairs* 16, no. 5.

"The New Surplus Era." 1999. *New York Times,* February 3.

Nichols, Len M., and Robert D. Reischauer. 2000. "Who Really Wants Price Competition in Managed Care?" *Health Affairs* 19, no. 5:30–43.

Nissenson, Allen R., and Richard A. Rettig. 1999. "Medicare's End-Stage Renal Disease Program: Current Status and Future Prospects." *Health Affairs* 18, no. 1:161–79.

Nitschke, Lori, and Bill Swindell. 2001. "Tax Law Signed, Its Sunset Chided." *Congressional Quarterly Weekly Report,* June 9, p. 1364.

Nordhaus, William D. 1998. "Quality Changes in Price Indexes." *Journal of Economic Perspectives* 12, no. 1.

Norton, Stephen. 2001. "Taxes: Bidding Begins in Tax Cut Sweepstakes." *National Journal,* January 27. Downloaded from PolicyCentral website, December 27, 2002.

Oberlander, Jonathan. 1995. "Medicare and the American State: The Politics of Federal Health Insurance, 1965–1994." Ph.D. diss., Yale University.

———. 1998. "Managed Care and Medicare Reform." In Mark A. Peterson, ed., *Healthy Markets?* Durham, N.C.: Duke University Press.

———. 2000. "Is Premium Support the Right Medicine for Medicare?" *Health Affairs* 19, no. 5:84–99.

OECD. *See* Organisation for Economic Cooperation and Development.

Office of Homeland Security. 2002. *The National Strategy for Homeland Security.* July 16. At <www.whitehouse.gov/homeland>.

Olsen, Kelly A. 1999. "Application of Experimental Poverty Measures to the Aged." *Social Security Bulletin* 62, no. 3:3–19.

Olsen, Kelly A., and Dallas Salisbury. 1998. "Individual Social Security Accounts: Issues in Assessing Administrative Feasibility and Costs." *EBRI Special Report and Issue Brief,* no. 203 (November).

Olsen, Kelly A., Jack VanDerHei, Dallas L. Salisbury, and Martin R. Holmer. 1998. "How Do Individual Social Security Accounts Stack Up? An Evaluation Using the EBRI/SSASIM2 Policy Simulation Model." *EBRI Issue Brief,* no. 195 (March).

Organisation for Economic Cooperation and Development (OECD). 1990. *Health Care Systems in Transition.* Paris: Organisation for Economic Cooperation and Development.

———. 1994. *Health Care Reform: Controlling Spending and Increasing Efficiency.* Working Party no. 1 of the Economic Policy Committee, Paris, Sept. 7. Paris: Organisation for Economic Cooperation and Development.

———. 1996. *Ageing in OECD Countries: A Critical Policy Challenge.* Social Policy Studies no. 20. Paris: Organisation for Economic Cooperation and Development.

Ornstein, Norman J. 1997. "A Bad Rap on the Budget Deal?" *Washington Post,* June 4, p. A23.

Orshansky, Mollie. 1968. "Living in Retirement: A Moderate Standard for an Elderly City Couple." *Social Security Bulletin,* October, pp. 3–17.

Orszag, Peter, Richard Kogan, and Robert Greenstein. 2002. "Social Security and the Tax Cut: The 75-Year Cost of the Tax Cut Is More than Twice as Large as the Long-Term Deficit in Social Security." Center on Budget and Policy Priorities Issue Brief, April 11. At <www.cbpp.org/4-9-02socsec.htm>.

Orszag, Peter R., and Joseph E. Stiglitz. 1999. "Rethinking Pension Reform: Ten Myths about Social Security Systems." Paper presented at World Bank conference, New Ideas about Old Age Security, Washington, D.C., September 14–15.

O'Sullivan, Jennifer, Celinda Fanco, Beth Fuchs, Bob Lyke, Richard Price, and Kathleen Swendiman. 1997. "Medicare Provisions in the Balanced Budget Act of 1997." *CRS Report for Congress* 97–802 EPW. U.S. Congress, Congressional Research Service, Washington, D.C.

Ota, Alan K. 2002. "Tax Cut Becomes Top Priority." *Congressional Quarterly Weekly Report,* November 9, p. 2895.

Page, Benjamin I. 1999. "Is Social Security Reform Ready for the American Public?" Paper presented at the annual conference of the National Academy of Social Insurance, Washington, D.C., January 27–28.

Panis, Constantijn W. A., and Lee A. Lillard. 1996. "Socioeconomic Differentials in the Returns to Social Security." RAND Labor and Population Program Working Paper Series, 96–05. RAND Corporation, Santa Monica, Calif.

Parks, Daniel J. 2000a. "Even GOP's Toughest Budget Hawks Perceive Fiscal Caps' Time Has Passed." *Congressional Quarterly Weekly Report,* January 29, p. 176.

———. 2000b. "Prompt and Parsimonious." *Congressional Quarterly Weekly Report,* April 8, pp. 822–24.

Parks, Daniel J., with Bill Swindell. 2001. "Tax Debate Assured a Long Life as Bush, GOP Press for New Cuts." *Congressional Quarterly Weekly Report,* June 2, pp. 1304–9.

Passell, Peter. 1996. "Trying to Slice the National Pie and Mend Social Security, Too." *New York Times,* December 27, p. D1.

———. 1997a. "Economic Scene." *New York Times,* March 6, p. B2.

———. 1997b. "Economic Scene: The Budget Deficit Problem Will Be Back, with a Vengeance." *New York Times,* May 8, p. D2.

Patashnik, Eric. 1997. "Trust Funds and the Politics of Precommitment." *Political Science Quarterly* 112, no. 3:431–52.

Paulin, Geoffrey, and Brian Riordon. 1998. "Making It on Their Own: The Baby Boom Meets Generation X." *Monthly Labor Review,* February, pp. 10–21.

Pear, Robert. 1997a. "Medicare Revamp Advances in Vote by Senate Panel." *New York Times,* June 19, p. A1.

———. 1997b. "Senate Backs Rise in Medicare Costs for Wealthy Aged." *New York Times,* June 25, p. A1.

————. 1997c. "Clinton Is 'Open' to Making the Well-Off Pay More for Medicare." *New York Times,* July 9, p. A14.

————. 1998. "Panel Says Administration Underestimates Medicare Costs." *New York Times,* June 3.

————. 1999. "Medicare Panel, Sharply Divided, Submits No Plan." *New York Times,* March 17, p. A1.

————. 2000. "More H.M.O.s Exit Medicare and Cite Its Unprofitability." *New York Times,* June 3, p. A1.

Penner, Rudolph G. 1989. *Social Security and National Saving.* Washington, D.C.: Committee for Economic Development.

————. 1994. *Dealing with the Retirement of the Baby Boomers.* Washington, D.C.: Urban Institute Press.

————. 1999. "A Budget Built on Subterfuges." *Newsday,* November 23.

Peterson, Peter G. 1996. *Will America Grow Up before It Grows Old?* New York: Random House.

Physician Payment Review Commission (PPRC). 1996. *1996 Annual Report.* Washington, D.C.: Physician Payment Review Commission.

————. 1997. *1997 Annual Report.* Washington, D.C.: Physician Payment Review Commission.

Pooley, Eric. 1997. "No Guts, No Glory." *Time,* January 20, pp. 23–26.

Poterba, James M. 1997. "The History of Annuities in the United States." *National Bureau of Economic Research Working Papers,* no. 6001.

Poterba, James M., and Mark J. Warshawsky. 1998. "The Cost of Annuitizing Retirement Payouts from Individual Accounts." Available at <www.mit.edu/~poterba/costs5.pdf>.

PPRC. *See* Physician Payment Review Commission.

"President Clinton's Social Security Package, the Federal Budget, and the National Debt: A Layman's Guide." 1999. Issue Brief no. 9. of the Social Security Network, <www.socsec.org>. The Century Foundation, New York.

President's Commission to Strengthen Social Security. 2001a. *Interim Report.* August. At <www.commtostrengthensocsec.gov/reports/Report-Interim.pdf>.

————. 2001b. *Strengthening Social Security and Creating Personal Wealth for All Americans: Report of the President's Commission.* December 21. At <www.commto strengthensocsec.gov>.

ProPAC. *See* Prospective Payment Assessment Commission.

Prospective Payment Assessment Commission (ProPAC). 1997a. *Report and Recommendations to the Congress.* Washington, D.C.: Prospective Payment Assessment Commission.

————. 1997b. *Medicare and the American Health Care System: Report to the Congress.* Washington, D.C.: Prospective Payment Assessment Commission.

Quadagno, Jill, and Joseph Quinn. 1997. "Does Social Security Discourage Work?" In Kingson and Schulz 1997a, 127–46.

Radner, Daniel B. 1998. "The Retirement Prospects of the Baby Boom Generation." *Social Security Bulletin* 61, no. 1:3–19.

Rauch, Jonathan. 1997. "Ducking the Challenge." *National Journal,* February 9.

Reischauer, Robert D. 1997a. "The Budget: Crucible for the Policy Agenda." In Reischauer 1997b.

———, ed. 1997b. *Setting National Priorities: Budget Choices for the Next Century.* Washington, D.C.: Brookings Institution.

———. 1997c. "The Unfulfillable Promise: Cutting Nondefense Discretionary Spending." In Reischauer 1997b.

———. 1997d. "Midnight Follies." *Washington Post,* June 22, C7.

Reischauer, Robert D., Stuart Butler, and Judith R. Lave, eds. 1997. *Medicare: Preparing for the Challenges of the Twenty-first Century.* Washington, D.C.: National Academy of Social Insurance.

Renwick, Trudi J., and Barbara R. Bergmann. 1993. "A Budget-Based Definition of Poverty: With an Application to Single-Parent Families." *Journal of Human Resources* 28, no. 1.

Riley, Gerald F., Melvin J. Ingber, and Cynthia G. Tudor. 1997. "Disenrollment of Medicare Beneficiaries from HMOs." *Health Affairs* 16, no. 5:117–24.

Robinson, James C., and Patricia E. Powers. 1997. "Restructuring Medicare: The Role of Public and Private Purchasing Alliances." In Reischauer, Butler, and Lave 1997.

Roos, N. P., and L. L. Roos. 1994. "Small Area Variations, Practice Style, and Quality of Care." In Robert G. Evans, Morris L. Barer, and Theodore R. Marmor, eds., *Why Are Some People Healthy and Others Not? The Determinants of Health of Populations.* New York: Aldine de Gruyter.

Rosenbach, Margo L., and JoAnn Lamphere. 1999. "Bridging the Gaps between Medicare and Medicaid: The Case of QMBs and SLMBs." AARP Public Policy Institute Report no. 9902, January. American Association of Retired Persons, Washington, D.C.

Rosenbaum, David E. 2002. "Hard Truths Are Avoided on Social Security." *New York Times,* December 22, p. BU4.

Rosenblatt, Robert A. 1999. "Medicare HMO Charges to Jump Next Year." *New Orleans Times-Picayune,* September 16, p. A14.

Rovner, Julie. 1995. "Congress' 'Catastrophic' Attempt to Fix Medicare." In Mann and Ornstein 1995.

Sabelhaus, John, and Joyce Manchester. 1995. "Baby Boomers and Their Parents: How Does Their Economic Well-Being Compare in Middle Age?" *Journal of Human Resources* 30, no. 4.

Samuelson, Paul. 1970. *Economics.* 8th ed. New York: McGraw-Hill.

Samuelson, Robert J. 1996a. "The Savings Gap: Mostly Make-Believe." *Washington Post,* June 12, p. A21.

———. 1996b. "A Hidden Agenda?" *Washington Post,* September 4, p. A19.

———. 1998. "Why We're All Married to the Market." *Newsweek,* April 27, p. 49.

———. 1999. "The Deficit in Leadership." *Washington Post,* August 4, p. A21.

———. 2000. "Social Insecurity." *Washington Post,* May 31, p. A27.

Samwick, Andrew. 1998. Testimony. In U.S. Senate Committee on Finance 1999.

Savage, James D. 1988. *Balanced Budgets and American Politics.* Ithaca: Cornell University Press.

Schick, Allen. 1980. *Congress and Money.* Washington, D.C.: Urban Institute.

———. 1995. *The Federal Budget: Policy, Process, and Politics.* Washington, D.C.: Brookings Institution.

Schieber, Sylvester J. 1997. "Retirement Income Security at Risk." In Schieber and Shoven 1997a.

Schieber, Sylvester J., and John Shoven, eds. 1997a. *Public Policy toward Pensions.* Cambridge: MIT Press.

Schieber, Sylvester J., and John B. Shoven. 1997b. "The Consequences of Population Aging on Private Pension Fund Saving and Asset Markets." In Schieber and Shoven 1997a.

Schneider, William A. 1997. "A Cure for Acute Deficit Disorder." *National Journal,* May 10, p. 1014.

Schrammel, Kurt. 1998. "Comparing the Labor Market Success of Young Adults from Two Generations." *Monthly Labor Review,* February, pp. 3–9.

Schultze, Charles L. 1989. "Of Wolves, Termites and Pussycats: Or, Why We Should Worry about the Budget Deficit." *Brookings Review* (summer): 26–33.

———. 1990. "Setting Long-Run Deficit Reduction Targets: The Economics and Politics of Budget Design." In Aaron 1990.

———. 1997. "Is Faster Growth the Cure for Budget Deficits?" In Reischauer 1997b, 35–74.

Schwarz, John E., and Thomas J. Volgy. 1992. *The Forgotten Americans.* New York: W. W. Norton & Co.

Serafini, Marilyn W. 1997. "Health Care Costs: Ready for Takeoff?" *National Journal,* April 26, pp. 819–21.

Shuman, Howard. 1984. *Politics and the Budget: The Struggle between the President and the Congress.* Englewood Cliffs, N.J.: Prentice-Hall.

Smith, David G. 1992. *Paying for Medicare: The Politics of Reform.* New York: Aldine de Gruyter.

Smith, Sheila, Mark Freeland, Stephen Heffler, David McKusick, and the Health Expenditures Projection Team. 1998. "The Next Ten Years of Health Spending: What Does the Future Hold?" *Health Affairs* 17, no. 5:128–40.

Social Security Advisory Board. 1998. "Social Security: Why Action Should Be Taken Soon." . Social Security Advisory Board, Washington, D.C.

"Social Security Illusion." 1998. *Washington Post,* December 29.

"Social Security Politics." 2000. *Washington Post,* May 8, p. A22.

"Social Security's Savings." 1997. Editorial. *Wall Street Journal,* January 8.

Solomon, Burt. 1996. "OK, Now What?" *National Journal,* November 9, pp. 2394–97.

"Special Report: Health—Can GOP Make Good on Medicare Drug Pledge?" 2002. *Congressional Quarterly Weekly Report.* November 23, pp. 3064–69.

SSA/ORES. *See* U.S. Department of Health and Human Services, Social Security Administration, Office of Research, Evaluation, and Statistics.

Stein, Herbert. 1996. "The Fiscal Revolution in America, Part II: 1964–1994." In W. Elliot Brownlee, ed., *Funding the Modern American State, 1941–1995.* Cambridge: Cambridge University Press.

Steuerle, C. Eugene. 1996. Contribution to "Four Views on the Role of Means-Testing." In Diamond, Lindeman, and Young 1996.

———. 1997. "Letter to the Editor." *Brookings Review* (winter).

Steuerle, C. Eugene, with Jon M. Bakija. 1994. *Retooling Social Security for the Twenty-first Century: Right and Wrong Approaches to Reform.* Washington, D.C.: Urban Institute Press.

Stevenson, Richard W. 1998. "SEC Chairman Is Cautious about Social Security Plans." *New York Times,* October 20.

Stewart, Kenneth J., and Joseph Pavalone. 1996. "Experimental Consumer Price Index for Americans 62 Years of Age and Older." Bureau of Labor Statistics, *CPI Detailed Report,* April.

Stone, Deborah. 1997. *Policy Paradox: The Art of Political Decision Making.* 2d ed. New York: W. W. Norton & Co.

Strunk, Bradley C., Paul B. Ginsburg, and Jon R. Gabel. 2002. "Tracking Health Care Costs: Growth Accelerates Again in 2001." *Health Affairs* web-based article, September 25. At <www.healthaffairs.org/WebExclusives/Strunk_Web_Excl_092502.htm>.

"Symposium on the 'Safety Net.'" 1997. *Health Affairs* 16, no. 4:7–63.

"Taking Stock: A Roundtable of Experts on Diversification of the Social Security Trust Funds." 1999. Social Security Network, <www.socsec.org/new/19martrans.pdf>. The Century Foundation, New York.

Tanner, Michael. 1996. "It's Time to Privatize Social Security." *Challenge,* November–December, p. 20.

———. 1998. "The Perils of Government Investing." Cato Institute Briefing Papers, no. 43. Cato Institute, Washington, D.C.

Taylor, Andrew. 1999a. "Special Report: Budget." *Congressional Quarterly Weekly Report,* October 16, pp. 2426–32.

———. 1999b. "GOP Finds Hastert Strategy Paying Off in Fiscal Showdown." *Congressional Quarterly Weekly Report*, October 23, pp. 2511–13.

———. 1999c. "Hill Digs Deeper than Ever into Bag of Budget Tricks." *Congressional Quarterly Weekly Report*, October 30, pp. 2575–78.

———. 1999d. "Clinton Gives Republicans a Gentler End-of-Year Beating." *Congressional Quarterly Weekly Report*, November 13, pp. 2698–2700.

Taylor, Andrew, with Alan K. Ota. 2002. "GOP Weighs Critical Staff Shifts to Grease the Legislative Gears." *Congressional Quarterly Weekly Report*, November 23, pp. 3079–80.

Technical Review Panel on the Medicare Trustees Reports. 2000. *Review of Assumptions and Methods of the Medicare Trustees' Financial Projections*. Baltimore, Health Care Financing Administration, December. At <www.cmms.gov/publications/technicalpanelreport/report.pdf>.

"The Text of the President's State of the Union Address to Congress." 1999. *New York Times*, Jan. 20, p A22.

Thompson, Lawrence H. 1990. "Discussion." In Aaron 1990.

———. 1998a. *Older and Wiser: The Economics of Public Pensions*. Washington, D.C.: Urban Institute Press.

———. 1998b. "The Predictability of Retirement Income." National Academy of Social Insurance Social Security Brief no. 3. National Academy of Social Insurance, Washington, D.C.

Thompson, Lawrence, and Melinda Upp. 1997. "The Social Insurance Approach and Social Security." In Kingson and Schulz 1997a.

Thompson, Tommy G. 2001. "Remarks by HHS Secretary Tommy G. Thompson at Press Conference Announcing Reforming Medicare and Medicaid Agency." U.S. Department of Health and Human Services, press release June 14, 2001. At <www.hhs.gov/news>.

Thorpe, Kenneth E. 1998. "Fiscal and Policy Issues Facing Medicare in the Twenty-first Century." Photocopy in author's possession.

———. 1999. "Options for Reforming Medicare." Testimony before the U.S. Senate Committee on Finance, May 26. Photocopy in author's possession.

Thorpe, Kenneth E., and Curtis Florence. 1998. "Covering Uninsured Children and Their Parents: Estimated Costs and Number of Newly Insured." Commonwealth Fund, New York.

U.S. Congressional Budget Office (CBO). 1980. *An Analysis of the President's Budgetary Proposals for Fiscal Year 1981*. Washington, D.C.: Congressional Budget Office.

———. 1983. *An Analysis of the President's Budgetary Proposals for Fiscal Year 1984*. Washington, D.C.: Congressional Budget Office.

———. 1985. *The Economic and Budget Outlook for Fiscal Years 1986–1990*. Washington, D.C.: Congressional Budget Office.

———. 1993. *The Economic and Budget Outlook: Fiscal Years 1994–1998.* Washington, D.C.: Congressional Budget Office.

———. 1994. "Is the Growth of the CPI a Biased Measure of the Changes in the Cost of Living?" CBO Papers, October. Congressional Budget Office, Washington, D.C.

———. 1995. *The Economic and Budget Outlook: Fiscal Years 1996–2000.* Washington, D.C.: Congressional Budget Office.

———. 1997a. *The Economic and Budget Outlook: Fiscal Years 1998–2007.* Washington, D.C.: Congressional Budget Office.

———. 1997b. *Long-Term Budgetary Pressures and Policy Options.* Washington, D.C.: Congressional Budget Office.

———. 1997c. Letter from June E. O'Neill, director, to the Honorable Pete V. Domenici providing preliminary cost estimate of the conference agreement on H.R. 2015, the Balanced Budget Act of 1997, July 30. Congressional Budget Office, Washington, D.C.

———. 1998a. *The Economic and Budget Outlook: Fiscal Years 1999–2008.* Washington, D.C.: Congressional Budget Office.

———. 1998b. *Long-Term Budgetary Pressures and Policy Options.* Washington, D.C.: Congressional Budget Office.

———. 1998c. Letter from June E. O'Neill, director, to the Honorable Bill Archer analyzing the Feldstein proposal for Social Security personal accounts, August 4. Congressional Budget Office, Washington, D.C.

———. 1998d. "Social Security and Private Saving: A Review of the Empirical Literature." CBO Memorandum. Congressional Budget Office, Washington, D.C.

———. 1999. *The Economic and Budget Outlook: Fiscal Years 2000–2009.* Washington, D.C.: Congressional Budget Office.

———. 2000. *The Economic and Budget Outlook: Fiscal Years 2001–2010.* Washington, D.C.: Congressional Budget Office.

———. 2000a. *The Long-Term Budget Outlook.* Washington, D.C.: Congressional Budget Office.

———. 2002a. "Letter from CBO Director Dan L. Crippen to the Honorable George V. Voinovich." December 4. At <www.cbo.gov>.

———. 2002b. "A 125-Year Picture of the Federal Government's Share of the Economy, 1950 to 2075." CBO Long-Range Fiscal Policy Brief, July 3. At <www.cbo.gov>.

U.S. Department of Health and Human Services, Health Care Financing Administration (HCFA). 1997. *Profiles of Medicare, 30th Anniversary.* Washington, D.C.: GPO.

U.S. Department of Health and Human Services, Office of Inspector General (HHS Inspector General). 2000. "Adequacy of Medicare's Managed Care Payments after the Balanced Budget Act of 1997." Report A-14-00-00212 (September). U.S. Department of Health and Human Services, Office of Inspector General, Washington, D.C.

U.S. Department of Health and Human Services, Social Security Administration, Office of Research, Evaluation, and Statistics (SSA/ORES). 1995. *Social Security Programs throughout the World, 1995*. SSA Publication no. 13-11805. Washington, D.C.: GPO.

——. 1997. *Fast Facts and Figures about Social Security*. Washington, D.C.: GPO.

——. 1998a. *Income of the Population 55 or Older, 1996*. SSA Publication no. 13-11871. Washington, D.C.: GPO.

——. 1998b. *Income of the Aged Chartbook, 1996*. SSA Publication no. 13-11727. Washington, D.C.: GPO.

U.S. General Accounting Office (GAO). 1995. *The Deficit and the Economy: An Update of Long-Term Simulations*. GAO/AIMD/OCE-95-119. Washington, D.C.: General Accounting Office.

——. 1998a. *Social Security Financing: Implications of Government Stock Investing for the Trust Fund, the Federal Budget, and the Economy*. GAO/AIMD/HEHS-98-74. Washington, D.C.: General Accounting Office.

——. 1998b. *Social Security: Implications of Extending Mandatory Coverage to State and Local Employees*. GAO/HEHS-98-196. Washington, D.C.: General Accounting Office.

——. 1999. *Medicare Contractors: Despite Its Efforts, HCFA Cannot Ensure Their Effectiveness or Integrity*. GAO/HEHS-99-116. Washington, D.C.: General Accounting Office.

——. 2002. "Budget Issues: Long-Term Fiscal Challenges." February 27. GAO-02-467T. Washington, D.C. General Accounting Office.

U.S. House of Representatives, Committee on Ways and Means. 1996. *1996 Green Book: Background Material and Data on Programs within the Jurisdiction of the Committee on Ways and Means*. Washington, D.C.: GPO.

——. 1998. *1998 Green Book: Background Material and Data on Programs within the Jurisdiction of the Committee on Ways and Means*. Washington, D.C.: GPO.

U.S. Senate Committee on Finance. 1996. *Final Report of the Advisory Commission to Study the Consumer Price Index*. 104th Cong., 2d sess., Committee Print 104-72.

——. 1997. "Summary: Health and Welfare Provisions of the Balanced Budget Act of 1997." July 31. U.S. Senate Committee on Finance, Washington, D.C.

——. 1999. *Retirement Security Policy: Proposals to Preserve and Protect Social Security: Hearing before the Committee on Finance*. 105th Cong., 2d sess., September 9, 1998.

Utthof, Andras W. 1993. "Pension System Reforms and Savings in Latin American and Caribbean Countries with Special Reference to Chile." In Yilmaz Akyuz and Gunther Held, eds., *Finance and the Real Economy*. Santiago, Chile: United Nations Economic Commission for Latin America and the Caribbean.

Valdivia, Victor H. 1997. "The Insurance Role of Social Security: Theory and Lessons for Policy Reform." IMF Working Paper 97/113, September. International Monetary Fund, Washington, D.C.

Vittas, Dimitri. 1995. "Strengths and Weaknesses of the Chilean Pension Reform." Financial Sector Development Department, World Bank, May. World Bank, Washington, D.C.

Vladeck, Bruce C. 1999. "Plenty of Nothing: A Report from the Medicare Commission." *New England Journal of Medicine* 340, no. 19:1503–6.

Vobejda, Barbara. 1997. "Bipartisan Concern about Medicare, Social Security." *Washington Post,* May 5, p. A6.

Waidmann, Timothy A. 1998. "Potential Effects of Raising Medicare's Eligibility Age." *Health Affairs* 17, no. 2.

Waldo, Daniel R., Sally T. Sonnefeld, David R. McKissick, and Ross H. Arnett III. 1989. "Health Expenditures by Age Group, 1977 and 1987." *Health Care Financing Review* 10, no. 4:111–20.

Walsh, Bill. 1999. "Social Security Plan Won't Fly, Critics Say." *New Orleans Times-Picayune,* January 21, p. A1.

Weaver, Carolyn. 1998. "Personal Security Accounts: A Means of Strengthening and Securing Social Security." In U.S. Senate Committee on Finance 1999.

Weaver, R. Kent. 1984. "Controlling Entitlements." In John E. Chubb and Paul E. Peterson, eds., *The New Direction in American Politics.* Washington, D.C.: Brookings Institution.

———. 1988. *Automatic Government: The Politics of Indexation.* Washington, D.C.: Brookings Institution.

———. 1999. "The Politics of Pension Reform: Lessons from Abroad." In R. Douglas Arnold, Michael Graetz, and Alicia Munnell, eds., *Framing the Social Security Debate.* Washington, D.C.: Brookings/NASI.

———. 2000. *Ending Welfare As We Know It.* Washington, D.C.: Brookings Institution.

Weaver, R. Kent, and William T. Dickens, eds. 1995. "Looking before We Leap: Social Science and Welfare Reform." Brookings Occasional Paper, August. Brookings Institution, Washington, D.C.

Weinstein, Michael M. 1998. "Social Insecurity: Poof! You Can Retire Rich." *New York Times,* December 20.

———. 1999a. "News Analysis: Debate over Social Security Proposal Misfires in Focus on Double Counting." *New York Times,* January 30.

———. 1999b. "Managed Care's Other Problem: It's Not What You Think." *New York Times,* February 28, p. C1.

Wennberg, John E. 1984. "Dealing with Medical Practice Variations: A Proposal for Action." *Health Affairs* 3, no. 4:6–31.

Wessel, David. 1997a. "The Outlook: Sometimes Stocks Go Nowhere for Years." *Wall Street Journal,* January 13, p. A1.

———. 1997b. "Agreement Seems to Cause Surprisingly Little Pain." *Wall Street Journal,* May 8, p. A12.

White, Joseph. 1994. "Paying the Right Price." *Brookings Review* 12, no. 2:6–11.

———. 1995a. *Competing Solutions: American Health Care Proposals and International Experience.* Washington, D.C.: Brookings Institution.

———. 1995b. "Fact and Fiction about Medical Savings Accounts." Brookings Working Paper, June. Brookings Institution, Washington, D.C.

———. 1997. "Which 'Managed Care' for Medicare?" *Health Affairs* 16, no. 5:73–82.

———. 1998a. "Making 'Common Sense' of Federal Budgeting." *Public Administration Review* 58, no. 2:101–8.

———. 1998b. "Entitlement Budgeting versus Bureau Budgeting." *Public Administration Review* 58, no. 6:510–21.

———. 1999a. "Budgeting for Entitlements." In Roy T. Meyers, ed., *Handbook of Government Budgeting.* San Francisco: Jossey-Bass.

———. 1999b. "Uses and Abuses of Long-Term Medicare Cost Estimates." *Health Affairs* 18, no. 1:63–79.

———. 1999c. "Understanding Long-term Medicare Cost Estimates." A Century Foundation White Paper. The Century Foundation, New York.

———. 1999d. "Targets and Systems of Health Care Cost Control." *Journal of Health Politics, Policy, and Law* 24, no. 4:653–96.

———. 2000. "Budgeting for Social Security: Or, When Are Savings Really Savings?" *Public Budgeting and Finance* 20, no. 3.

———. 2001. "Looking in the Wrong Place: Why Chile Provides No Evidence for Social Security Privatization." *Public Budgeting and Finance* 20, no. 4.

———. 2002. "The Entitlement Crisis That Never Existed." In Stuart H. Altman and David I. Shactman, eds., *Policies for an Aging Society.* Baltimore: Johns Hopkins University Press.

White, Joseph, and Aaron Wildavsky. 1991. *The Deficit and the Public Interest: The Search for Responsible Budgeting in the 1980s.* Berkeley: University of California Press; New York: Russell Sage Foundation.

Wildavsky, Aaron. 1964. *The Politics of the Budgetary Process.* Boston: Little, Brown & Co.

———. 1979. "Strategic Retreat on Objectives: Learning from Failure in American Public Policy." In Aaron Wildavsky, *Speaking Truth to Power: The Art and Craft of Policy Analysis.* Boston: Little, Brown & Co.

Wildavsky, Ben. 1998. "Working Solutions." *National Journal,* July 4, p. 1561.

Wilensky, Gail, and Joseph Newhouse. 1999. "Medicare Reform: What's Right, What's Wrong, What's Next?" *Health Affairs* 18, no. 1.

Woodward, Bob. 1994. *The Agenda: Inside the Clinton White House.* New York: Simon & Schuster.

————. 2002. *Bush at War.* New York: Simon & Schuster.

World Bank. 1994. *Averting the Old Age Crisis: Policies to Protect the Old and Promote Growth.* A World Bank Policy and Research Report. New York: Oxford University Press.

Yates, John. 1987. *Why Are We Waiting? An Analysis of Hospital Waiting Lists.* New York: Oxford University Press.

Zachary, G. Pascal. 1996. "U.S. Savings Worries May Be Overdone." *Wall Street Journal,* June 7, p. B7A.

Zelman, Walter A., and Robert A. Berenson. 1998. *The Managed Care Blues and How to Cure Them.* Washington, D.C.: Georgetown University Press.

Zweifel, P., S. Feleder, and Markus Meier. 1995. "Ageing of Population and Health Care Expenditure: A Red Herring?" Paper presented to International Conference on Ageing and Old-Age Econometrics, University of Athens, May 18–19.

INDEX

Page numbers in italics indicate figures; those in boldface refer to tables.